AF584295

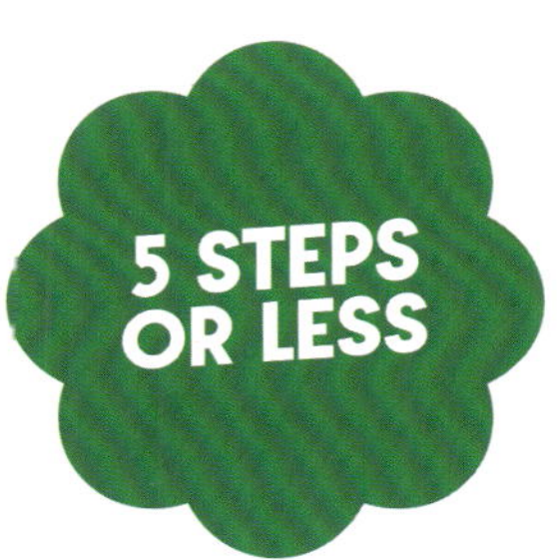

Making cooking simple.

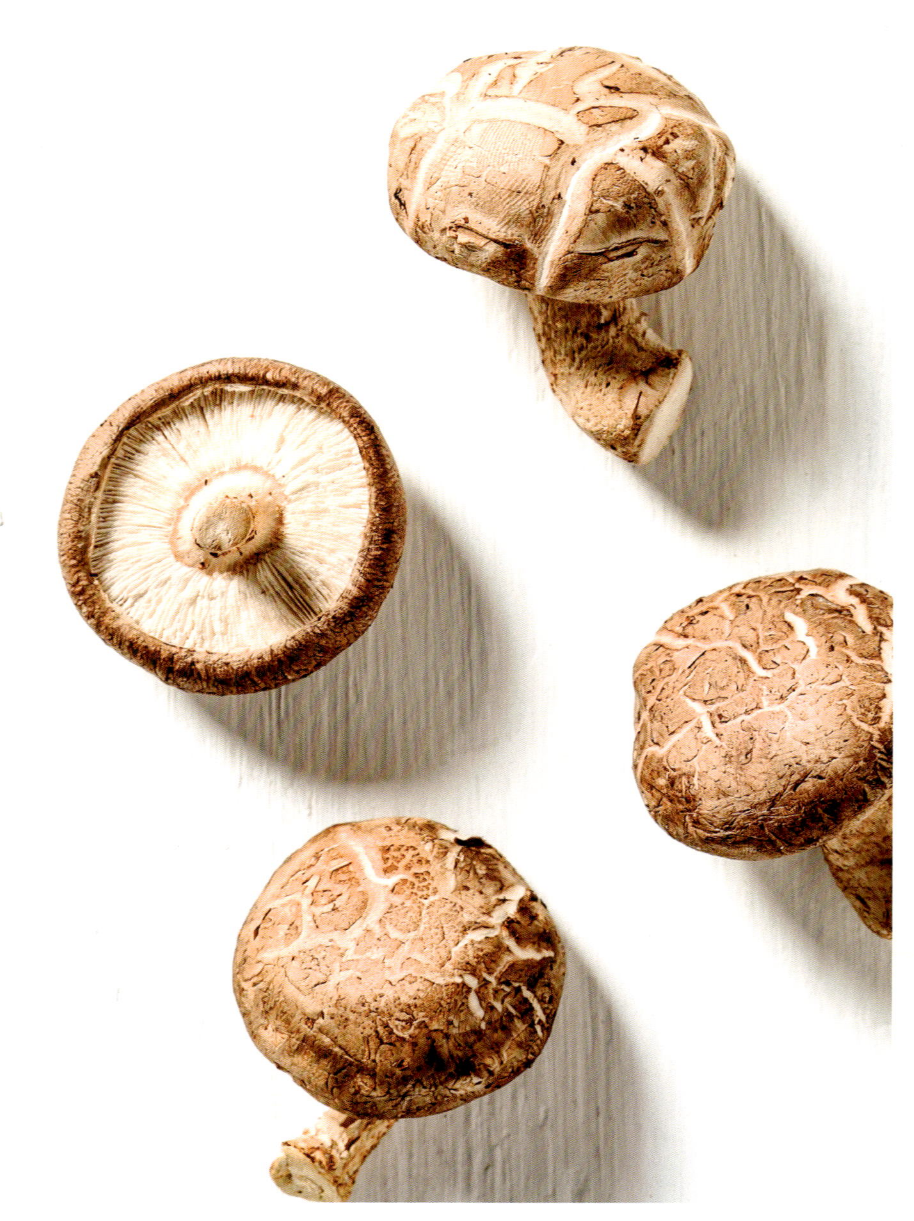

With this book you can enjoy all your favourite takeaway-style meals from the comfort of your own kitchen. Bursting with flavoursome curries, stews, soups, stir-fries and rice dishes, it contains a delicious recipe for every meal of the day, every day of the week, and then some. Or, for something different, explore Asian-inspired street-food snacks, treats and desserts. Affordable, easy to prepare and fun to eat, here are the flavours of Asia on a plate: easy, doable, delicious.

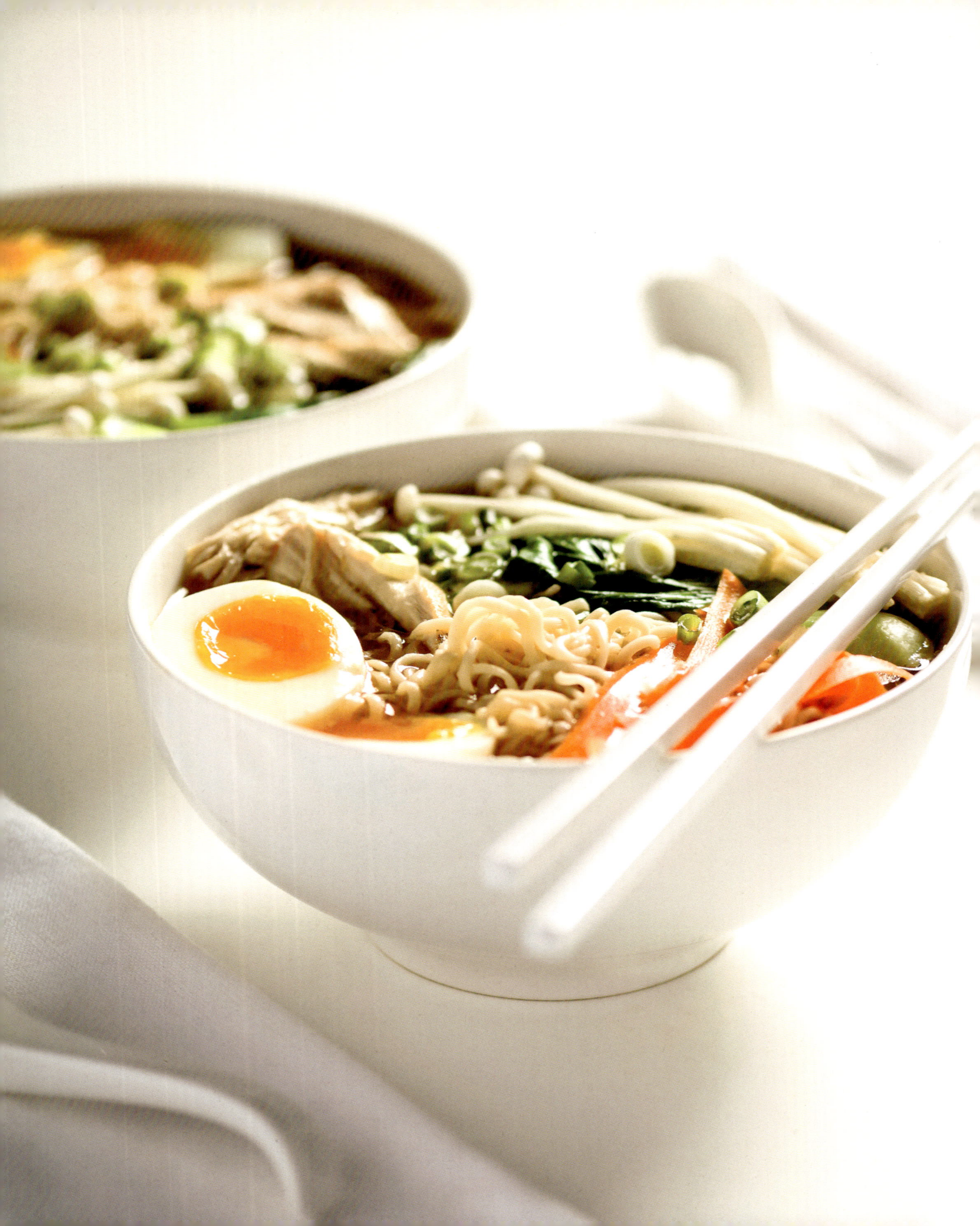

EAT EASY

Asian

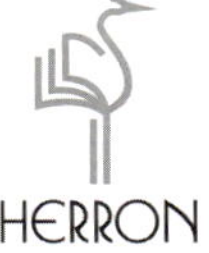

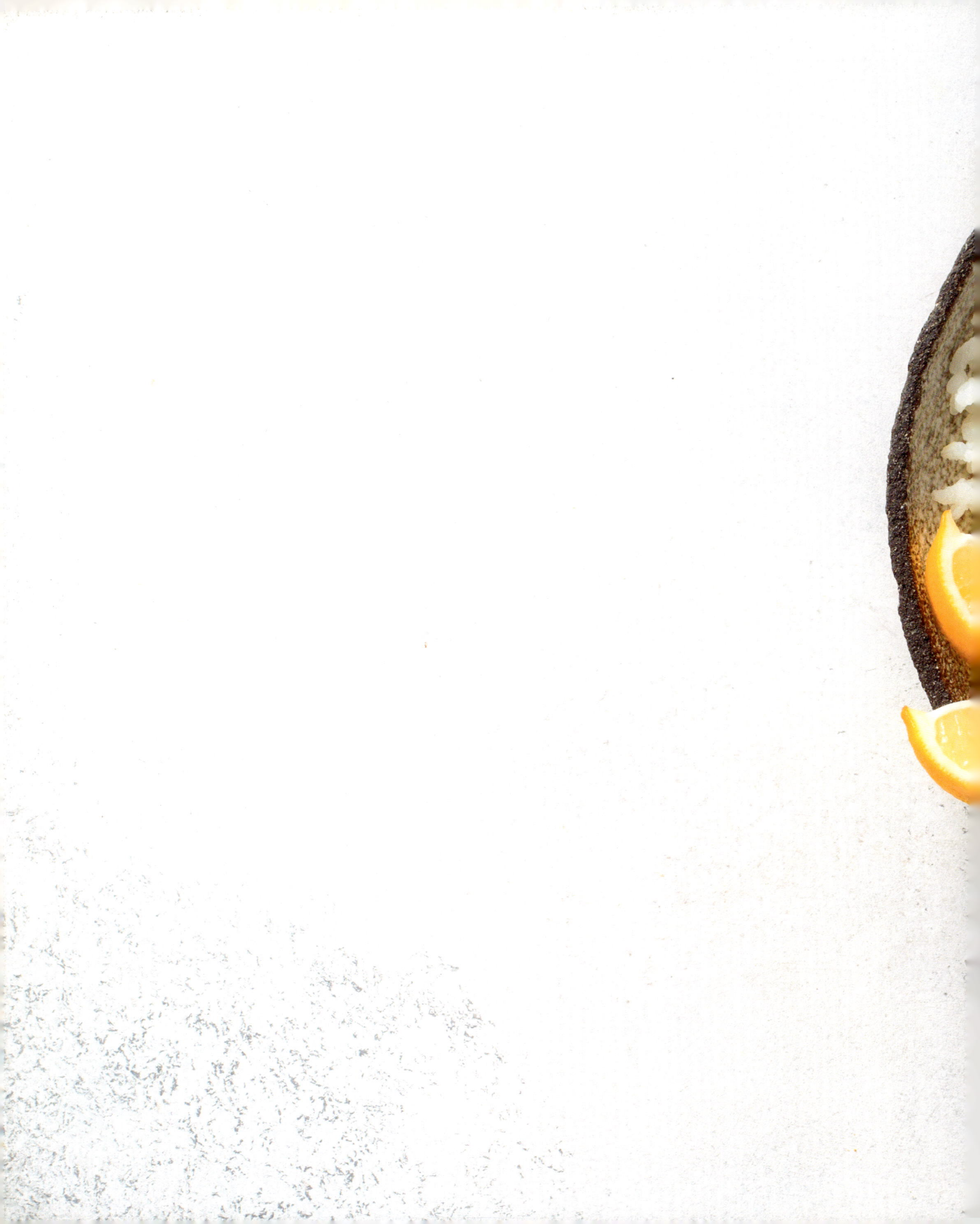

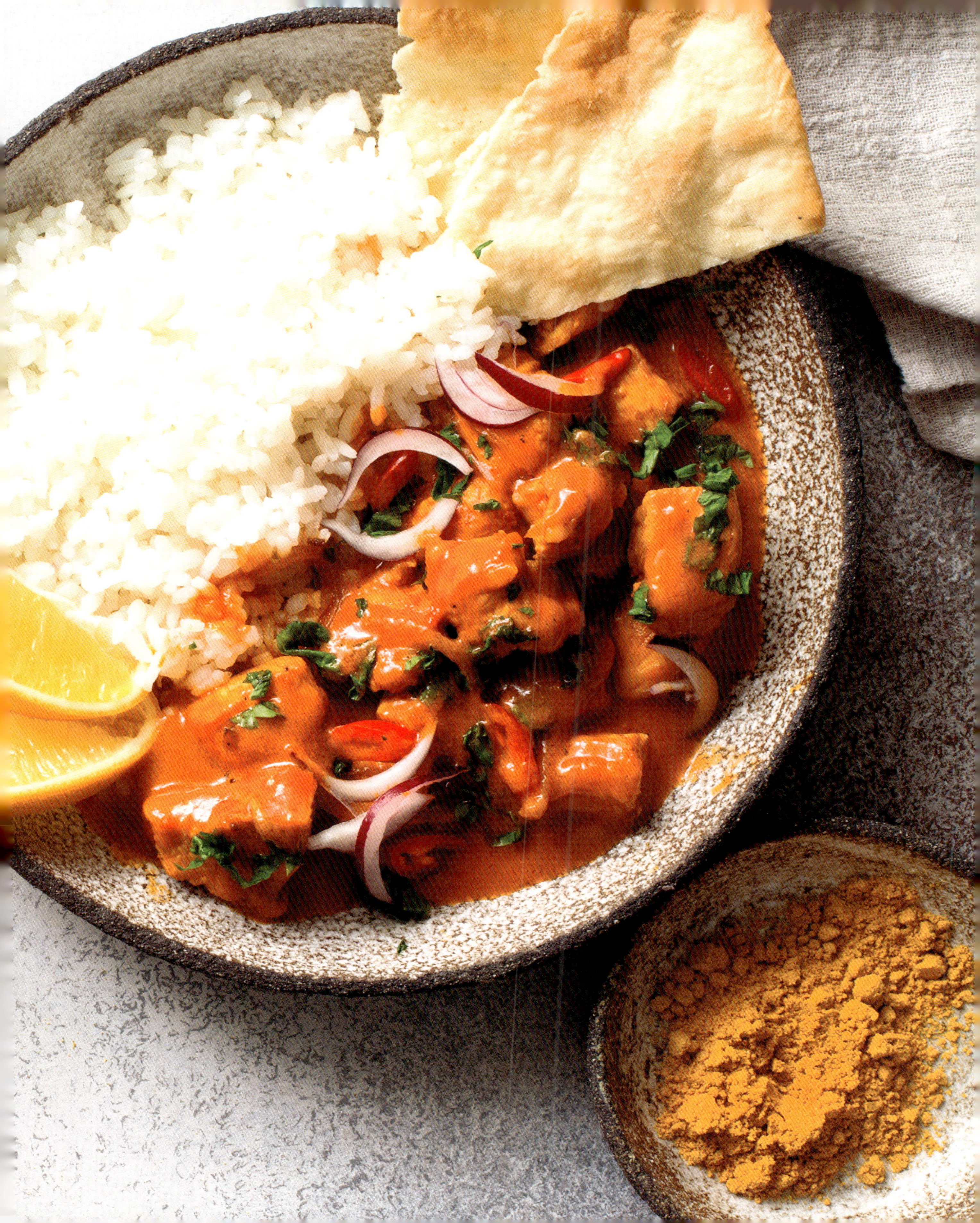

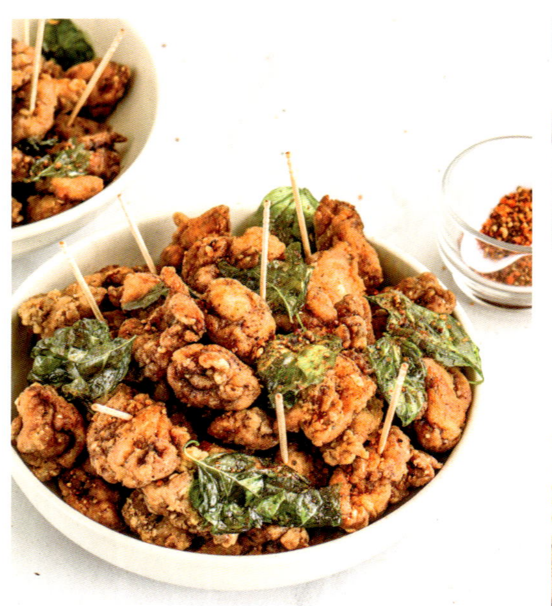
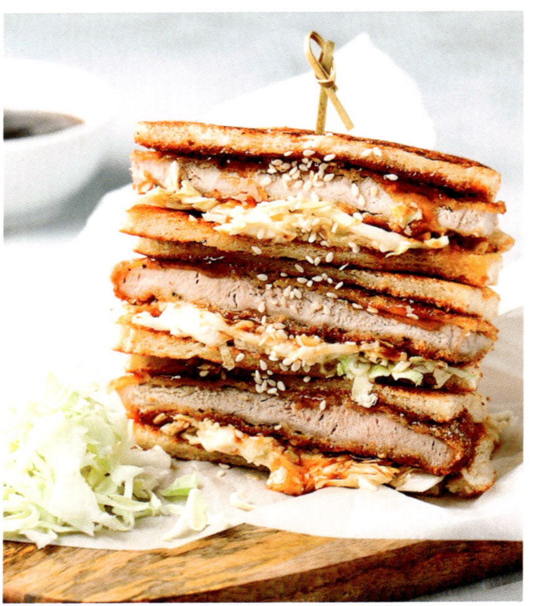
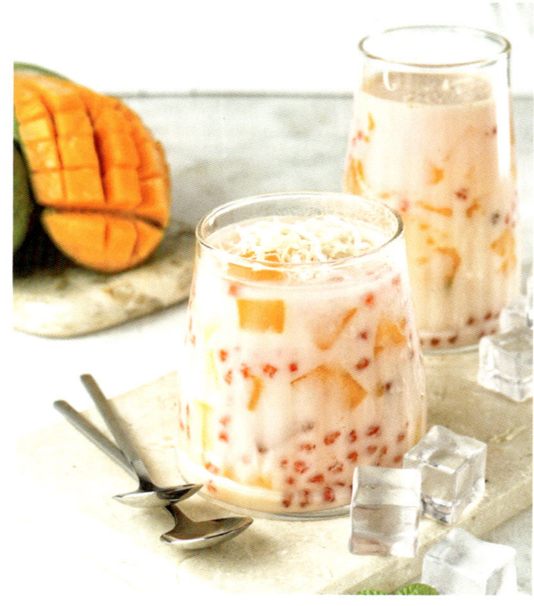
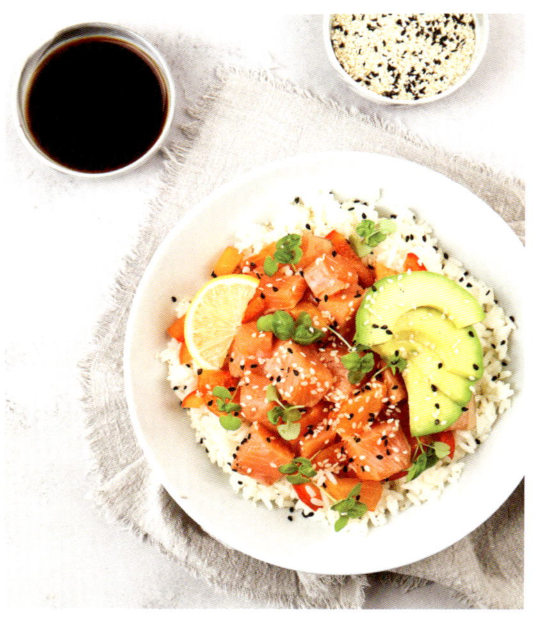

CONTENTS

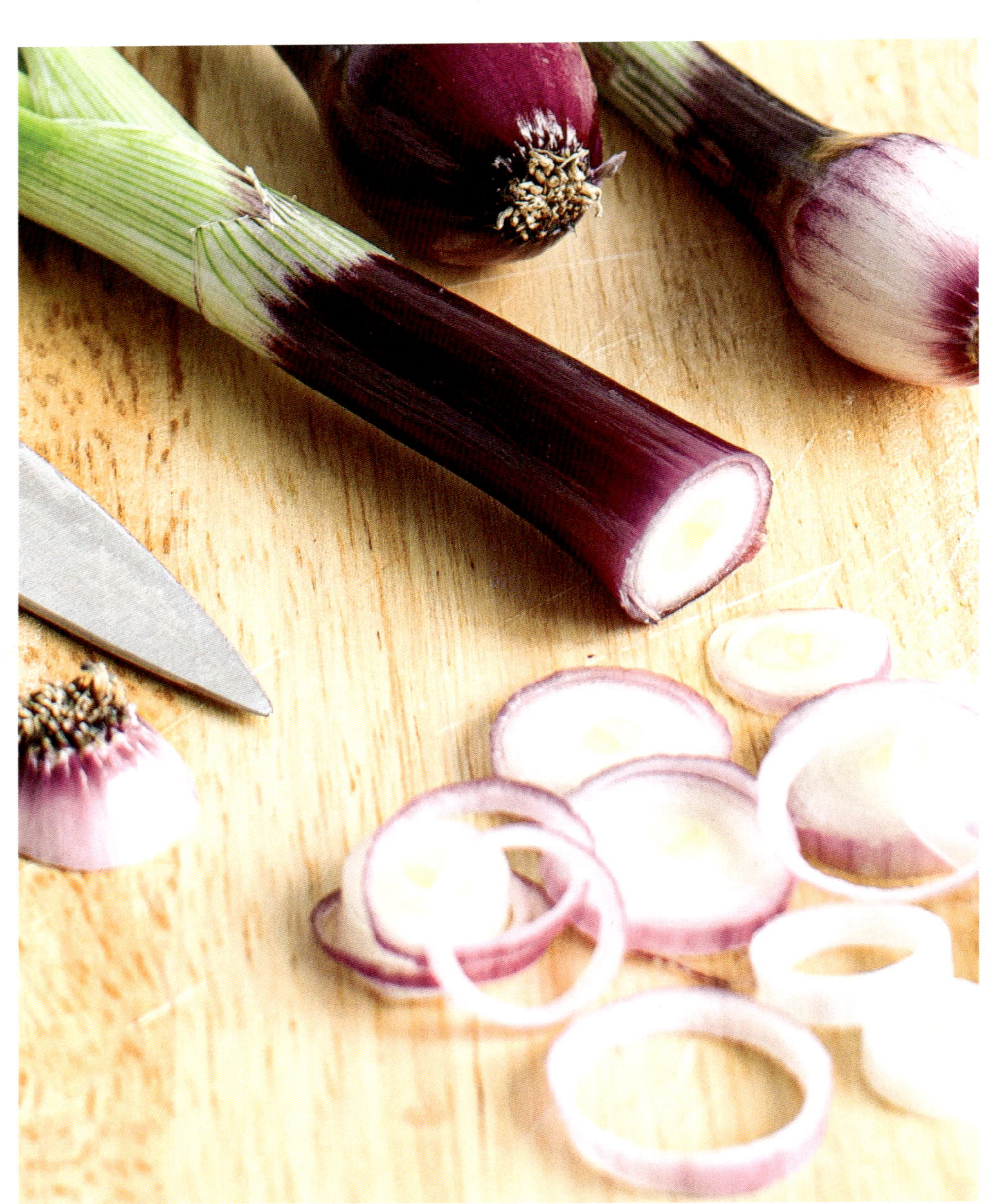

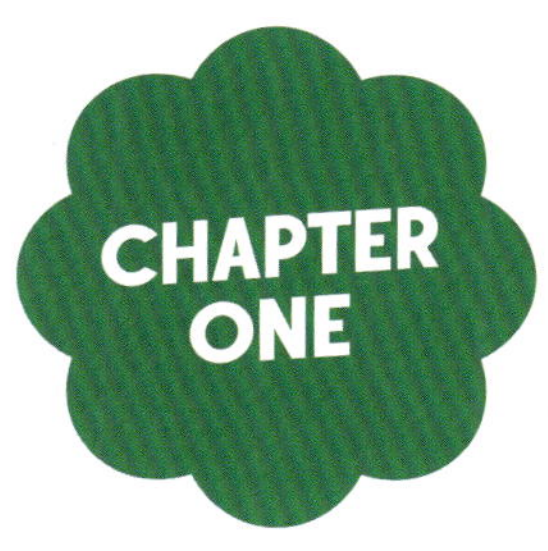

BOWLS & SALADS

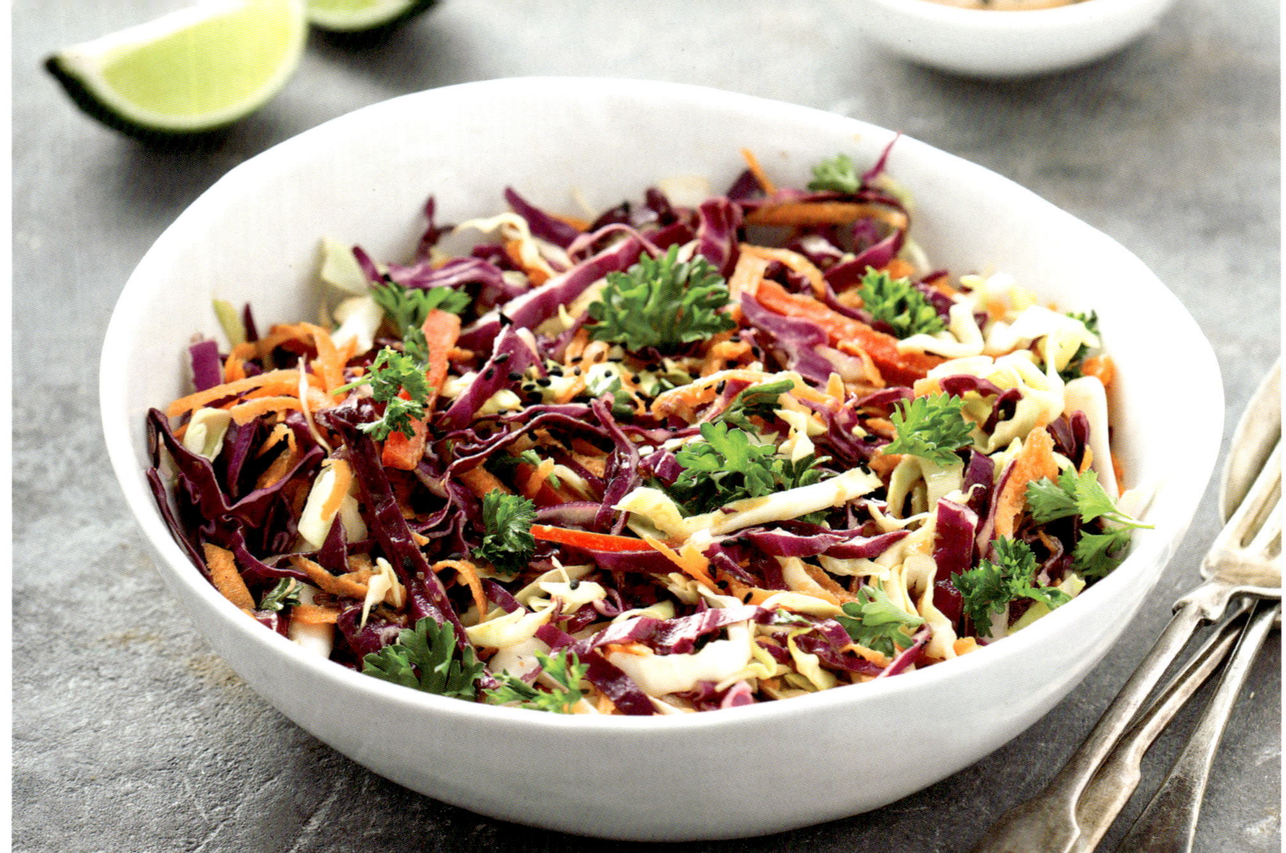

SERVES 4 | PREP + COOK TIME: 20 MINS | VEG | GLUTEN FREE | DAIRY FREE |

CABBAGE SLAW WITH CITRUS DRESSING

CITRUS DRESSING

1 Asian shallot, minced

1 orange, juiced and zested

2 tbsps apple cider vinegar

2 tbsps maple syrup

¼ tsp salt

¼ tsp pepper

¼ tsp cayenne pepper

3 tbsps olive oil

SALAD

1 small red cabbage, shredded

½ small white cabbage, shredded

1 carrot, shredded

1 red capsicum, thinly sliced

1 apple, very finely sliced

¼ cup (5g) parsley leaves

1 tbsp toasted sesame seeds

STEPS

1. Place the shallot, orange juice and zest, apple cider vinegar, maple syrup, salt, pepper and cayenne pepper into a small jug or bowl. Whisk to combine. Continue to whisk as you slowly pour in the olive oil. When all the oil is incorporated set aside.
2. Place the red and white cabbage in a large serving bowl along with the carrot, capsicum and apple. Add the parsley and toss to combine.
3. Top with toasted sesame seeds. Drizzle with dressing to serve.

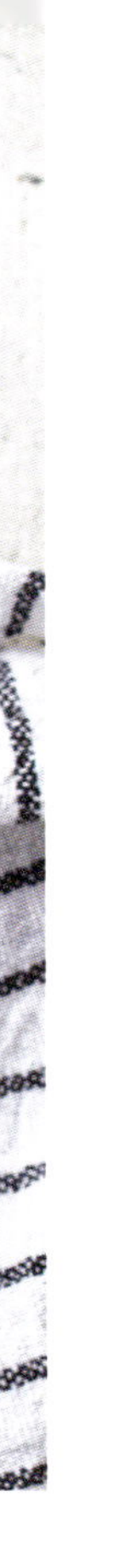

KALE & MANGO SALAD BOWL

SALAD

1 bunch curly kale, leaves torn and tough stems removed

2 mangos, cubed

200g mixed sprouts

2 tbsps sesame seeds

balsamic vinaigrette

DRESSING

¼ cup (60ml) balsamic vinegar

1 tsp dark brown sugar (optional)

1 clove garlic, minced

½ tsp salt

½ tsp pepper

¾ cup (185ml) olive oil

STEPS

1. Prepare the salad ingredients and arrange in serving bowls.
2. Combine the balsamic vinegar, sugar (if using), garlic, salt and pepper in a small mixing bowl. Gradually add the olive oil and whisk until emulsified.
3. Dress the salad and serve immediately.

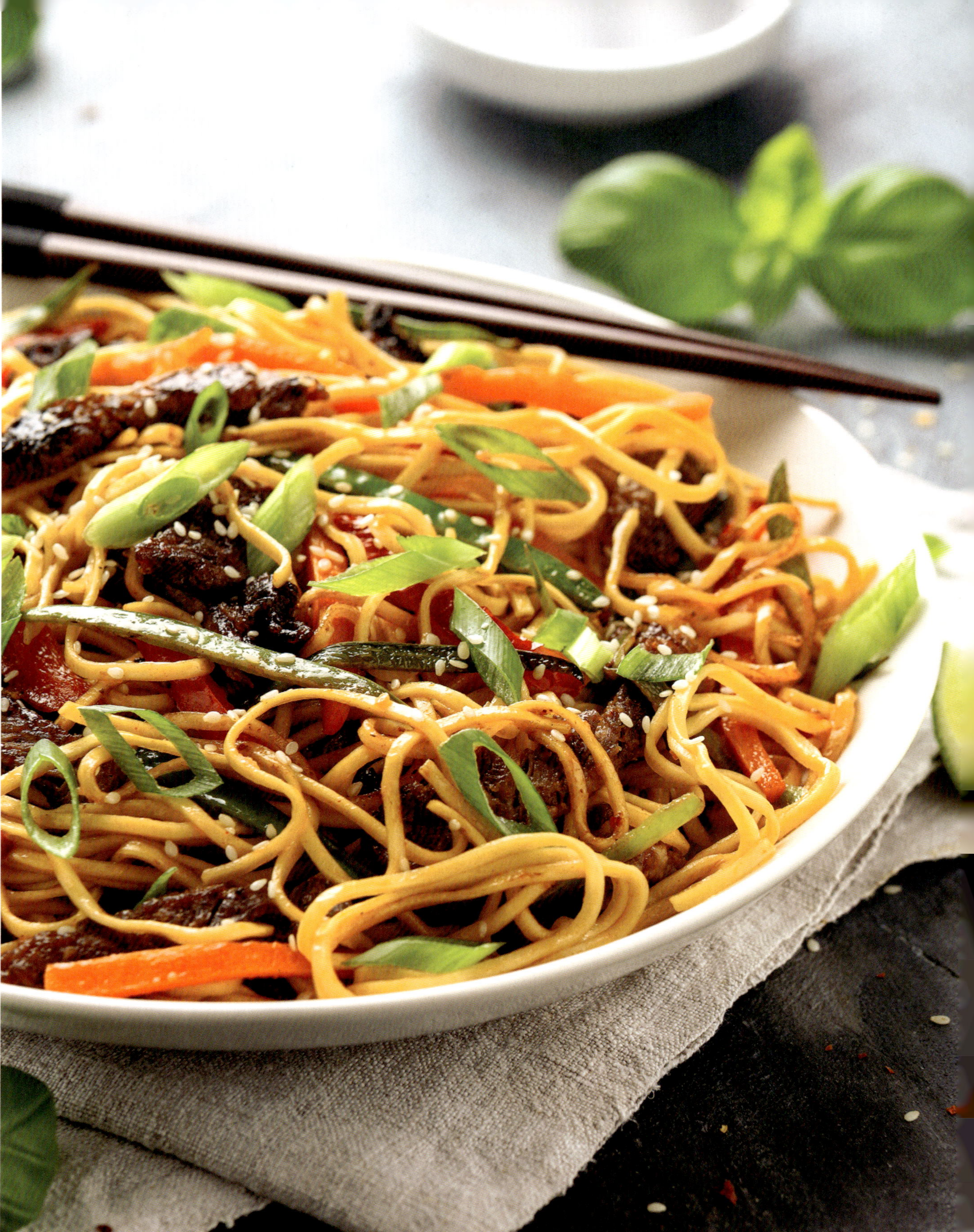

BEEF CHOW MEIN

150g egg noodles

3 tbsps sunflower oil

300g sirloin, skirt or flank steak, thinly sliced against the grain

1 small onion, peeled and sliced

2 cloves garlic, peeled and minced

1 carrot, cut into thin 5cm batons

1 green capsicum, thinly sliced

1 red capsicum, thinly sliced

1 cup (100g) bean sprouts

SAUCE

1 tbsp cornflour

2 tbsps soy sauce

1 tbsp Chinese rice wine

2 tbsps kecap manis (sweet soy sauce)

2 tbsps hoisin sauce

⅓ cup (90ml) beef stock

1 tbsp sesame oil

¼ tsp white pepper

TO SERVE

2 spring onions, chopped

2 tsps toasted sesame seeds

STEPS

1. Cook the noodles in boiling water according to the packet instructions, then run under cold water.
2. In a small bowl, mix together the sauce ingredients. Set aside.
3. Heat 2 tablespoons of the oil in a wok or large frying pan over a high heat. Add the steak to the pan and stir-fry for 2-3 minutes until the steak is just cooked. Remove the steak from the pan with a slotted spoon, place on a plate and set aside.
4. Add the remaining oil to the pan. Add the onion, garlic and carrot and stir-fry for 3 minutes, then add the capsicums and bean sprouts and stir-fry for a further 2 minutes.
5. Return the steak to the pan, along with the noodles and the sauce. Toss everything together for 2-3 minutes until everything is heated through. Scatter with spring onions and sesame seeds to serve.

SERVES 4 | PREP + COOK TIME: 30 MINS | DAIRY FREE |

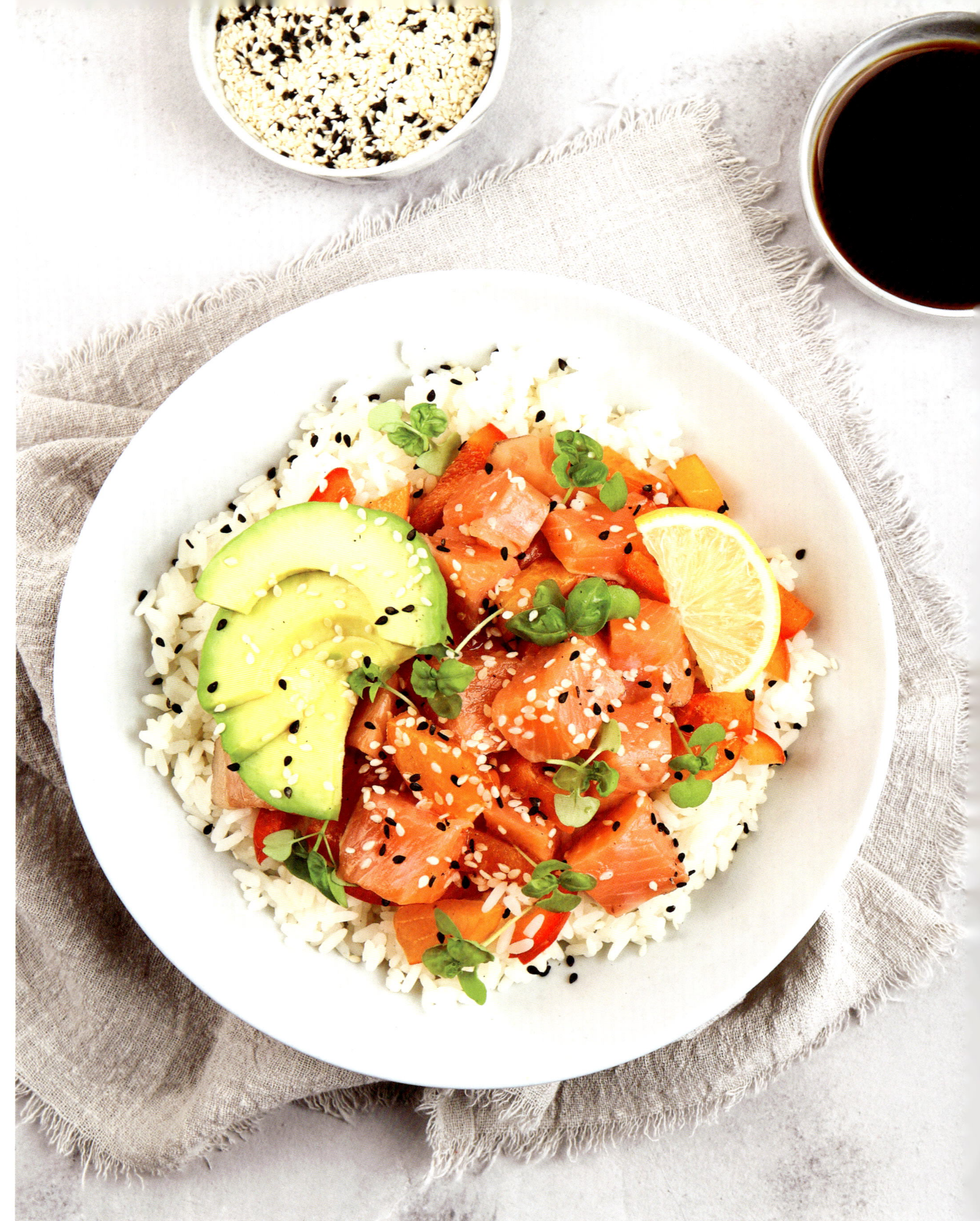

SPICY SALMON POKE BOWL

500g sashimi-grade salmon, cut into 2cm cubes

¼ cup (60ml) tamari

1 tsp rice wine vinegar

1 tsp Sriracha

1 tsp sesame oil

1 cup (155g) sushi rice

1½ cups (375ml) water

1 red capsicum, sliced

1 avocado, sliced

1 tsp black and white sesame seeds

Handful of micro herbs (optional)

Lemon wedges to serve

STEPS

1. In a medium-sized bowl combine diced salmon, tamari, vinegar, Sriracha and sesame oil. Cover and refrigerate for 15-45 minutes but no longer than 1 hour.

2. Combine rice and water in a saucepan over medium-high heat and bring to a boil. Reduce heat to low, cover and cook until rice is tender and all the water is absorbed, about 20 minutes.

3. Divide the cooked rice between bowls and top with marinated salmon, sliced capsicum and avocado. Sprinkle with sesame seeds and micro herbs, if desired, and serve with lemon wedges.

SERVES 4 | PREP + COOK TIME: 30 MINS + MARINATING | GLUTEN FREE | DAIRY FREE |

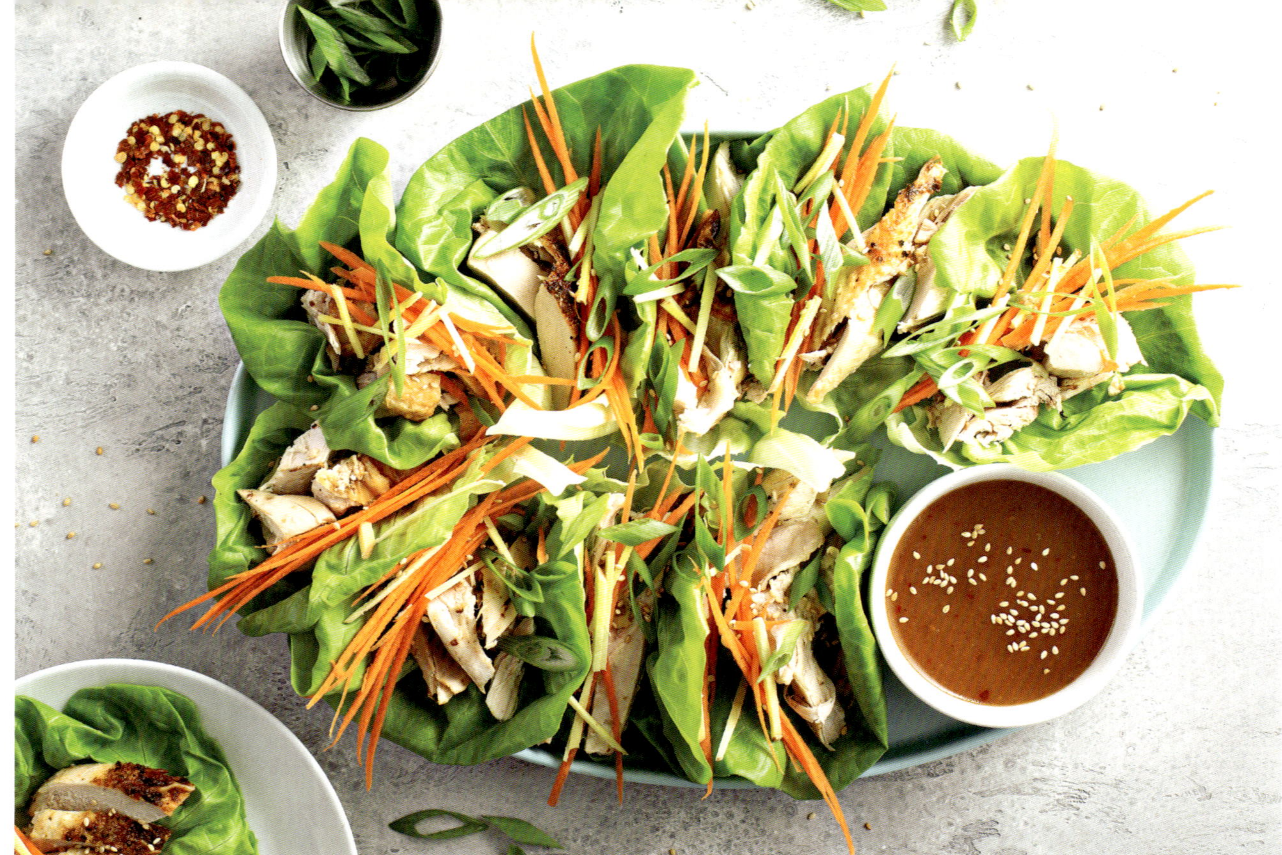

SALAD CUPS WITH PEANUT SUACE

2 little gem lettuces or 1 butter lettuce, leaves separated

2 cooked chicken breasts, cut into bite-sized pieces

4 spring onions, thinly sliced on the diagonal

1 Lebanese cucumber, cut into very fine matchsticks

1 medium carrot, cut into very fine matchsticks

2 tsps toasted sesame seeds

3 tbsps crunchy peanut butter

3 tbsps boiling water

1 tbsp sweet chilli sauce

Juice of ½ lime

Medium piece ginger, grated

STEPS

1. Arrange the lettuce leaves on a large serving platter. Fill with chicken pieces, spring onion, cucumber and carrot strips.
2. Put the peanut butter in a small bowl and stir in the boiling water until smooth. Add the sweet chilli sauce, lime juice and ginger. Mix well to combine.
3. Serve the lettuce cups with peanut sauce and scatter with sesame seeds.

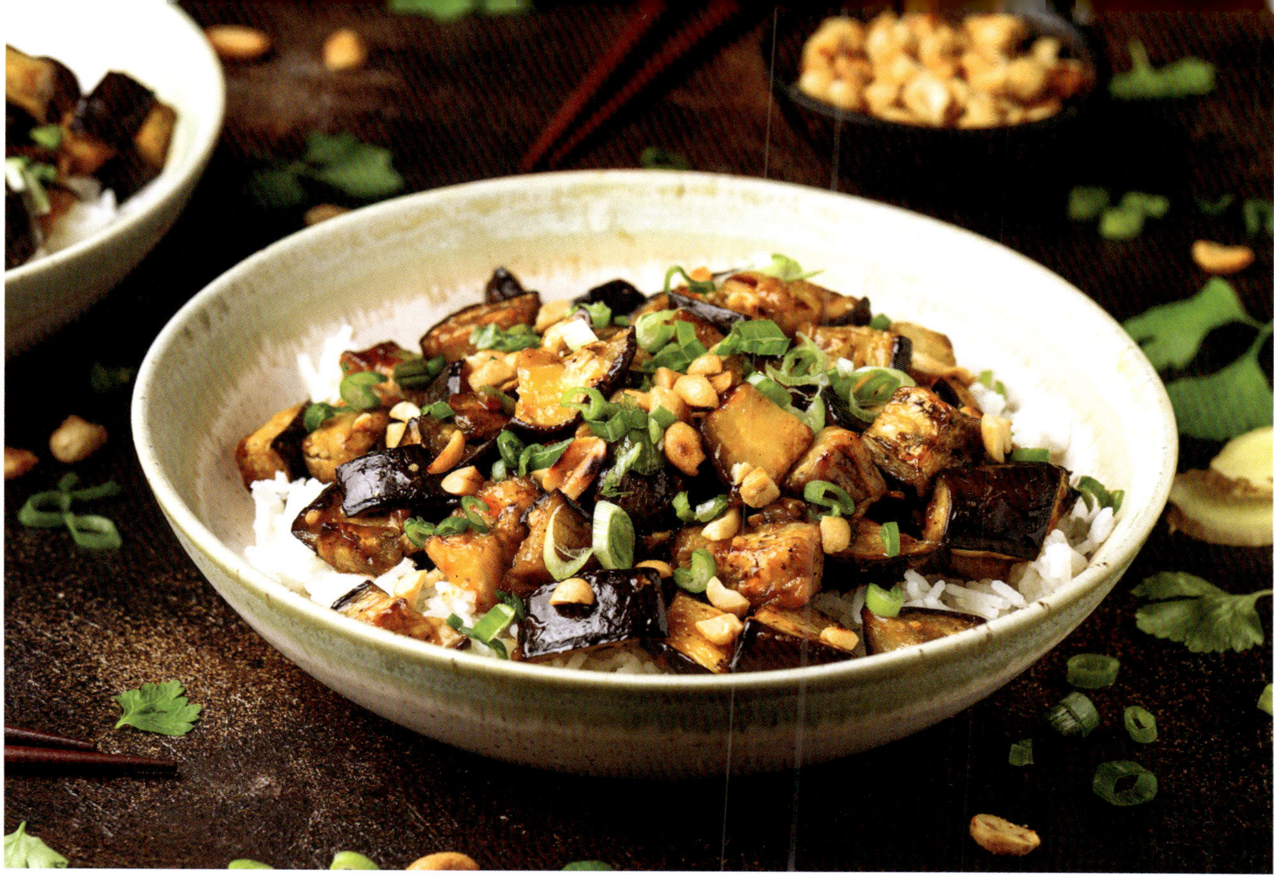

SESAME EGGPLANT BOWL

⅓ cup (40g) raw peanuts

3 tbsps soy sauce

4 tsps rice wine vinegar

1 tbsp maple syrup

1 tbsp toasted sesame oil

3 tbsps water

1 tbsp peanut oil

3 large eggplants, cut into 3cm pieces

3 cloves garlic, minced

½ tbsp cornflour + 2 tbsps water, combined to make a slurry

Steamed rice to serve

1 tsp dried chilli flakes

2 spring onions, chopped, to serve

STEPS

1. Place peanuts in a dry frying pan over medium-high heat and cook, stirring regularly, for 3-5 minutes until toasted and fragrant. Remove from the pan immediately and set aside.
2. In a small bowl, combine soy sauce, rice wine vinegar, maple syrup, sesame oil and 3 tablespoons of water. Set aside.
3. Heat the oil in a large frying pan or wok over medium-high heat. Add the eggplant and garlic and stir-fry for 8-10 minutes until eggplant is soft.
4. Pour in soy sauce mixture, followed by cornflour slurry. Bring to a simmer and thicken.
5. Serve over steamed rice and scatter with toasted peanuts, chilli flakes and chopped spring onions.

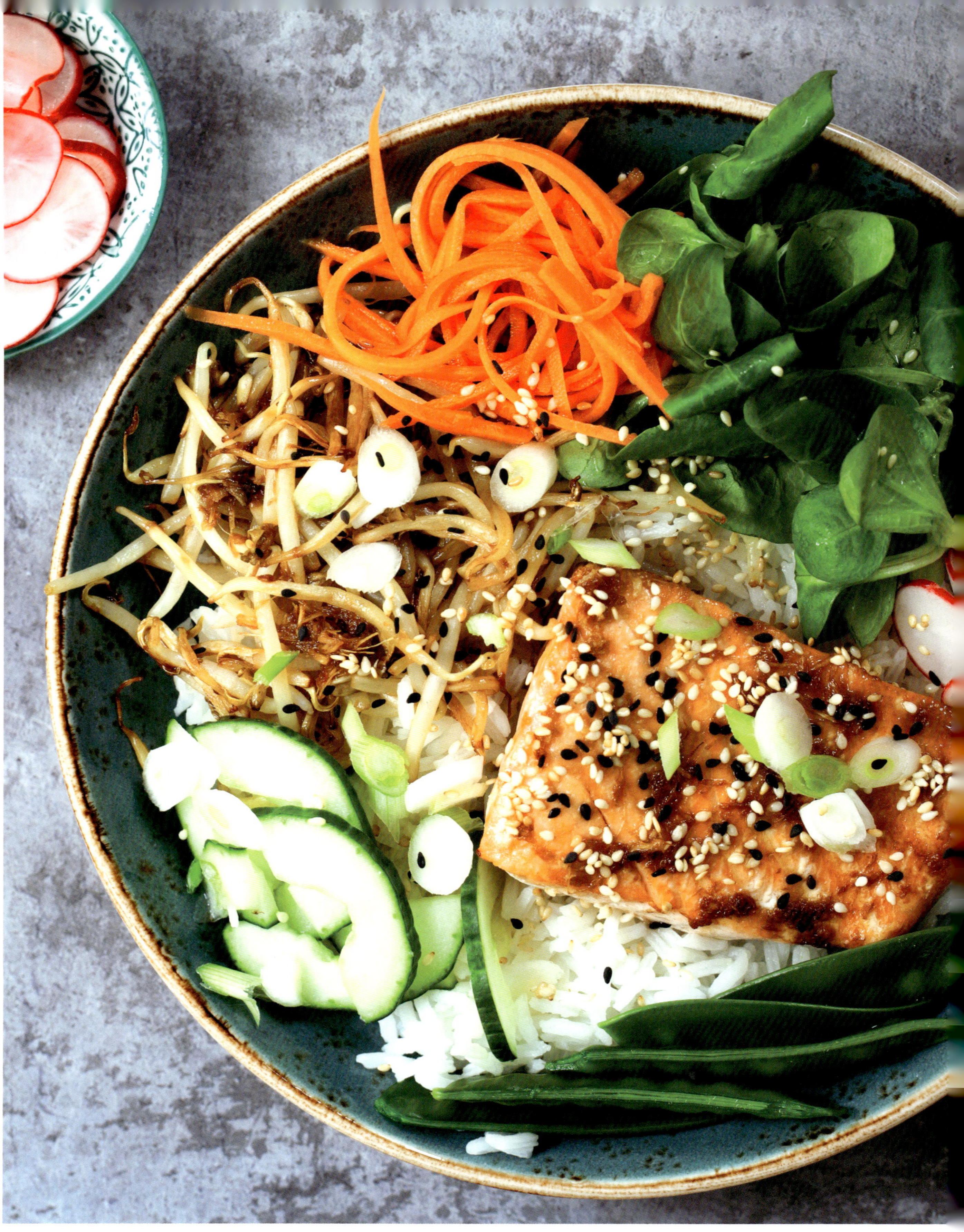

MISO-GLAZED SALMON BOWL

1½ cups (235g) medium-grain white rice

3 cups (750ml) cold, salted water

¼ cup (40g) packed brown sugar

2 tbsps + 2 tsps tamari

2 tbsps hot water

2 tbsps white miso

4 x 150g salmon fillets, about 2cm thick

2 tbsps peanut oil

2 cloves garlic, minced

3½ cups (350g) bean sprouts

1 cup (100g) snow peas, trimmed

½ cucumber, deseeded and sliced

8 radishes, thinly sliced

2 carrots, julienned

100g lamb's lettuce

1 tbsp sesame oil

1 tbsp black and white sesame seeds, to garnish

2 spring onions, thinly sliced, to garnish

STEPS

1. Combine the rice with the water in a large saucepan over a medium-high heat and bring to the boil. Cover the pan and reduce the heat to low. Cook for 20 minutes, then remove from the heat and let the pan stand for a further 5 minutes.

2. Meanwhile in a medium-sized bowl combine the brown sugar, 2 tablespoons tamari, hot water and miso. Stir with a whisk.

3. Arrange the fish on a shallow baking tray lined with greaseproof paper. Spoon the miso glaze evenly over the fish fillets. Place the salmon under a hot grill for 7-9 minutes, until the fish flakes easily with a fork, basting with the miso glaze halfway through cooking. Set aside to rest.

4. Heat the peanut oil in a wok over high heat. Add the garlic and fry for 1 minute until fragrant. Add the bean sprouts and 2 teaspoons tamari and cook for 2 minutes until the bean sprouts soften. Remove from the heat and set aside.

5. Divide the rice into four bowls. Add the snow peas, cucumber slices, radishes, carrots, lamb's lettuce and cooked bean sprouts. Top with the salmon, drizzle with the sesame oil and garnish with sesame seeds and spring onion.

SERVES 4 | PREP + COOK TIME: 45 MINS | DAIRY FREE |

VIETNAMESE PRAWN NOODLE BOWL

1kg shell-on, raw king prawns

Medium piece ginger, sliced

1 tsp black peppercorns

2 cloves garlic, chopped

2 large fresh red chillies, deseeded and thinly sliced

1 stalk lemongrass, sliced

8 cups (2L) water

350g shiitake mushrooms, sliced

250g rice noodles

3 tbsps lemon juice

3 tbsps fish sauce

2 spring onions, sliced thinly

⅓ cup (5g) coriander leaves

¼ cup (5g) mint leaves

Lime wedges to serve

STEPS

1. Peel and devein prawns; discard heads.
2. Place prawn shells, ginger, peppercorns, garlic, half the chilli, lemongrass and water in a large pan. Bring to the boil. Reduce heat and simmer, uncovered, for 20 minutes. Strain stock and return to pan.
3. Add prawns and mushrooms to stock. Simmer, covered, for 3 minutes, or until prawns are pink.
4. Meanwhile cook noodles according to packet directions.
5. Add lemon juice and fish sauce to soup. Divide noodles and soup evenly among four bowls. Top with spring onions, herbs, remaining chilli and lime wedges.

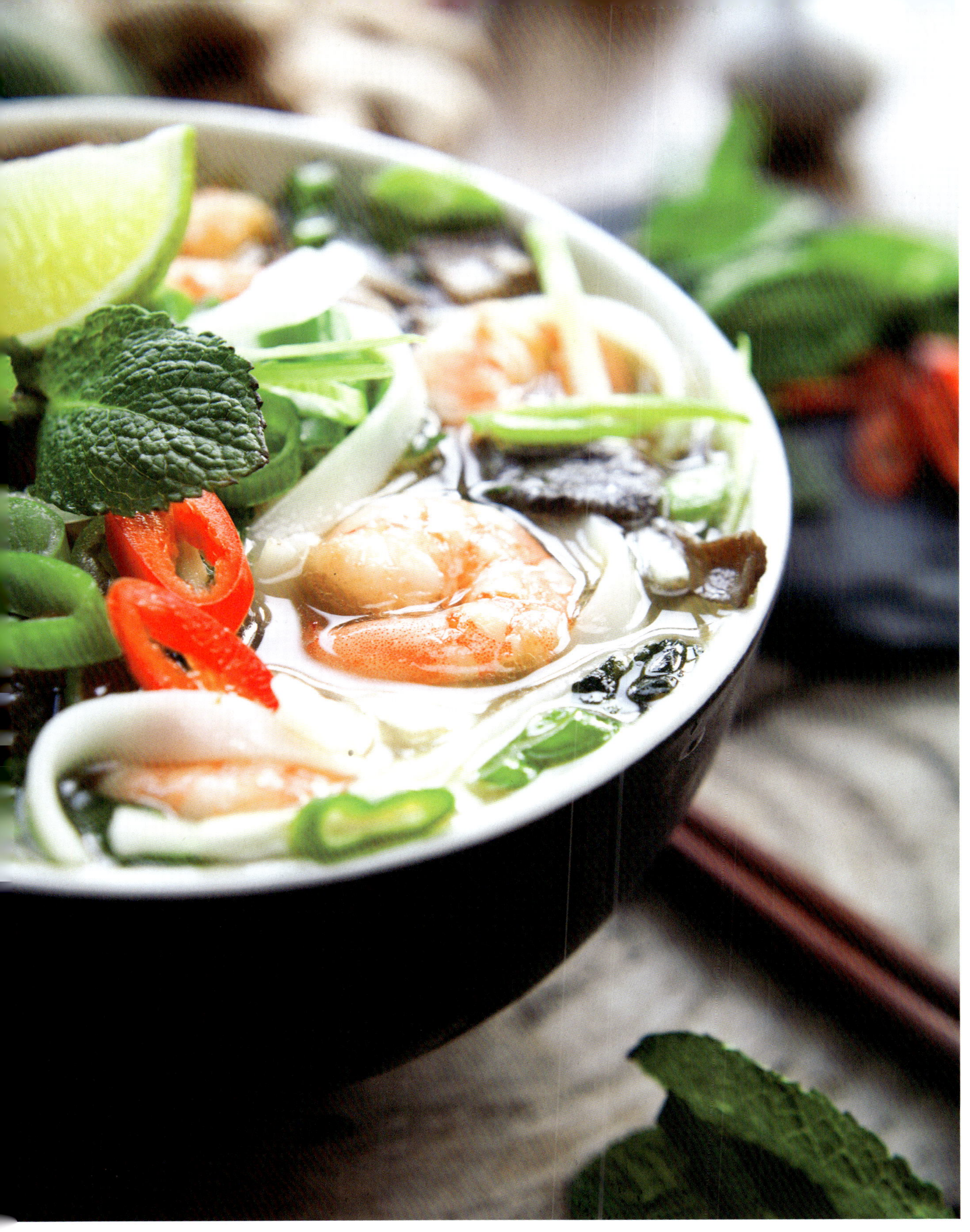

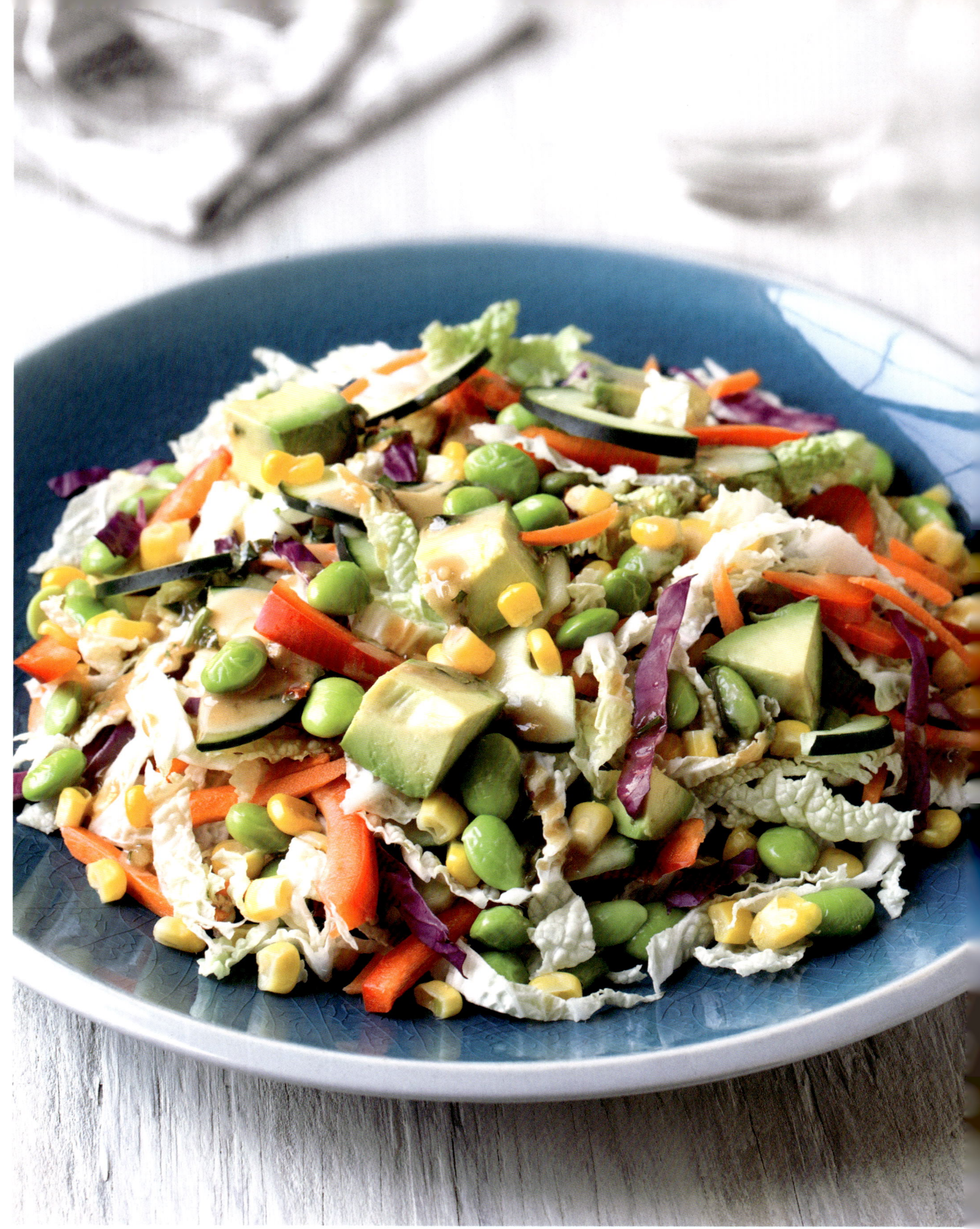

VEGETARIAN THAI SALAD

SERVES 4 | PREP + COOK TIME: 20 MINS | VEG | GLUTEN FREE | DAIRY FREE |

DRESSING

2 tbsps peanut butter

1 tbsp agave syrup

1 tbsp lemon juice

1 tbsp tamari

1 tbsp water

1 tsp garlic powder

1 tsp Sriracha

SALAD

1 cup (175g) corn kernels

1 cup (180g) edamame beans

3 cups (300g) shredded Chinese cabbage (wombok)

1 cup (100g) shredded red cabbage

1 carrot, julienned

1 red capsicum, thinly sliced

1 Lebanese cucumber, sliced into thin half moons

1 avocado, diced

STEPS

1. Whisk all the dressing ingredients together in a small bowl. Set aside.
2. Cook the corn and edamame beans in a pan of boiling salted water for 1-2 minutes until tender. Drain and run under cold water to cool.
3. Add sweetcorn and edamame beans to a large bowl along with the remaining salad ingredients. Pour over the dressing and toss to coat. Serve immediately.

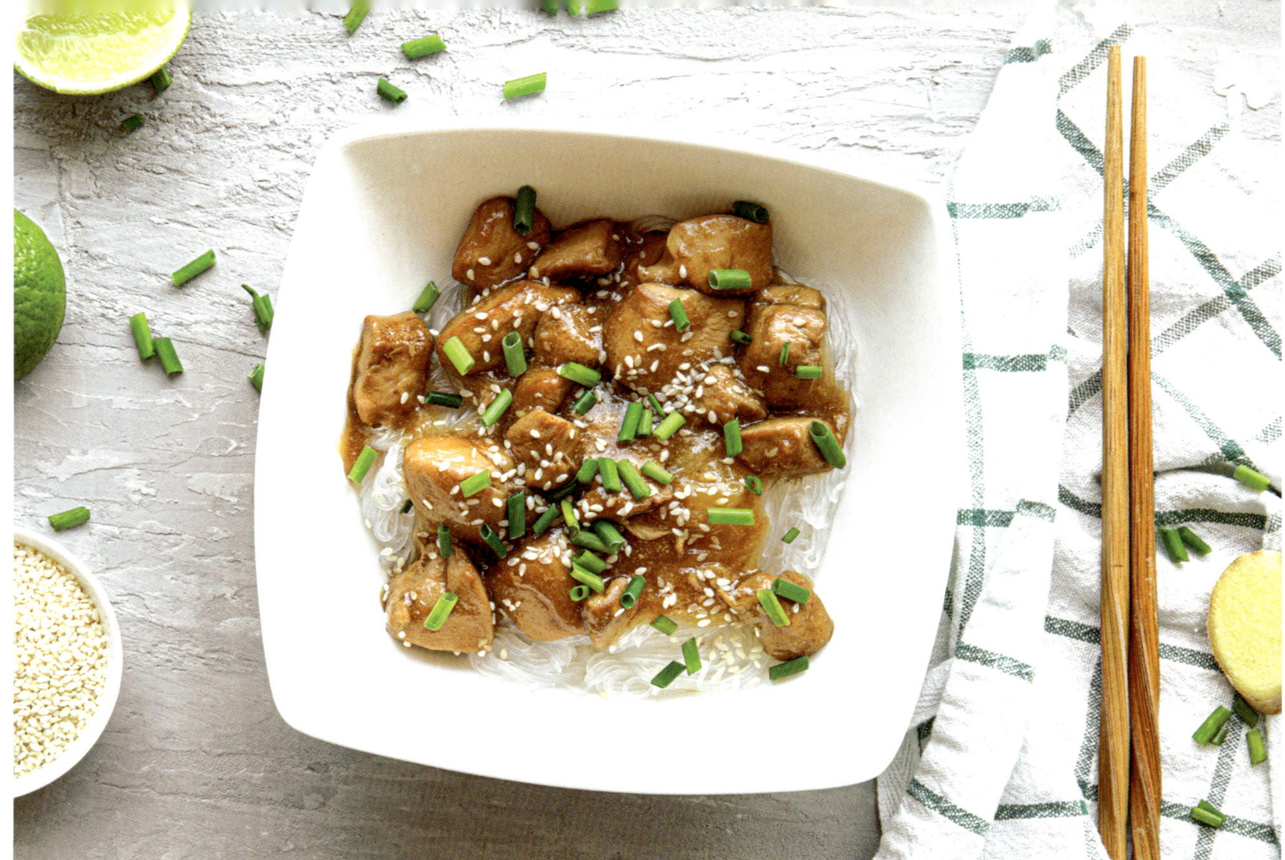

SESAME CHICKEN WITH GLASS NOODLES

1 large egg

2 tbsps cornflour

Pinch each of salt and pepper

500g chicken thigh fillets, cut into 3cm pieces

2 tbsps peanut oil

200g glass noodles, cooked

1 tsp sesame seeds

2 spring onion tops, chopped

SAUCE

¼ cup (60ml) soy sauce

2 tbsps water

1 tbsp toasted sesame oil

3 tbsps brown sugar

1 tbsp rice wine vinegar

Small piece fresh ginger, grated

2 cloves garlic, minced

1 tbsp sesame seeds

½ tbsps cornflour

STEPS

1. In a small bowl stir together the sauce ingredients. Set aside.
2. In a large bowl, whisk together the egg, cornflour, salt and pepper. Toss the chicken in the mixture.
3. Heat the peanut oil in a large frying pan or wok over medium-high heat. Add the coated chicken and spread out in a single layer. Allow the chicken to cook, undisturbed, for 2 minutes until golden brown on the bottom. Carefully flip the chicken and continue to cook until golden brown all over, turning the chicken as necessary.
4. Pour the sauce into the pan and stir to coat chicken in sauce. Bring to simmer and allow the sauce to thicken.
5. Serve the chicken over a bed of noodles and sprinkle with sesame seeds and spring onions.

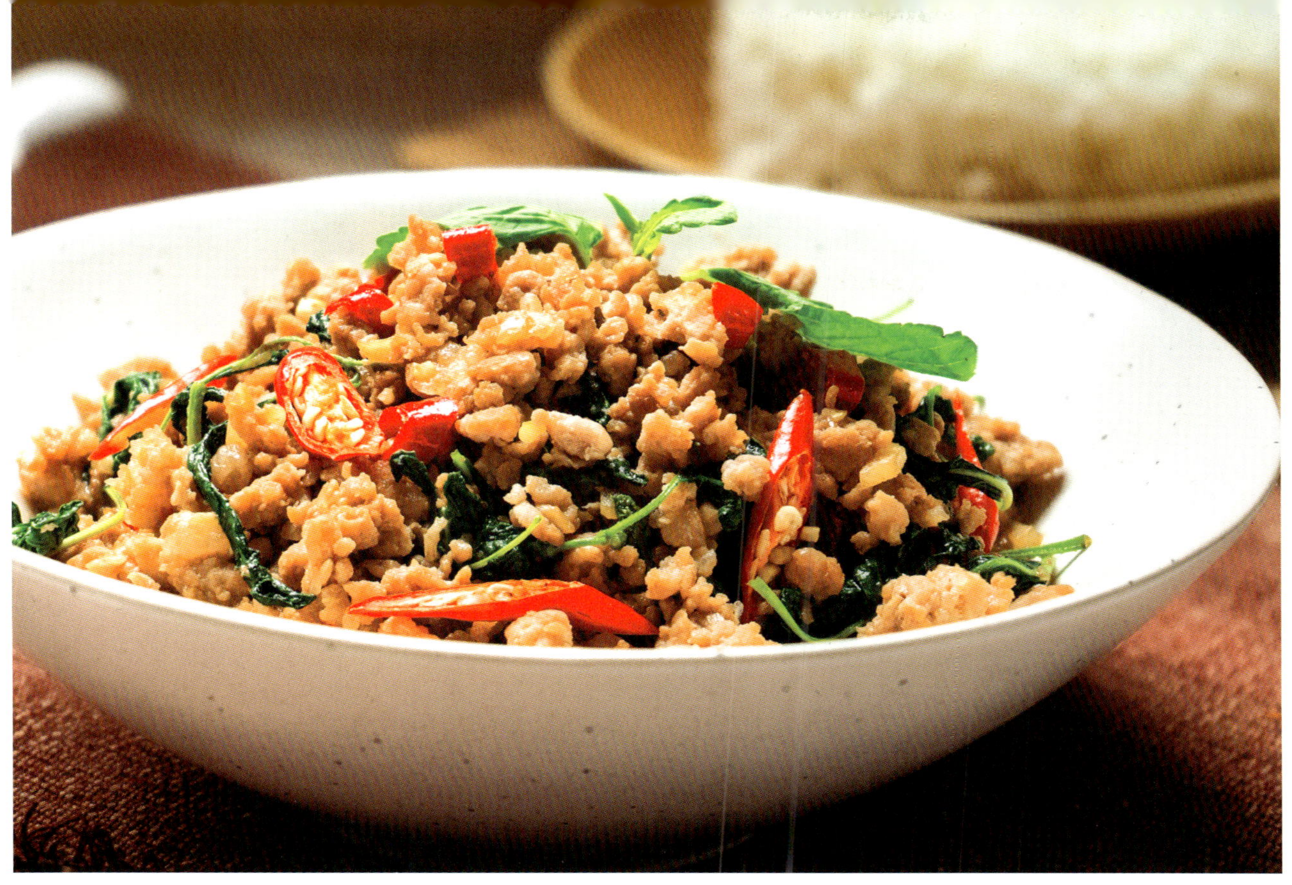

SPICY CHICKEN THAI BASIL

3 tbsps vegetable oil

2 Asian shallots, thinly sliced

7 cloves garlic, sliced

3 red Thai chillies, thinly sliced

500g chicken mince

1 tsp sugar

1 tbsp fish sauce

1 tbsp soy sauce

1 tsp dark soy sauce (optional)

2 tsps oyster sauce

⅓ cup (80ml) chicken stock or water

1½ cups (65g) packed Thai basil leaves

STEPS

1. Heat oil in a wok over medium-high heat. Add the shallots and garlic and fry for 3 minutes. Add the chillies and cook for another minute.
2. Increase heat to high and add the chicken mince. Cook for 3-4 minutes, breaking it up with a wooden spoon, until crispy.
3. Add the sugar, fish sauce, soy sauce, dark soy sauce and oyster sauce. Stir-fry for another minute and deglaze the pan with the stock or water.
4. Add the basil, and stir-fry until wilted. Serve immediately.

NOTE: Pork mince can be used in place of chicken for this recipe, if preferred.

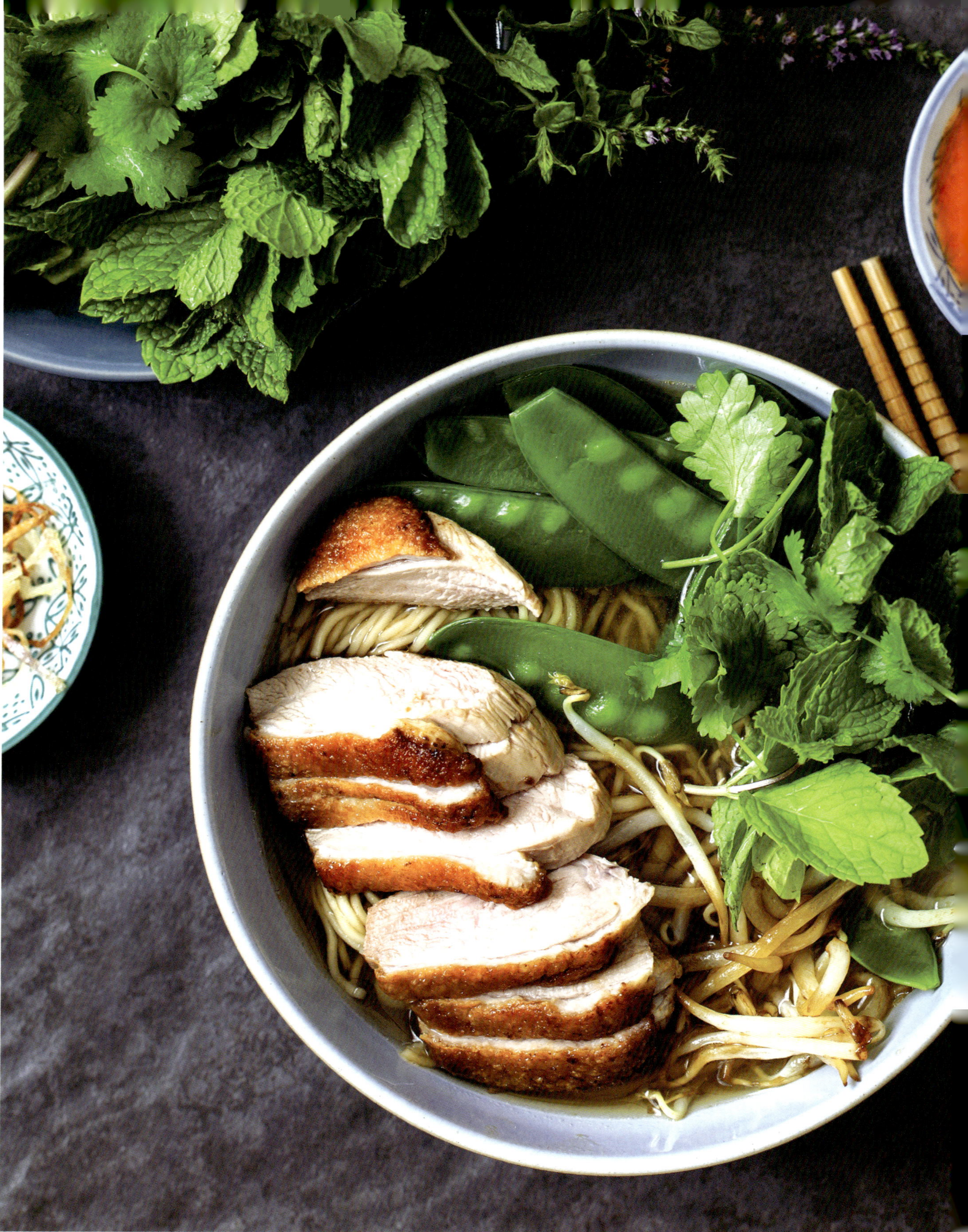

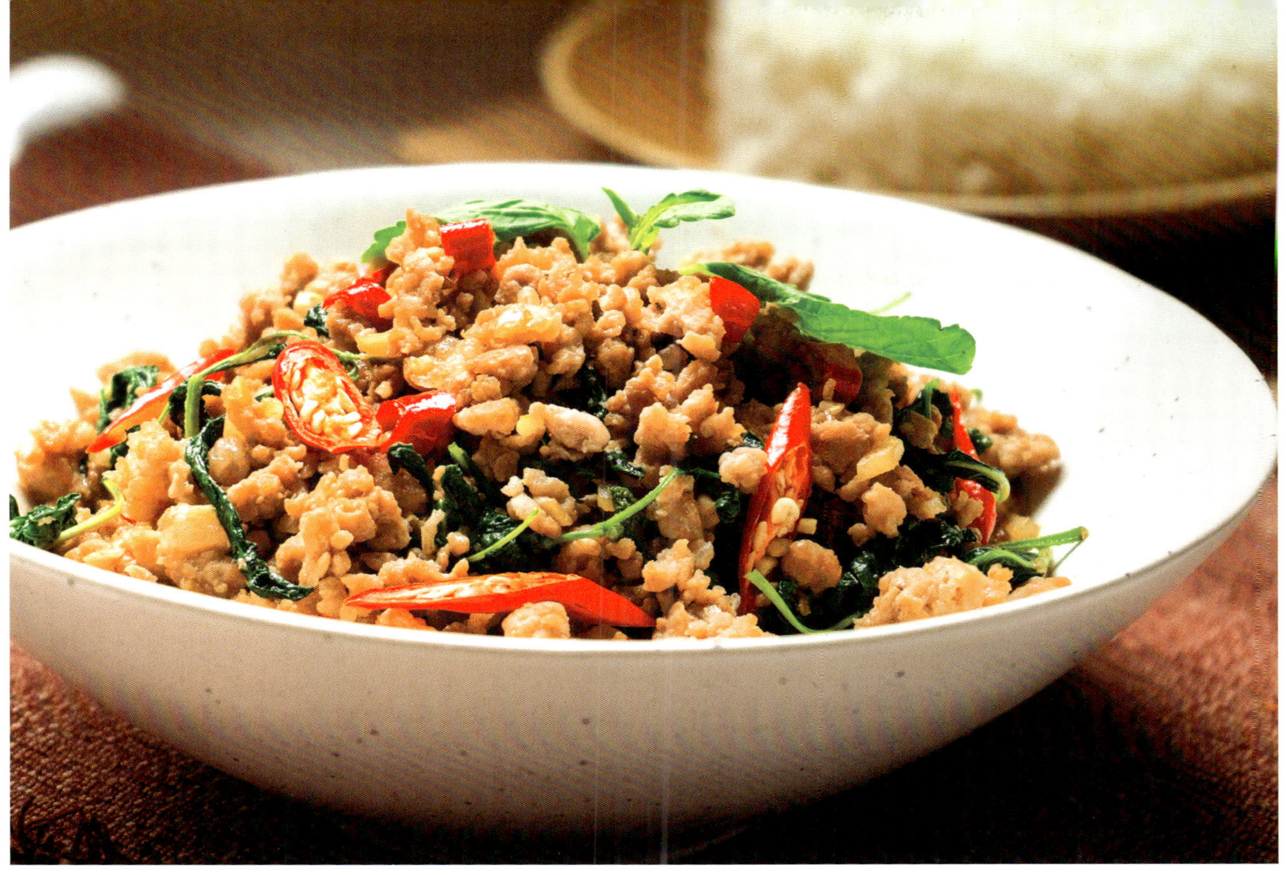

SPICY CHICKEN THAI BASIL

3 tbsps vegetable oil
2 Asian shallots, thinly sliced
7 cloves garlic, sliced
3 red Thai chillies, thinly sliced
500g chicken mince
1 tsp sugar
1 tbsp fish sauce
1 tbsp soy sauce
1 tsp dark soy sauce (optional)
2 tsps oyster sauce
⅓ cup (80ml) chicken stock or water
1½ cups (65g) packed Thai basil leaves

STEPS

1. Heat oil in a wok over medium-high heat. Add the shallots and garlic and fry for 3 minutes. Add the chillies and cook for another minute.
2. Increase heat to high and add the chicken mince. Cook for 3-4 minutes, breaking it up with a wooden spoon, until crispy.
3. Add the sugar, fish sauce, soy sauce, dark soy sauce and oyster sauce. Stir-fry for another minute and deglaze the pan with the stock or water.
4. Add the basil, and stir-fry until wilted. Serve immediately.

NOTE: Pork mince can be used in place of chicken for this recipe, if preferred.

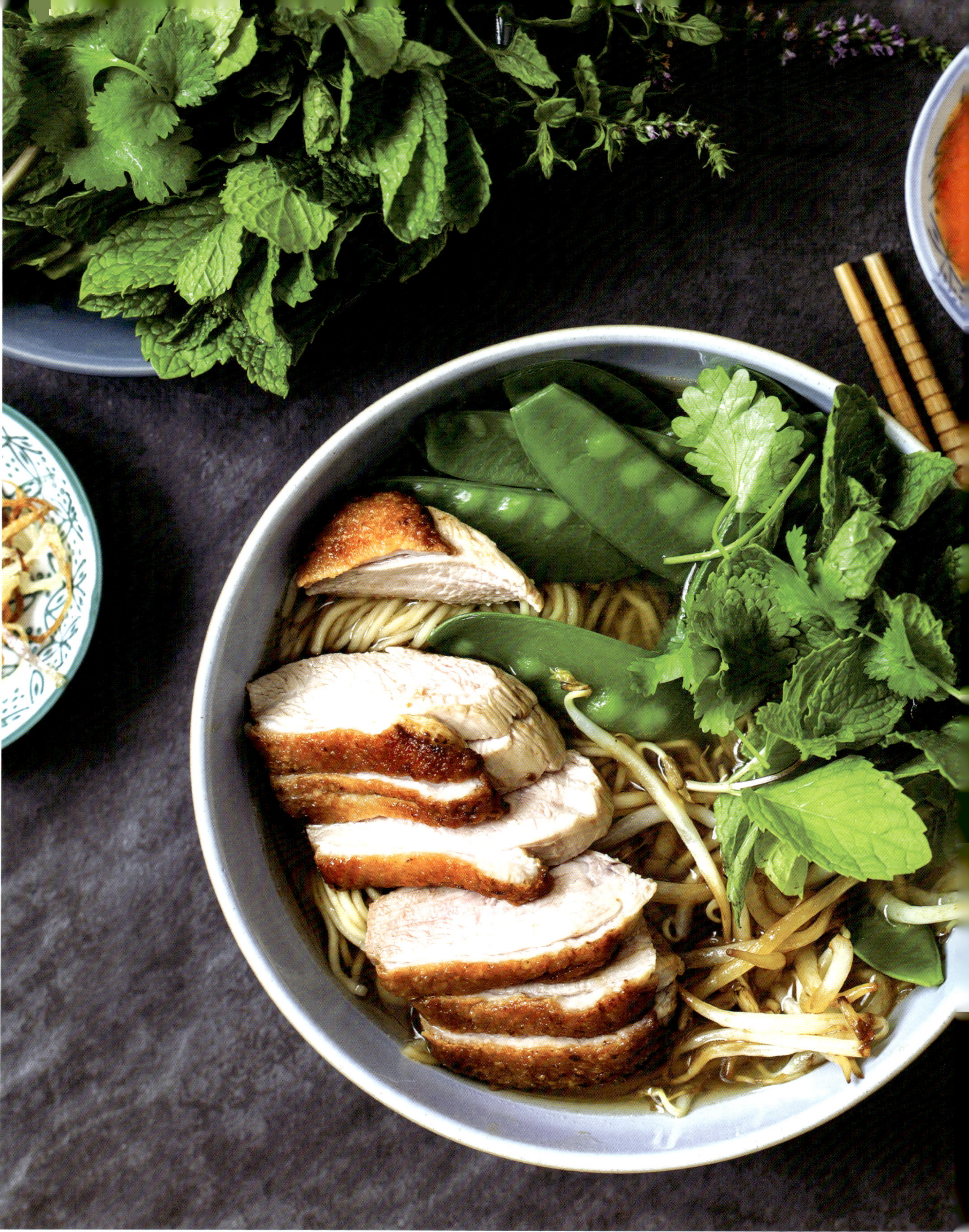

DUCK PHO

300g egg noodles
4 duck breasts
1 tbsp salt
1 tbsp whole black peppercorns
1 tbsp coriander seeds
4 star anise
Large piece fresh ginger, minced
1 bunch spring onions, chopped
12 cups (3L) chicken stock
1 cup (220g) sugar snap peas
1 cup (110g) bean sprouts
¼ cup (60ml) fish sauce
½ cup (10g) fresh mint leaves
½ cup (10g) fresh coriander leaves
Chilli sauce, such as Sriracha, to serve

STEPS

1. Cook the noodles according to packet directions, drain and set aside.
2. Heat a large frying pan over medium heat until very hot. Rub duck skin with salt then add duck breasts to the pan, skin-side down. Cook for 4-5 minutes until the skin is a deep golden colour. Turn over the duck breasts and cook for a further 3 minutes for medium. Remove from the pan and let the duck rest for at least 10 minutes. Then slice.
3. While the duck is resting heat a large saucepan over medium-high heat. Toast the black peppercorns, coriander seeds and star anise pods for 2 minutes, until fragrant. Add the ginger and spring onion and cook for 2 minutes, or until fragrant.
4. Add the chicken stock. Increase the heat to high, cover, and bring to a simmer. Cook for 5 minutes. Add the sugar snap peas and bean sprouts. Cook for 1 minute more. Remove from the heat. Add fish sauce.
5. Divide the noodles between four bowls. Pour over the hot stock. Top with sliced duck, sugar snap peas and bean sprouts. Scatter with fresh herbs and serve with chilli sauce.

SERVES 4 | PREP + COOK TIME: 30 MINS | DAIRY FREE |

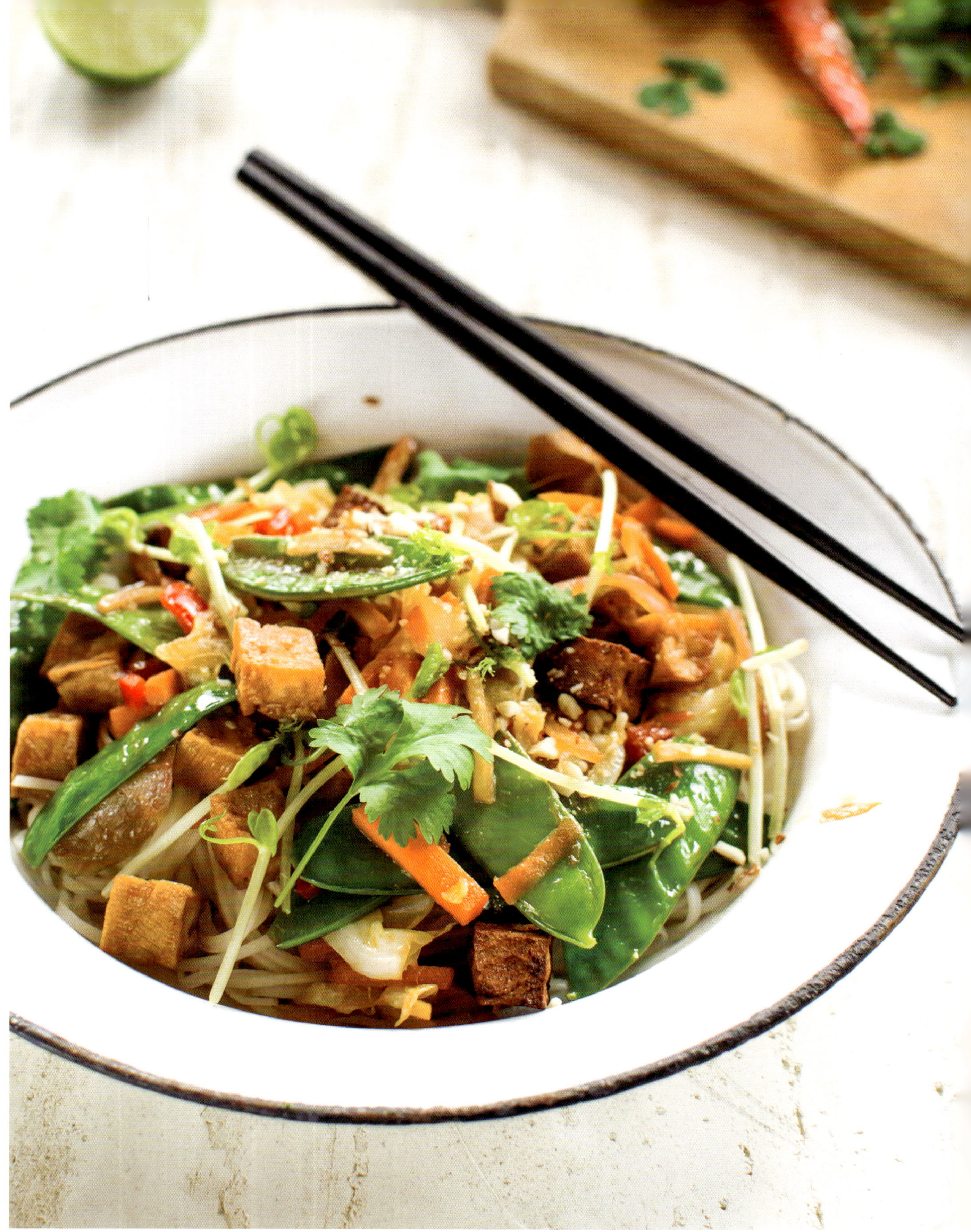

STIR-FRY WITH TOFU & SNOW PEAS

2 tbsps kecap manis (sweet soy sauce)

2 tbsps soy sauce

2 cloves garlic, crushed

320g firm tofu, drained and cut into cubes

Vegetable oil, for frying

1 onion, halved and finely sliced

Medium piece ginger, cut into thin strips

1 red capsicum, cut into thin strips

1 carrot, cut into thin strips

1¾ cups (200g) snow peas

¼ cup (60ml) water

450g noodles, cooked according to packet instructions

2 cups (200g) bean sprouts

¾ cup (90g) peanuts, chopped, to serve

Coriander leaves to serve

STEPS

1. Combine kecap manis, soy sauce and garlic in a shallow dish. Add the tofu and toss with the marinade to coat on all sides. Cover with plastic wrap and transfer to the fridge to marinate for 1 hour. Drain, reserving the marinade.
2. Add oil to a wok or large frying pan. Cook the tofu in batches until golden and crisp. Transfer to a plate.
3. Heat a splash more oil in the wok. Add the onion, ginger, capsicum and carrot and stir-fry for 2 minutes. Add the snow peas and water. Cover and cook for 1 minute or until vegetables are just tender.
4. Add the noodles, bean sprouts and remaining marinade to the pan. Cook, tossing, until well combined and the sauce coats the noodles. Add the tofu and toss gently to combine.
5. Serve in bowls garnished with chopped peanuts and coriander leaves.

SERVES 4 | PREP + COOK TIME: 30 MINS + MARINATING | VEG | DAIRY FREE |

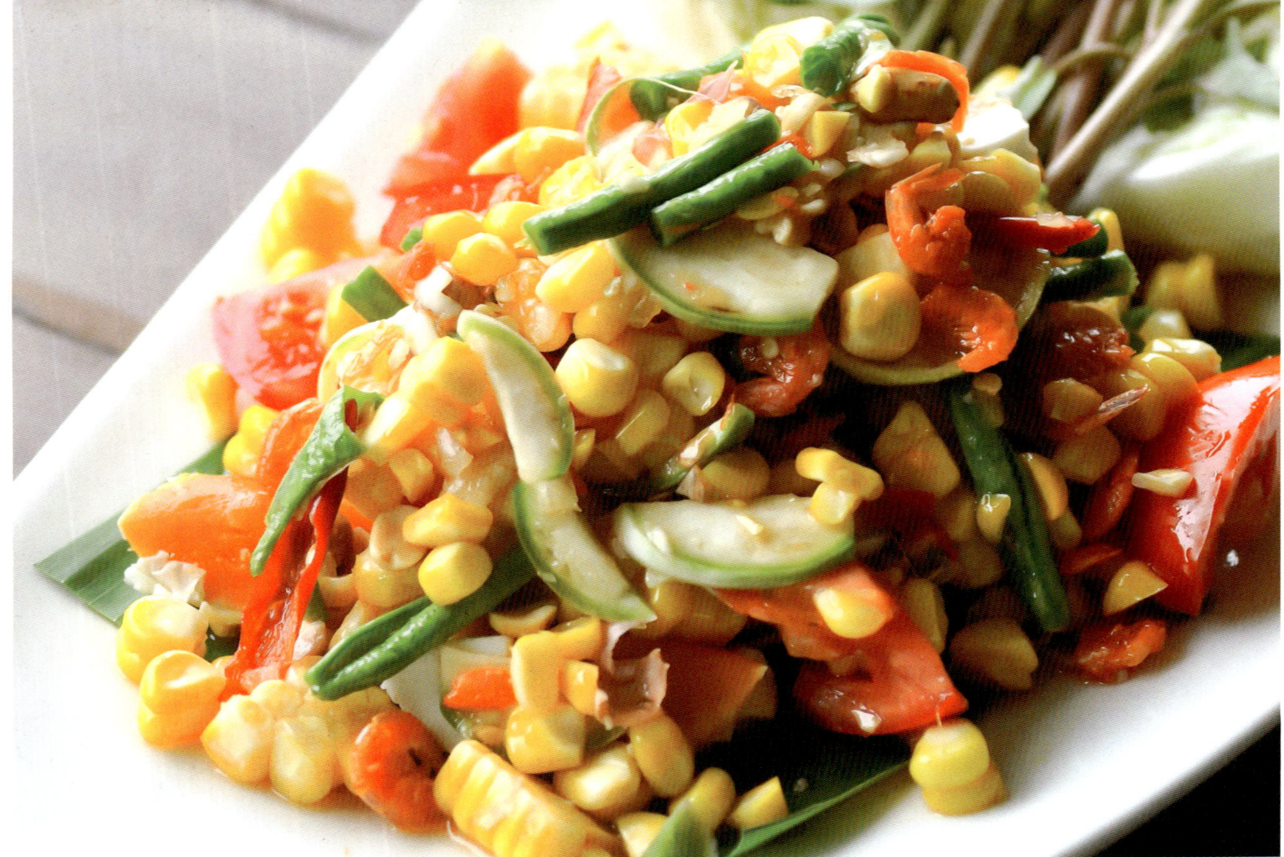

THAI CORN & PEANUT SALAD

½ cup (75g) sliced snake beans (or green beans)

6 cloves garlic

3 small bird's-eye chillies

4 tbsps roasted peanuts

3½ tbsps fish sauce

1 tbsp palm sugar

Juice of 2 limes

150g tomatoes, cut into eighths

3 cups (525g) raw corn kernels cut from the cob

¼ green papaya, thinly sliced (optional)

1 large red chilli, sliced

STEPS

1. Cook beans in a medium saucepan of boiling salted water for about 5 minutes until tender-crisp. Rinse under cold water. Cut into 3cm pieces.
2. Use a mortar and pestle to pound the garlic, bird's-eye chillies and half the peanuts. Then add the fish sauce, palm sugar and lime juice. Mix together.
3. Place the beans, tomatoes, corn, green papaya, if using, and sliced chilli in a large bowl. Add the garlic mixture and toss well to combine.
4. Scatter with remaining peanuts to serve.

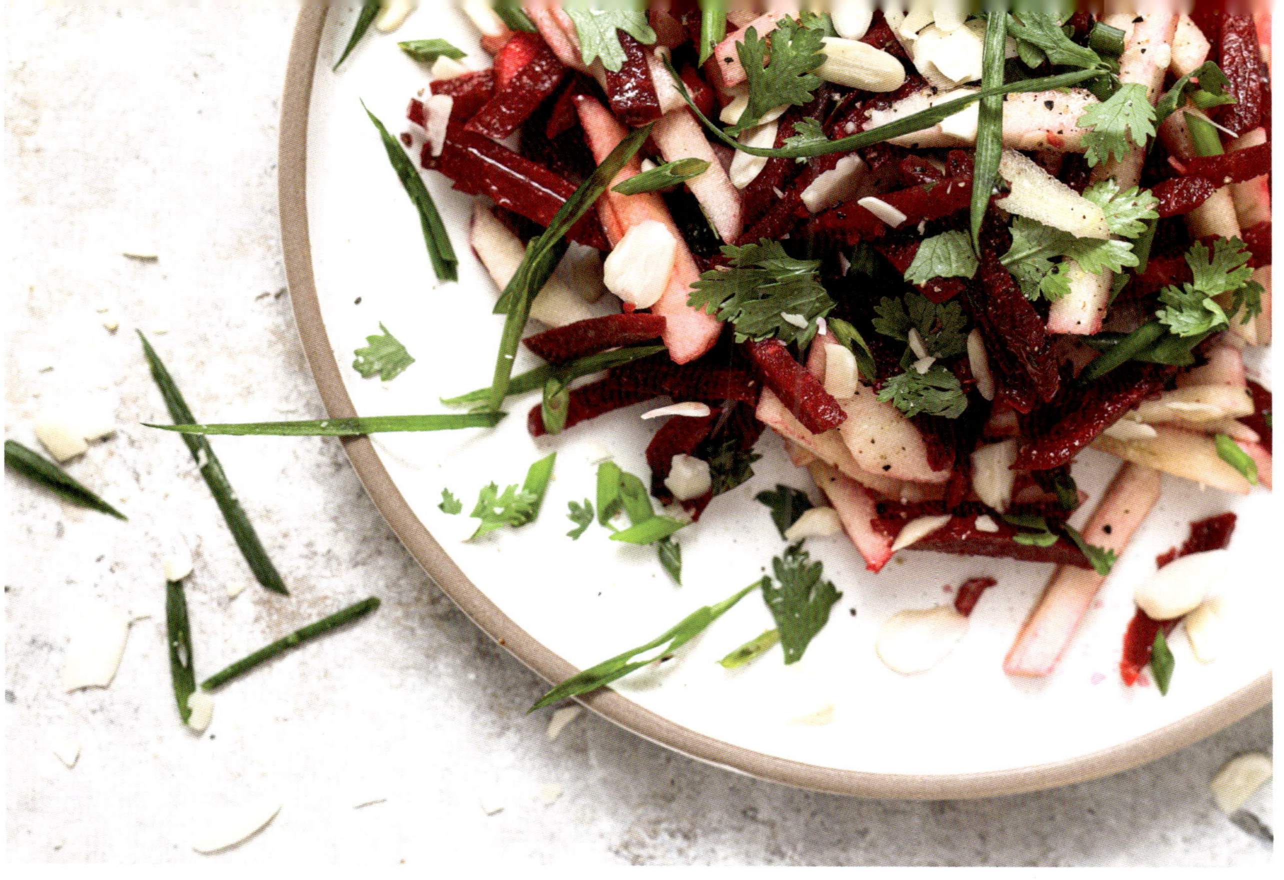

SERVES 4 | PREP + COOK TIME: 20 MINS | VEG | GLUTEN FREE | DAIRY FREE |

BEETROOT, APPLE & CORIANDER SALAD

3-4 large beetroots, peeled

3 apples

3 tbsps olive oil

Juice of 1 orange

Juice of ½ lemon

Salt and pepper to taste

Handful of fresh coriander leaves

1 spring onion, green part only, roughly chopped

¼ cup (30g) flaked almonds

STEPS

1. Cut the beetroot and apple into thin batons using a sharp knife or mandoline.
2. Transfer to a large bowl and drizzle with olive oil, orange and lemon juice. Season with salt and pepper. Toss to combine.
3. Scatter with coriander, spring onion and flaked almonds before serving.

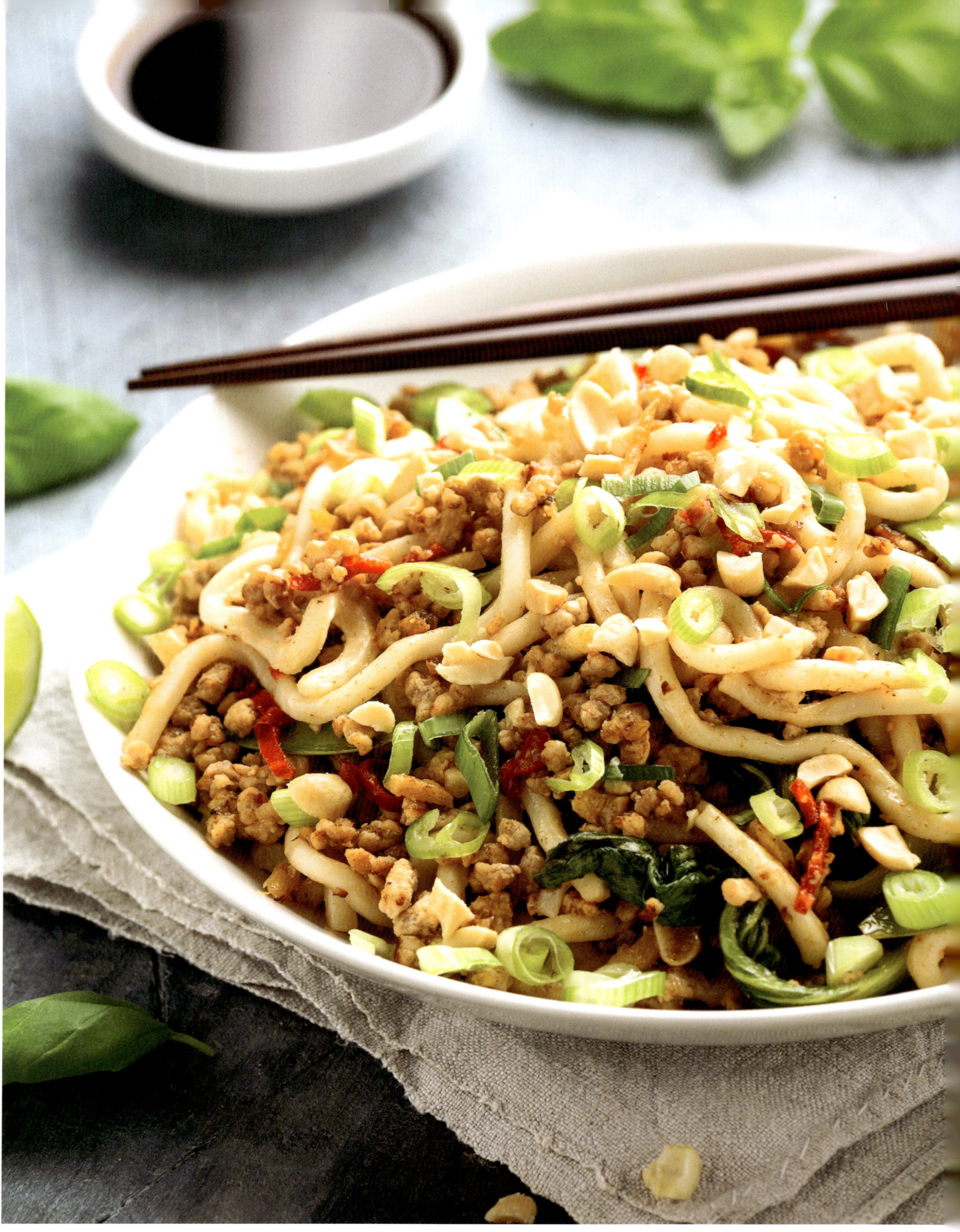

PORK UDON STIR-FRY

440g fresh udon noodles
1 tsp neutral-flavoured oil
2 tbsps peanut oil
500g pork mince
¼ cup (60ml) soy sauce
1 long red chilli, sliced
2 cloves garlic, minced
3 heads bok choy, chopped
1 tbsp oyster sauce
1 tbsp rice wine vinegar
1 tsp sesame oil
½ cup (50g) chopped spring onions
¼ cup (30g) chopped peanuts

STEPS

1. Prepare the noodles in boiling water, according to the packet directions. Drain and toss with the teaspoon of oil to prevent them from sticking.
2. Heat 1 tablespoon peanut oil in a large frying pan or wok over medium-high heat. When hot add pork and cook, breaking up with a wooden spoon, until browned. Add a small splash of the soy sauce, stir to coat, then transfer the pork to a plate.
3. Add another tablespoon peanut oil to the pan, then add the chilli and garlic. Cook for 1 minute until fragrant, then add the bok choy. Cook for another minute, then add the noodles to the pan. Stir for 1 minute.
4. Return the pork to the pan along with the soy sauce, oyster sauce, rice wine vinegar, sesame oil and most of the spring onions, reserving a few for serving. Toss everything together until the sauce.
5. Scatter with peanuts and the remaining spring onions to serve.

SERVES 4 | PREP + COOK TIME: 30 MINS | DAIRY FREE |

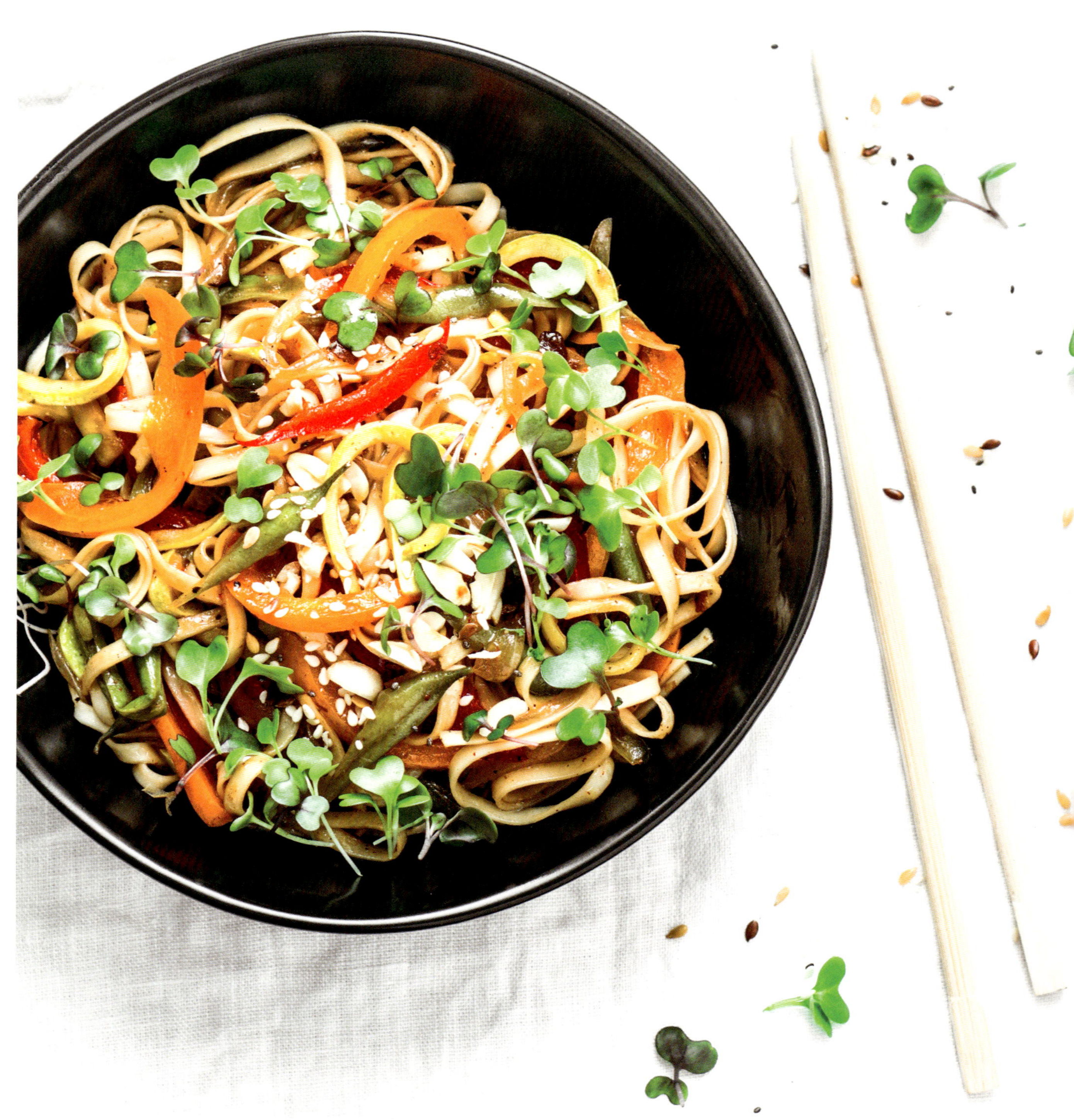

VEGETABLE PAD THAI

- 350g pad thai rice noodles or flat egg noodles
- 3 tbsps soy sauce
- 1 tbsp fish sauce
- 1 tbsp sambal oelek
- 2 tbsps lime juice
- 1 tbsp olive oil
- 2 tbsps brown sugar
- 1 tbsp peanut oil
- 1 large onion, thinly sliced
- 1 red capsicum, sliced
- 1 orange capsicum, sliced
- 1 green capsicum, sliced
- 1 cup (150g) green beans, cut into 5cm lengths
- 1 carrot, julienned
- ¼ cup (30g) peanuts, chopped
- 1 tsp sesame seeds
- 1 tbsp micro herbs, to garnish

STEPS

1. Bring a large pot of salted water to a boil. Cook the noodles according to the directions on the packet. Drain and rinse.
2. In a small bowl, mix together the soy sauce, fish sauce, sambal oelek, lime juice, olive oil and brown sugar. Whisk until the sugar has dissolved.
3. Heat the peanut oil in a large frying pan or wok over a medium heat. Add the onion and cook, stirring, for 3-5 minutes until soft and translucent. Add the capsicums, green beans and carrot and stir-fry for 4-5 minutes until tender.
4. Add noodles and soy dressing to the pan and stir until well combined and heated through.
5. Spoon into bowls and top with peanuts and sesame seeds. Garnish with micro herbs to serve.

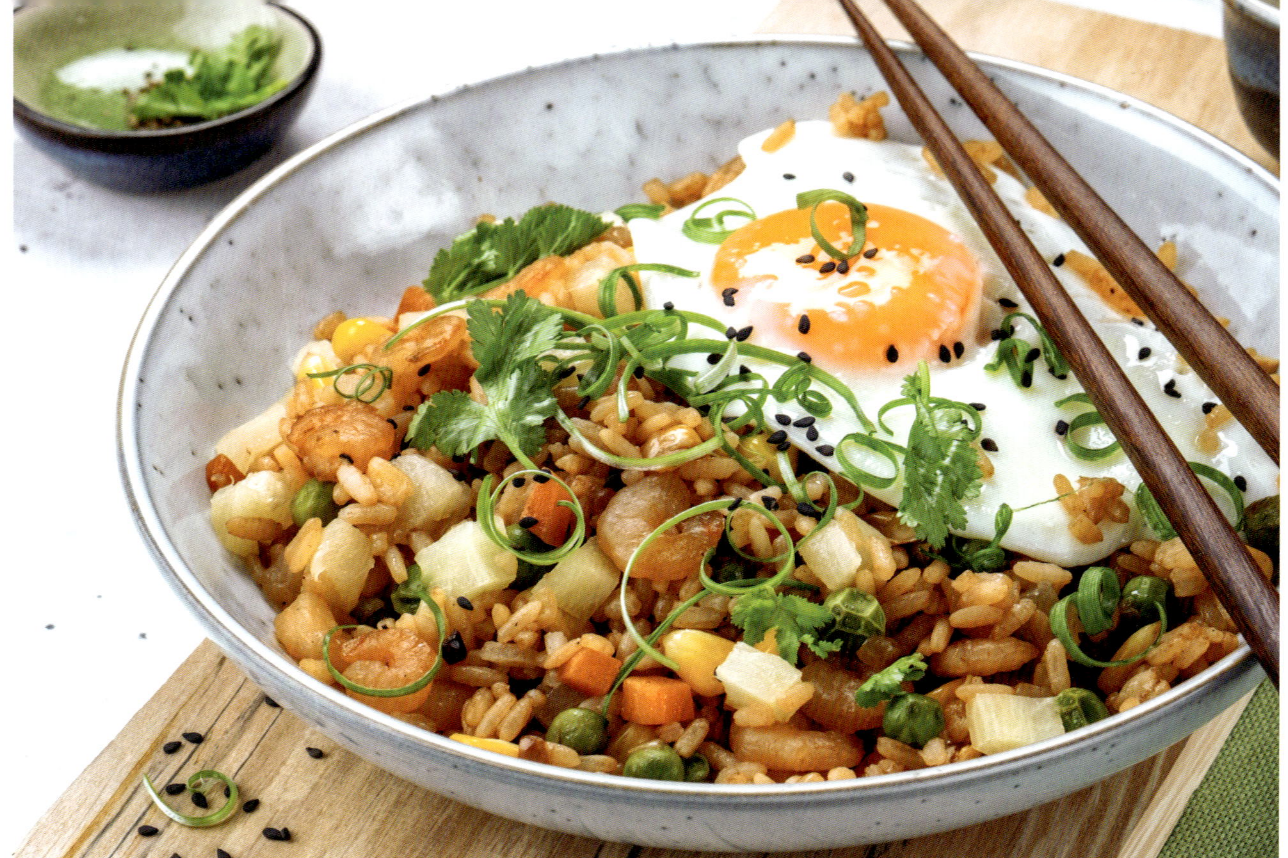

NASI GORENG

- 2 cups (310g) white long-grain rice
- 2½ tbsps kecap manis (sweet soy sauce)
- 1 tbsp dark soy sauce or tamari
- 1 tbsp sweet chilli sauce
- 4 tbsps peanut oil
- 1 onion, diced
- Medium piece ginger, sliced into thin strips
- 1 tsp sambal oelek
- 3 cloves garlic, minced
- 1 tsp shrimp paste
- 3 carrots, diced
- 200g school prawns, peeled
- 3 spring onions, thinly sliced
- 1 cup (170g) peas
- ½ cup (85g) corn kernels
- 4 eggs
- Handful fresh coriander leaves to serve
- 1 tsp black sesame seeds to serve

STEPS

1. Cook rice according to packet directions until just tender. Drain.
2. Combine kecap manis, soy sauce or tamari and sweet chilli sauce in a jug. Set aside.
3. Heat a wok over high heat until hot. Add 2 tablespoons oil and swirl to coat. Add onion, ginger, sambal oelek, garlic, shrimp paste and carrot. Stir-fry for 1 minute until fragrant.
4. Add prawns. Stir-fry for 1-2 minutes until just cooked then add rice, soy sauce mixture, spring onions, peas and corn. Stir-fry for 3-4 minutes or until rice is heated through. Spoon into bowls.
5. Heat 2 tablespoons oil in a large frying pan over medium-high heat. Crack eggs one at a time into the pan. Cook eggs for 3 minutes until white is cooked. Serve eggs on top of the rice and scatter with coriander leaves and sesame seeds.

SERVES 4 | PREP + COOK TIME: 30 MINS | GLUTEN FREE | DAIRY FREE |

THAI PORK BOWL

1 tbsp peanut oil
1 red onion, finely diced
1 stalk lemongrass, finely chopped
1 kaffir lime leaf
1 long red chilli, finely chopped
Small piece ginger, finely chopped
2 cloves garlic, finely chopped
1 green capsicum, finely chopped
500g pork mince
2 tbsps massaman curry paste
1½ tbsps fish sauce
2 tbsps lime juice
1 tbsp brown sugar
1 cup (15g) Thai basil leaves, shredded
Steamed rice to serve (optional)

STEPS

1. Heat oil in a wok over medium-high heat. Cook the onion, lemongrass, kaffir lime leaf, chilli, ginger and garlic for 1 minute or until fragrant. Add capsicum and cook for a further 2 minutes until just starting to soften. Add the pork and cook for 4-5 minutes, until cooked through.

2. Stir in the curry paste and cook for 1-2 minutes, until fragrant. Add the fish sauce, lime juice and sugar and cook, stirring, for 2 minutes.

3. Stir in the basil and serve immediately with steamed rice, if desired.

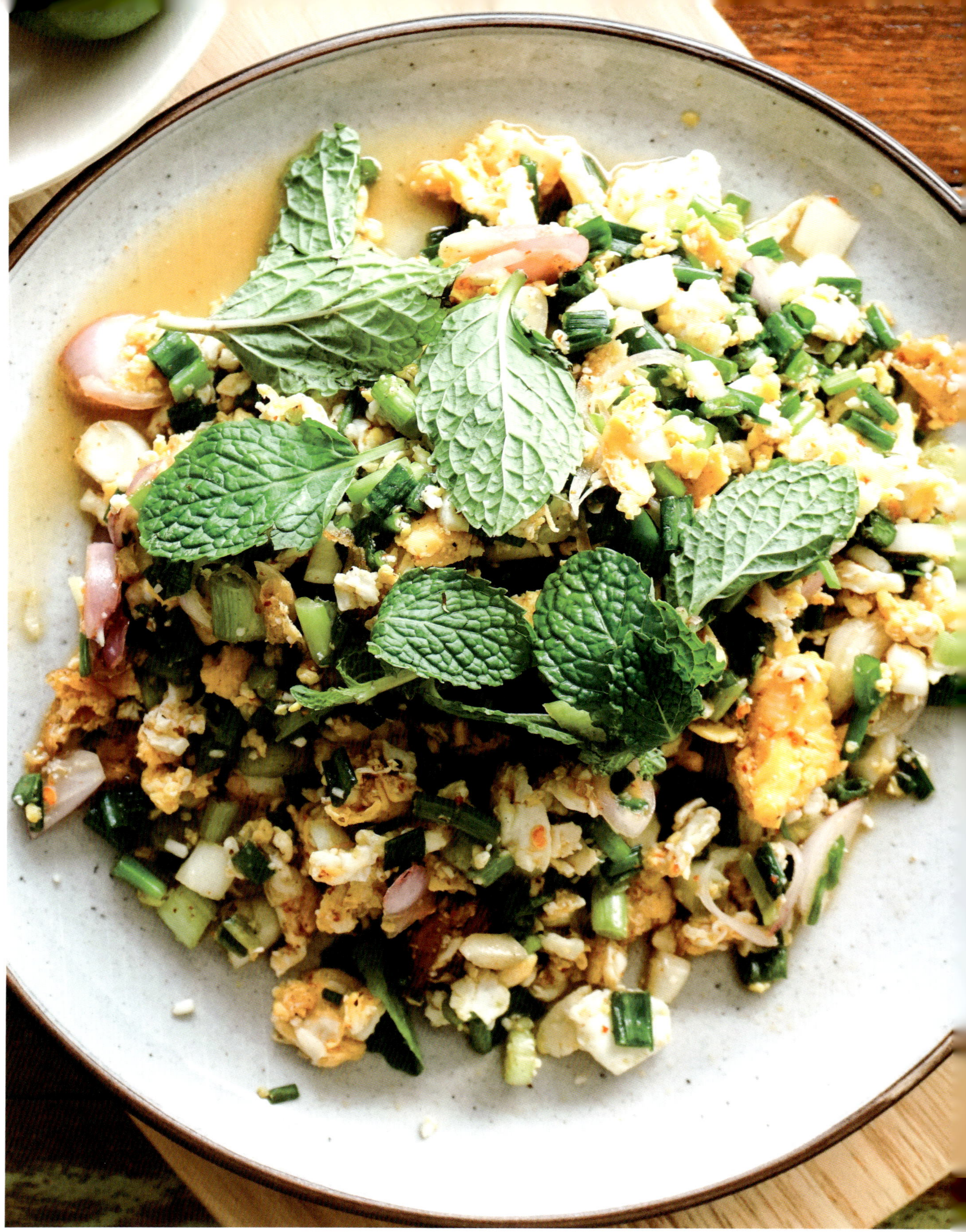

THAI SCRAMBLED EGG SALAD

SERVES 4 | PREP + COOK TIME: 15 MINS | GLUTEN FREE | DAIRY FREE |

1 tsp chilli flakes

½ tbsp crushed palm sugar or coconut sugar

2 tbsps fish sauce

¼ cup (60ml) lime juice + extra lime wedges to serve

1 tbsp peanut oil

8 eggs, beaten

2 Asian shallots, thinly sliced

4 spring onions, sliced

¼ cup (10g) mint leaves, torn + extra leaves to serve

STEPS

1. In a medium bowl mix together the chilli flakes, sugar, fish sauce and lime juice. Set aside.
2. Heat peanut oil in a large frying pan or wok over medium heat. When hot, pour in the egg. Wait for the egg to almost set and then break it into small pieces with a spatula or chopsticks; stir-fry for another 30 seconds until cooked. Remove from the heat.
3. Add the shallots, spring onions and mint to the pan. Pour over the sauce and toss to combine.
4. Serve immediately, garnished with extra mint leaves.

SERVES 4 | PREP + COOK TIME: 20 MINS | DAIRY FREE

SOBA NOODLE SALAD JARS

200g soba noodles
½ tsp sesame oil
1 tsp toasted sesame seeds
1⅓ cups (100g) torn lettuce leaves
2 carrots, julienned
1⅓ cups (130g) shredded red cabbage
1⅓ cups (160g) sliced cooked chicken

DRESSING

2 tbsps rice wine vinegar
1½ tbsps lime juice
4 tbsps soy sauce
2 tbsps honey
½ tsp dried chilli flakes
2 tbsps sesame oil
1 tsp sesame seeds

STEPS

1. Bring a medium pot of water to the boil and cook the soba noodles according to the packet directions. Once cooked, drain and rinse under cold water. Drain again then stir through sesame oil and sesame seeds.
2. Mix together the dressing ingredients and divide between four 500ml jars.
3. Layer lettuce, carrot and cabbage into the jars. Top with chicken and noodles.
4. Seal jars and refrigerate until ready to serve.
5. To serve, turn jars upside-down and allow the dressing to drain through the salad.

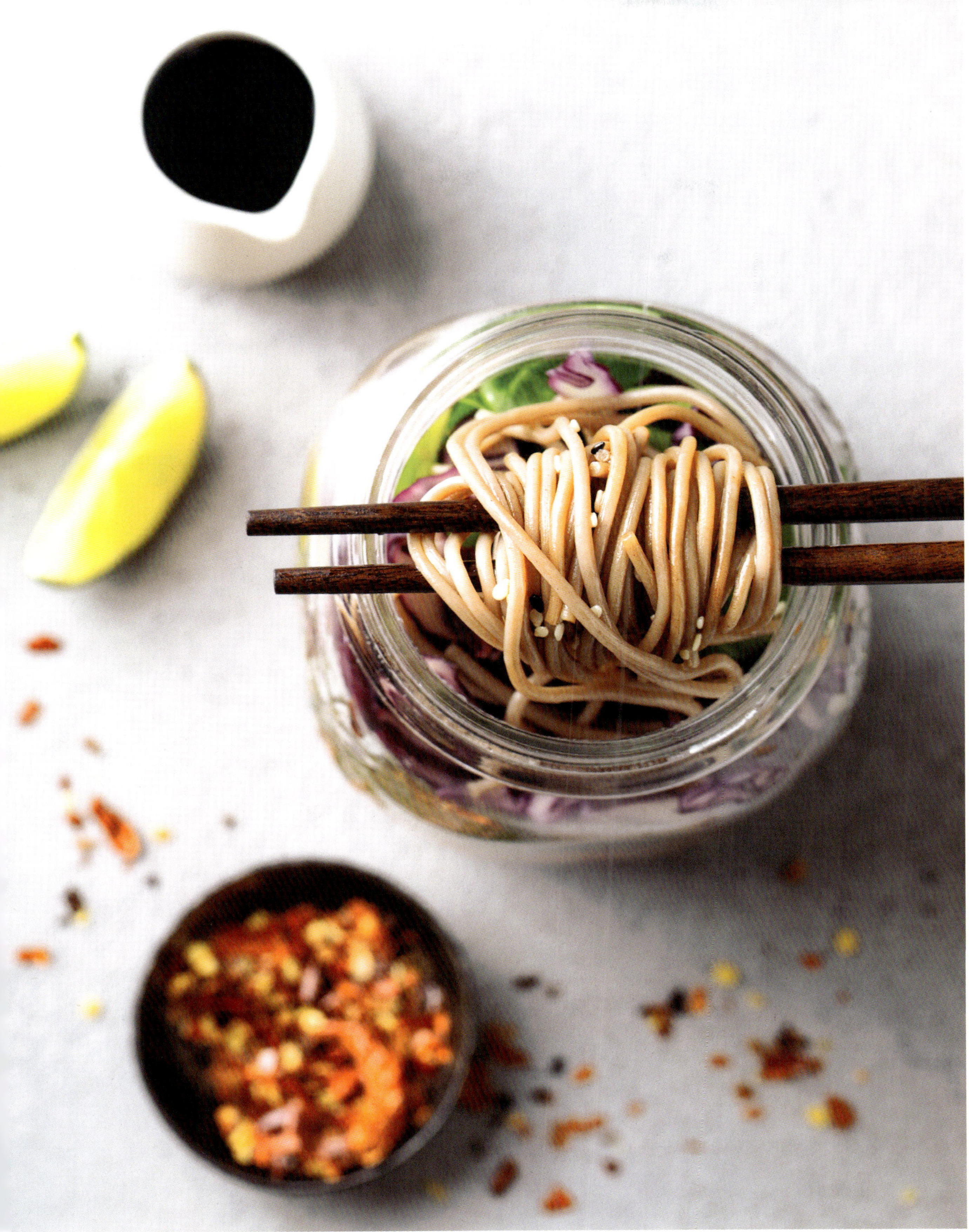

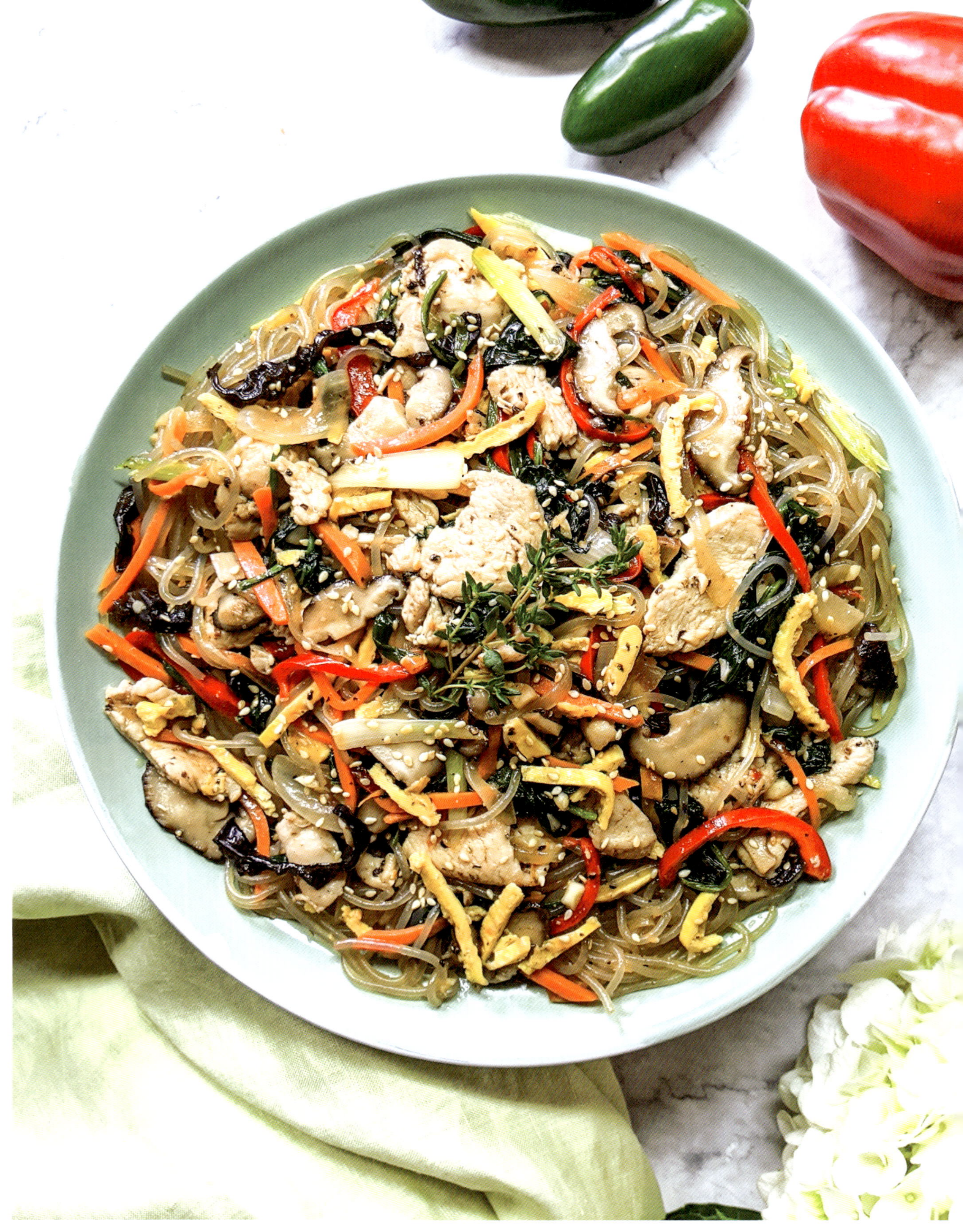

CHICKEN & MUSHROOM SOY NOODLES

500g chicken breast, sliced
1 tsp + 2 tbsps fish sauce
¼ tsp pepper
300g glass noodles
2 tbsps peanut oil
2 eggs, beaten
1 onion, sliced
Medium piece ginger, sliced
3 cloves garlic, minced
2 spring onions, cut into 5cm pieces
1 red capsicum, sliced
100g shiitake mushrooms
2 tbsps oyster sauce
1 tsp soy sauce
½ tsp sugar
1 tbsp toasted sesame seeds to serve

STEPS

1. Combine the chicken with 1 teaspoon fish sauce and pepper and allow to marinate for 15 minutes.
2. In a medium bowl, cover the noodles with boiling water. Let them sit for 15 minutes. Drain and set aside.
3. Meanwhile, heat 1 tablespoon peanut oil in a wok or large frying pan. Pour in the eggs. Swirl the pan gently to spread the eggs into a thin layer. Do not stir. When the eggs are set, remove from pan. Roll and slice the omelette into strips. Set aside.
4. Heat the remaining peanut oil in a wok or large frying pan. Add the onion and stir-fry for 3 minutes until softened. Add the ginger and garlic and fry for another minute until fragrant. Add spring onions, capsicum and shiitake mushrooms and stir-fry for 4 minutes until tender. Add the chicken and stir-fry for 3-4 minutes or until the chicken is cooked through.
5. Pour the noodles, remaining fish sauce, oyster sauce, soy sauce and sugar into the pan, along with the sliced omelette. Toss well to combine. Scatter with sesame seeds to serve.

SERVES 4 | PREP + COOK TIME: 30 MINS | DAIRY FREE |

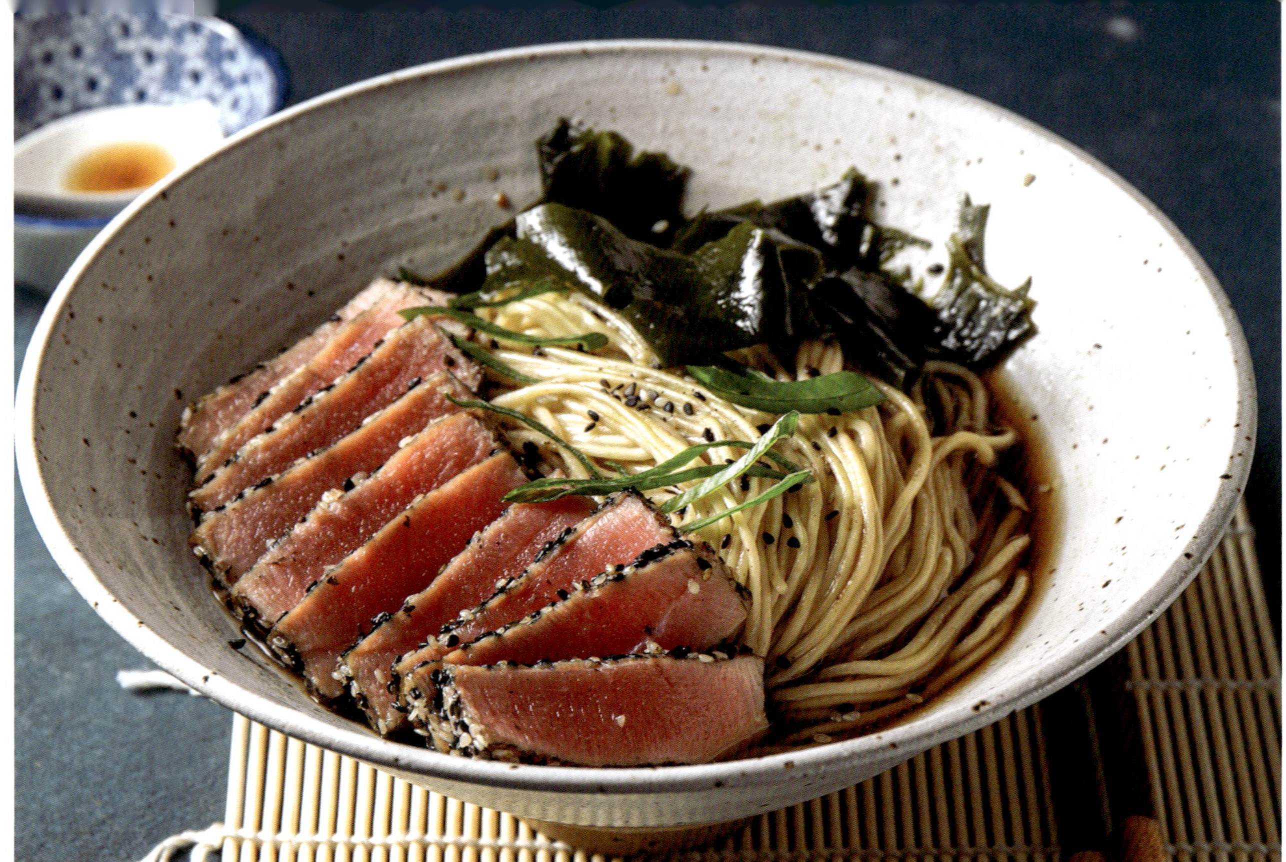

TUNA TATAKI WITH MISO NOODLES

4 cups (1L) vegetable stock

1 cup (250ml) water

380g somen noodles

1 tbsp dark miso

400g sashimi-grade tuna, cut into large rectangular blocks

1 tsp salt

1 tbsp vegetable oil

1 tbsp olive oil

2 tsps white sesame seeds

2 tsps black sesame seeds

1 tsp sesame oil

TO SERVE

2 spring onions, sliced

1 tsp black sesame seeds

STEPS

1. Combine stock and water in a saucepan. Bring to a boil. Add noodles to the pan and cook until almost done, according to the packet directions.
2. Add the miso to the pan. Stir to combine, then simmer for 3 minutes until the noodles are cooked.
3. Sprinkle tuna with salt. Brush with vegetable and olive oil. Place the sesame seeds in a shallow dish. Roll tuna in the sesame seeds, pressing to stick.
4. In a medium frying pan, heat the sesame oil over medium heat. Sear the tuna quickly for 20 seconds on each side. Remove from the pan, slice into thin slices of about 1cm and set aside.
5. Divide the noodles and miso soup between four bowls. Top with sliced tuna, spring onions and sesame seeds

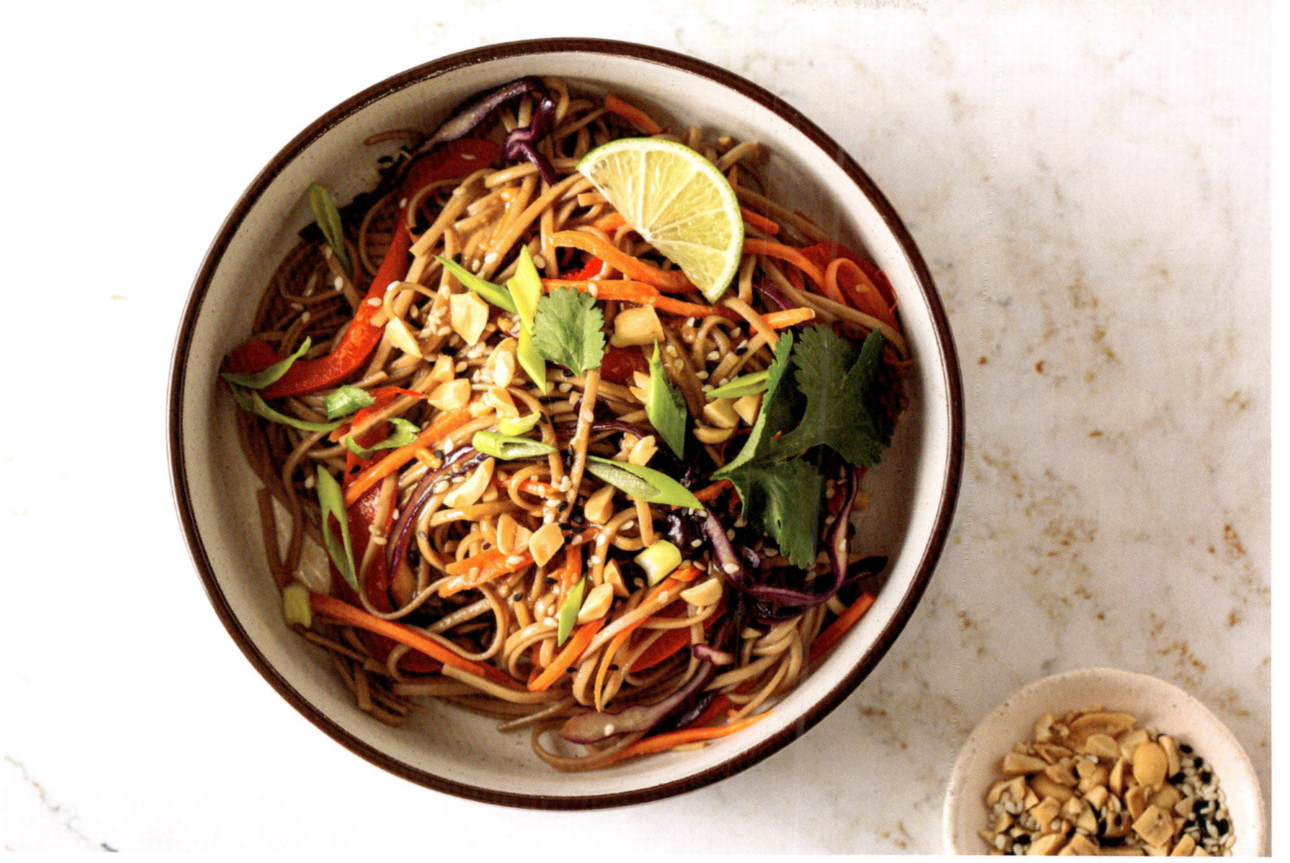

SERVES 3-4 | PREP + COOK TIME: 20 MINS | VEG | DAIRY FREE |

SOBA NOODLE STIR-FRY

500g soba noodles

2 tbsps peanut or vegetable oil

2 cloves garlic, sliced

Small piece ginger, grated

½ red onion, sliced

2 cups (200g) red cabbage, shredded

2 red capsicums, sliced

1 spring onion, sliced, green and white parts separated

2 tbsps toasted sesame oil

3 tbsps tamari or soy sauce

⅛ tsp cayenne pepper

1 tbsp sesame seeds

¼ cup (30g) toasted peanuts, chopped

Handful of coriander leaves

Lime wedges to serve

STEPS

1. Cook noodles according to package instructions. Drain and set aside.
2. Heat oil in a wok over high heat. Add garlic, ginger and onion and stir-fry for 5 minutes, until tender. Add cabbage and capsicum and stir-fry for a further 5 minutes until tender, then add white parts of spring onion and fry for another 3-4 minutes until just soft. Remove vegetables from wok and set aside.
3. Place noodles in the hot wok. Add sesame oil, tamari and cayenne pepper and toss for 5 minutes until the noodles absorb the sauce. Return the vegetables to the wok and toss to combine.
4. Sprinkle with sesame seeds, chopped peanuts, coriander leaves and spring onion tops. Serve with lime wedges.

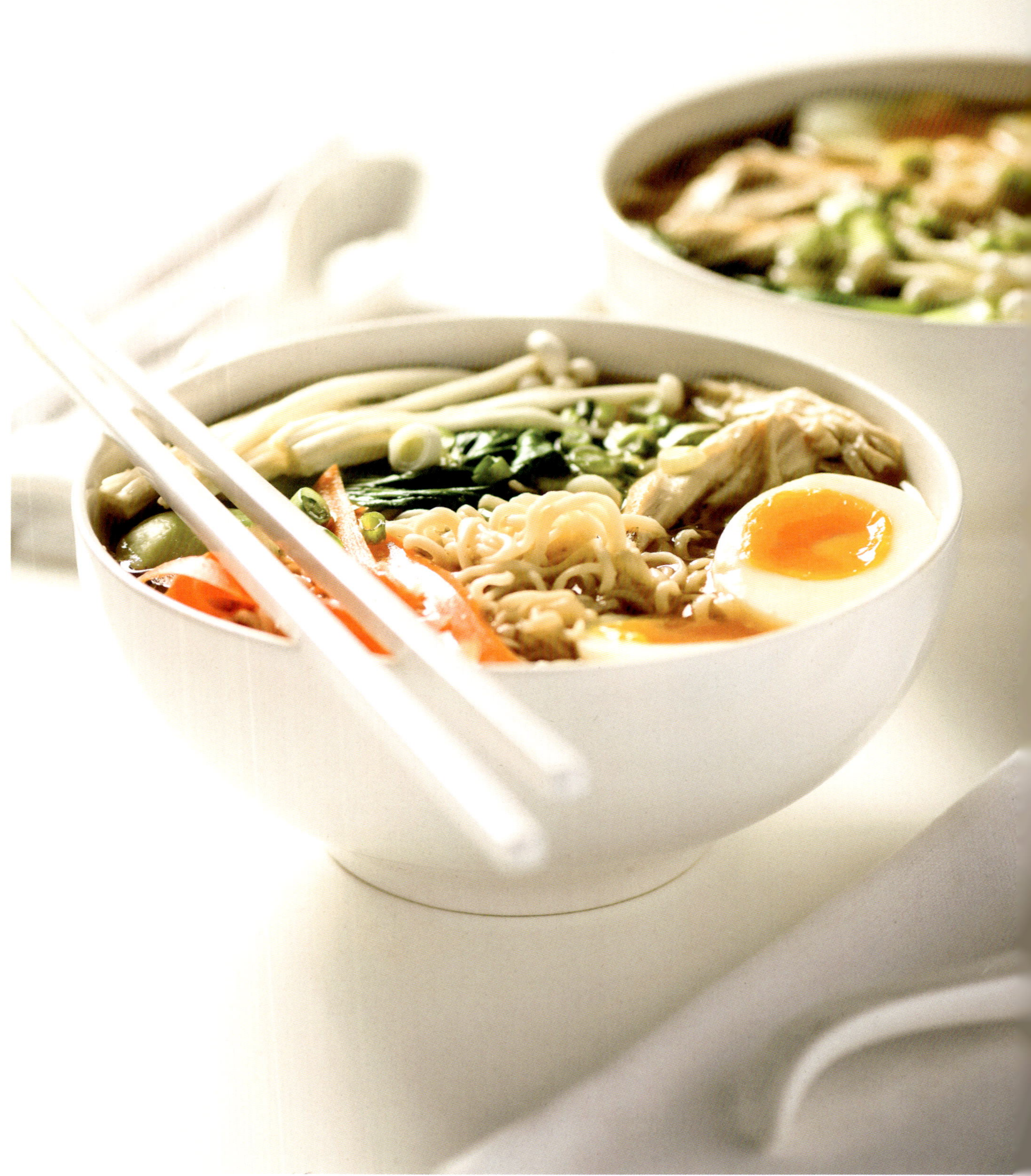

HOT JAPANESE RAMEN BOWL

2 chicken breasts

2 tsps sesame or vegetable oil

3 tsps minced garlic

2 tsps minced ginger

3 tbsps soy sauce

2 tbsps mirin

4 cups (1L) chicken stock

½ tsp chilli powder

1 cup (25g) dried shiitake mushroom (see note)

1 head bok choy, cut in half lengthwise

½ cup (35g) enoki mushrooms (see note)

Salt to taste

180g ramen noodles (dried or fresh)

½ cup (50g) spring onions, sliced

1 carrot, cut into thin ribbons

2 eggs, soft boiled

STEPS

1. Place chicken in a covered steamer basket over a pan of simmering water. Steam for 12-14 minutes until chicken is cooked through. Set aside to rest.
2. Meanwhile heat the oil in a large pot cver medium heat, until shimmering. Add the garlic and ginger and cook until softened. Add the soy sauce and mirin and stir to combine. Cook for another minute. Add the stock and chilli powder, cover and bring to the boil.
3. Remove the lid and let simmer uncovered for 5 minutes, then add the shiitake mushrooms. Simmer gently for 5 minutes, then add bok choy and enoki mushrooms. Simmer for a further 5 minutes and season with salt to taste.
4. Add the ramen noodles to a saucepan of boiling water. Cook for 2-3 minutes until soft, then drain and divide the noodles into two large bowls.
5. Pour the hot stock mixture over the noodles in the bowls. Slice the chicken and add to the bowls along with enoki mushrooms and bok choy. Garnish with spring onions, carrot ribbons and soft-boiled egg halves. Serve immediately.

NOTE: You can substitute enoki and shiitake mushrooms with button mushrooms, if preferred.

SERVES 2 | PREP + COOK TIME: 45 MINS | DAIRY FREE |

THAI CHICKEN SALAD

¼ cup (60ml) lime juice

1½ tbsps brown sugar

1 tbsp fish sauce

2 tsps lemongrass paste

1 tsp sesame oil

2 chicken breast fillets

2 Lebanese cucumbers, sliced into quarter moons

1 red capsicum, thinly sliced

1 carrot, grated

¼ red onion, thinly sliced

1 cos lettuce, roughly chopped

¼ white cabbage, finely shredded

1 cup (15g) coriander leaves

½ cup (70g) peanuts, toasted, roughly chopped

2 tsps sesame seeds

STEPS

1. Combine lime juice, sugar, fish sauce, lemongrass paste and sesame oil in a small bowl. Place chicken in a glass or ceramic dish. Pour over 1 tablespoon of the lime juice mixture, reserving the rest for use later. Set aside for 10 minutes to marinate.

2. Place chicken in a covered steamer basket over a saucepan of boiling water and steam for 12-14 minutes or until the chicken is cooked through. Set aside for 5 minutes to rest.

3. Combine the cucumber, capsicum, carrot, onion, lettuce, cabbage and coriander in a large bowl. Drizzle with the remaining lime juice mixture and toss to combine.

4. Cut the chicken into bite-size pieces. Add to the salad along with peanuts and toss to combine. Sprinkle with sesame seeds to serve.

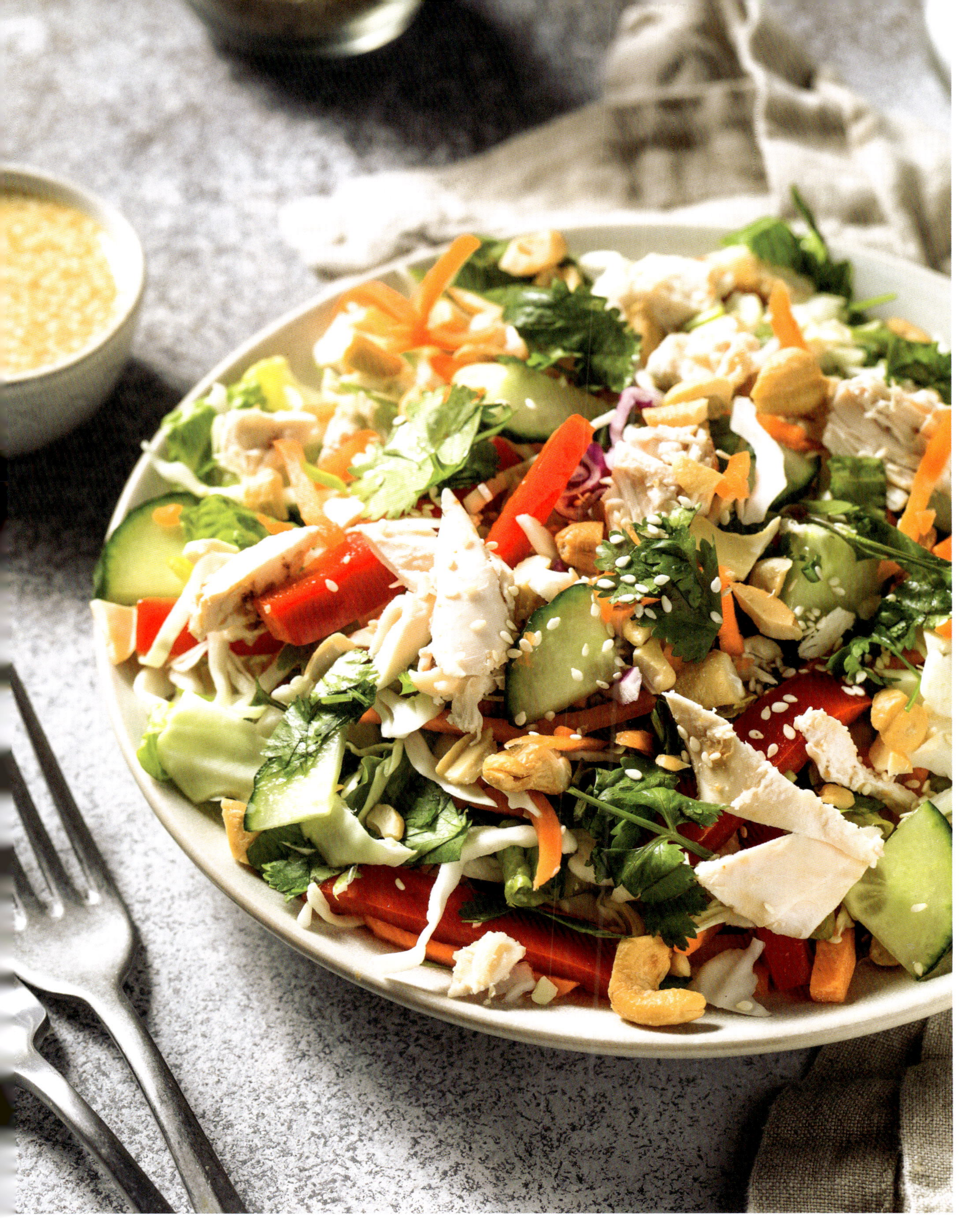

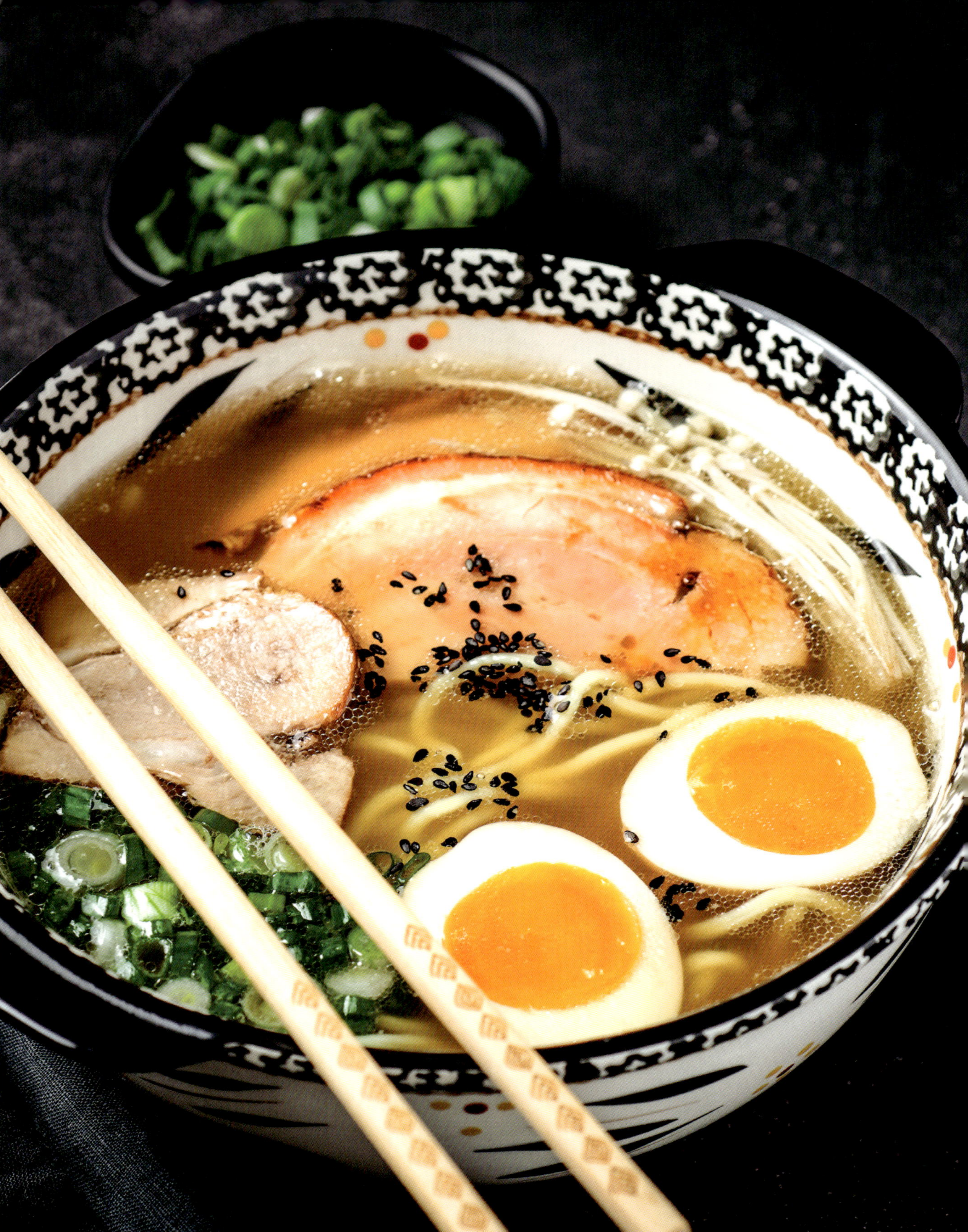

UDON NOODLES WITH PORK & MUSHROOMS

1 tbsp peanut oil
4 spring onions, thinly sliced
2 cloves garlic, crushed
2 tsps ginger, finely grated
4 cups (1L) chicken stock
2 tbsps light soy sauce
2 tsps sesame oil
Salt to taste
400g udon noodles
200g enoki mushrooms (see note)
4 eggs
500g piece Chinese barbecue pork, thinly sliced
2 spring onions, chopped
2 tsps black sesame seeds

STEPS

1. Heat oil in a large saucepan over medium heat, add spring onion, garlic and ginger and stir occasionally for 2 minutes or until fragrant.

2. Add stock, soy sauce, sesame oil and salt and bring to a simmer.

3. Meanwhile, cook udon noodles in boiling salted water according to packet directions. Drain, add to stock mixture with enoki mushrooms and simmer for 3 minutes.

4. Meanwhile fill a pot with sufficient water to cover the eggs and bring to a boil. Gently lower the eggs into the boiling water and simmer for 7 minutes. Drain eggs and rinse in cold water. When cool enough to handle, peel away the shells and slice in half.

5. Divide noodles and stock between bowls and top with pork slices, enoki mushrooms, boiled egg halves and spring onions. Serve scattered with sesame seeds.

NOTE: You can substitute enoki mushrooms with button mushrooms, if preferred.

SERVES 4 | PREP + COOK TIME: 25 MINS | DAIRY FREE |

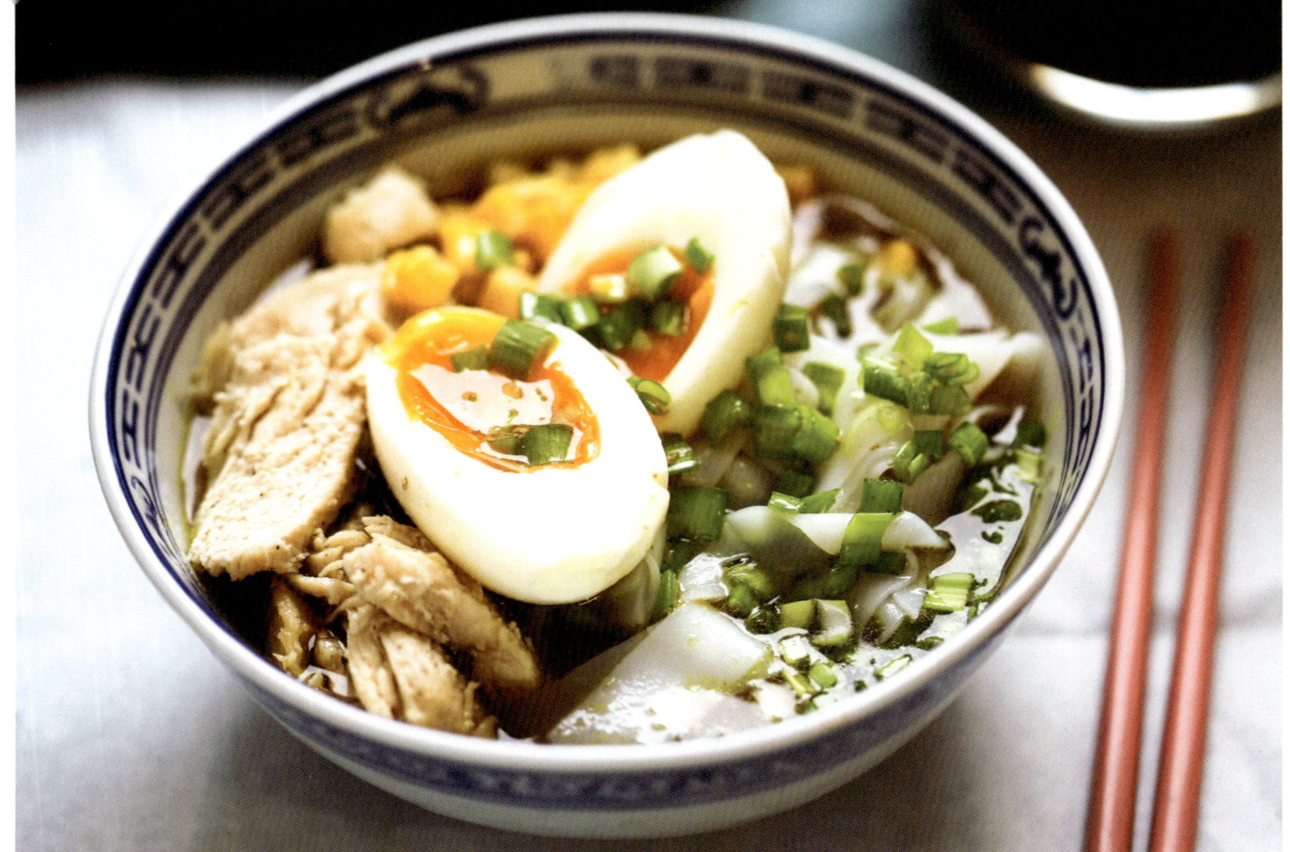

SERVES 4 | PREP + COOK TIME: 25 MINS | DAIRY FREE

CHICKEN NOODLE BOWL

6 cups (1.5L) chicken stock

4 cloves garlic, smashed

Medium piece ginger, sliced

3 tbsps soy sauce

3 tsps sugar

3 tbsps Shaoxing wine

1 tsp toasted sesame oil

360g rice stick noodles

4 eggs

2 cups (250g) shredded cooked chicken

2 spring onions, green part only, finely sliced

STEPS

1. Place stock, garlic, ginger, soy sauce, sugar, Shaoxing wine and sesame oil in a saucepan over high heat. Cover and bring to a boil then reduce to medium and simmer for 8-10 minutes to allow the flavours to infuse.

2. Meanwhile, cook noodles according to packet directions.

3. Bring another pan of water to a boil. Add the eggs and cook for 6 minutes, then drain. Peel and cut into halves.

4. Strain garlic and ginger from the soup, and discard.

5. Divide noodles between four bowls. Ladle over soup. Top with chicken, soft boiled egg halves and spring onions.

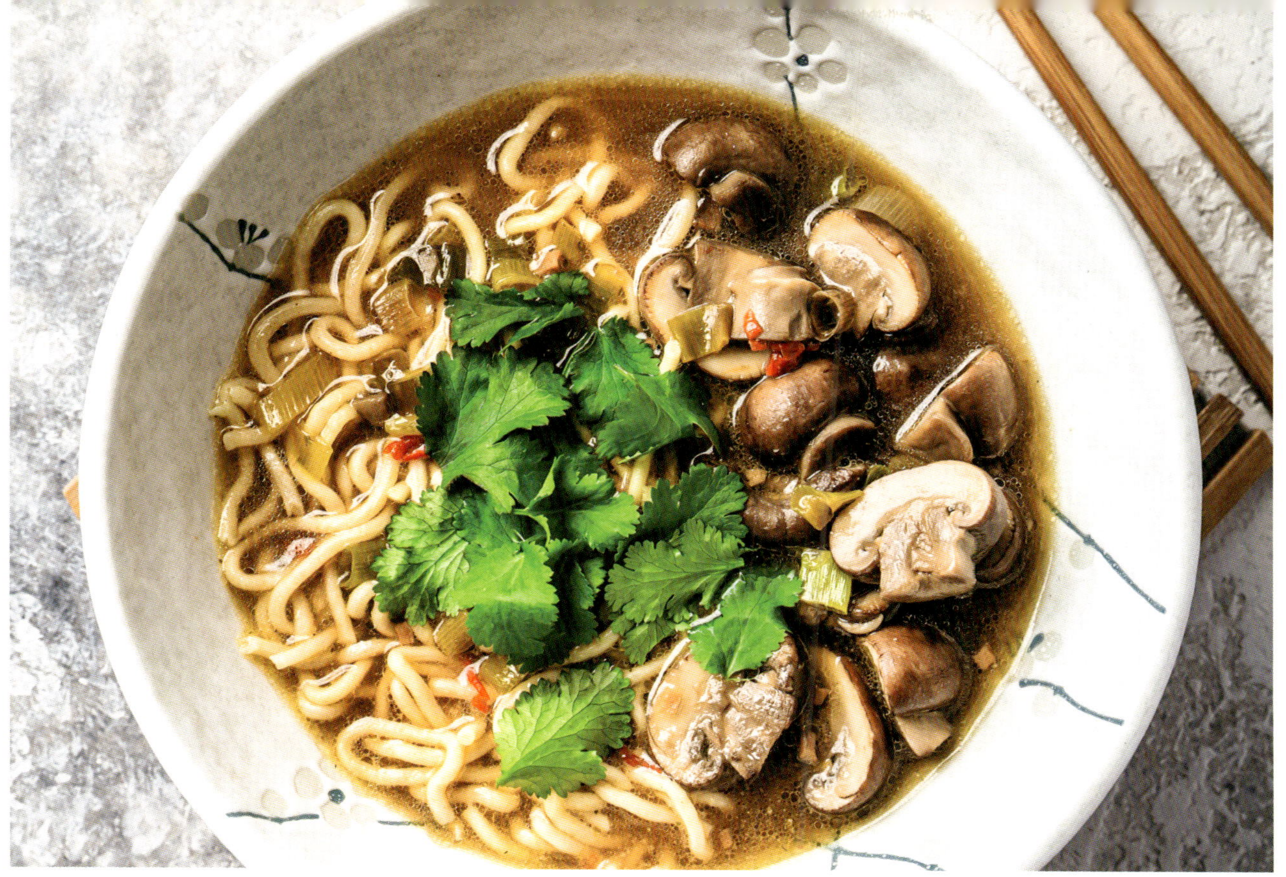

MUSHROOM MISO RAMEN

1 tbsp neutral-flavoured oil
3 leeks, thinly sliced
3 cloves garlic, minced
Medium piece ginger, grated
½ long red chilli, finely chopped
6 cups (1.5L) vegetable stock
5 tbsps red miso paste
350g mushrooms, sliced
400g ramen noodles
Handful of fresh coriander leaves

STEPS

1. Heat oil in a large saucepan over medium heat. Add leek and cook, stirring occasionally, for 3-5 minutes until the leek is softened. Add garlic, ginger and chilli and stir to combine. Cook for 1 minute until fragrant. Add stock and bring to a simmer.
2. Place the miso in a small bowl and add ½ cup of the hot stock. Stir to dissolve paste and then add it back to the pan, whisking to dissolve completely. Keep miso under the boiling point.
3. Add sliced mushrooms to miso broth, cover pan and simmer at a low temperature for 5 minutes or until mushrooms are cooked through.
4. Cook noodles according to the packet directions. Drain and divide between four bowls.
5. Top the noodles with mushrooms, stock and coriander leaves.

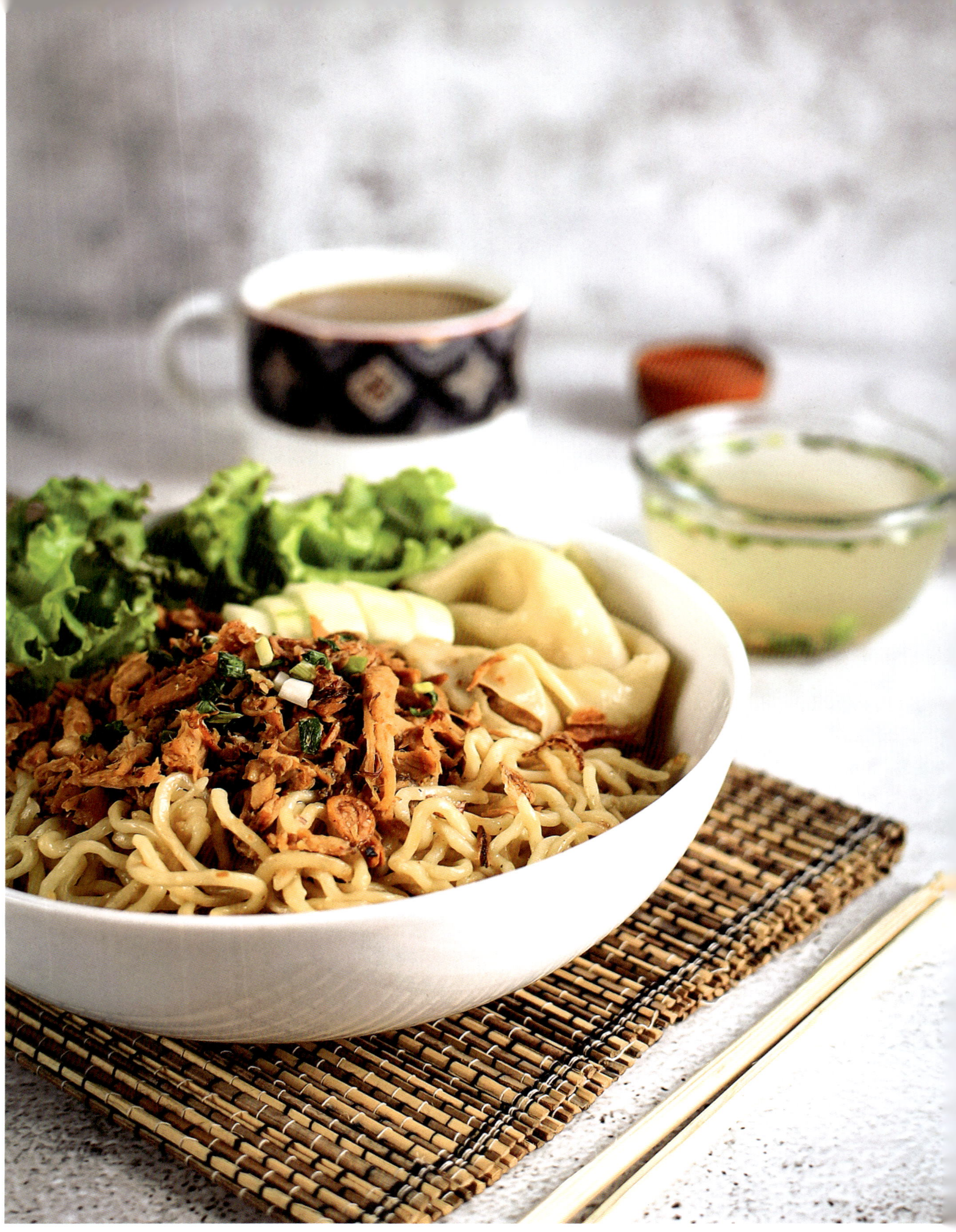

SHREDDED CHICKEN RAMEN BOWL

1 tsp sesame oil

2 tbsps unsalted butter

4 cloves garlic, minced

Small piece ginger, minced

3 cooked chicken breasts, shredded

5⅔ cups (1.4L) chicken stock

4 tbsps soy sauce

1-2 tbsps Sriracha or to taste

1 tbsp Shaoxing wine

1 tbsp light brown sugar

¼ tsp white pepper

8 frozen pork or chicken dumplings

210g ramen noodles

TOPPINGS:

4 spring onions, chopped

2 cups (150g) torn lettuce leaves

STEPS

1. Heat the oil and butter in a large saucepan, over a medium heat, until the butter melts. Add the garlic and ginger, and fry for 1 minute, stirring, until fragrant. Add the shredded chicken and fry for 5-7 minutes until golden brown and crispy. Set aside.

2. Add the stock, soy sauce, Sriracha, wine, brown sugar and white pepper. Increase the heat to high, and bring to the boil, then simmer for 3 minutes.

3. Add the dumplings. Bring back to the boil then simmer for 5 minutes, then add the noodles and simmer for 3 minutes, stirring a couple of times to separate the noodles.

4. Use a set of tongs to divide the noodles between four bowls. Ladle over the sauce and add the pieces of chicken and dumplings.

5. Top each bowl with torn lettuce and chopped spring onion.

SERVES 4 | PREP + COOK TIME: 25 MINS | DAIRY FREE |

EASY CHICKEN NOODLE STIR-FRY

½ cup (125ml) + 2 tbsps soy sauce
1 tbsp chilli paste
2 tbsps brown sugar
Medium piece ginger, minced
3 cloves garlic, minced
2 tbsps coconut oil
2 carrots, thinly sliced
4 cups (300g) broccoli florets, cut bite-size
250g mushrooms, sliced
1 red capsicum, sliced
750g chicken thighs, cut into bite-size pieces
2 tbsps cornflour
350g ramen noodles, cooked according to packet instructions
2 tbsps chopped coriander leaves

STEPS

1. In a small bowl mix together ½ cup soy sauce, chilli paste, sugar, ginger and garlic. Set aside.
2. Heat ½ tablespoon oil in a large frying pan or wok over high heat. When hot, add carrots and stir-fry for 1 minute. Add the broccoli, stir, cover with lid and cook for 1 minute. Add the mushrooms and capsicum and the remaining 2 tablespoons of soy sauce. Stir-fry for 2-3 minutes until the vegetables are just tender. Transfer to a bowl and set aside.
3. Add another tablespoon oil to pan over high heat. Add the chicken and sprinkle with cornflour. Stir well to coat. Continue to cook for 2 minutes, stirring frequently, until chicken is browned. Add sauce and cook for 1-2 minutes to thicken.
4. Add the noodles. Toss to coat. Cook, stirring frequently, for 2 minutes.
5. Return the vegetables back to the pan. Toss to coat. Scatter with chopped coriander to serve.

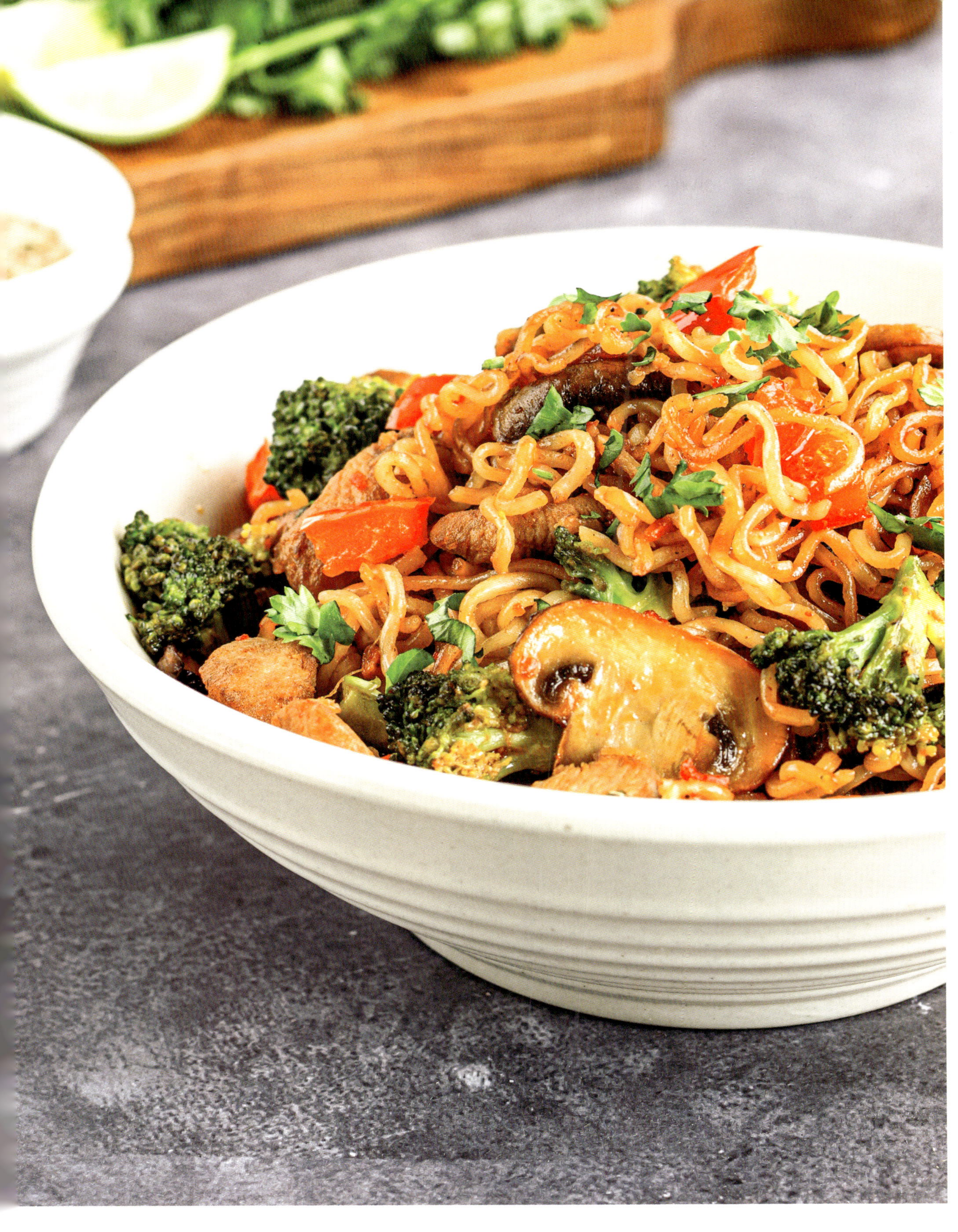

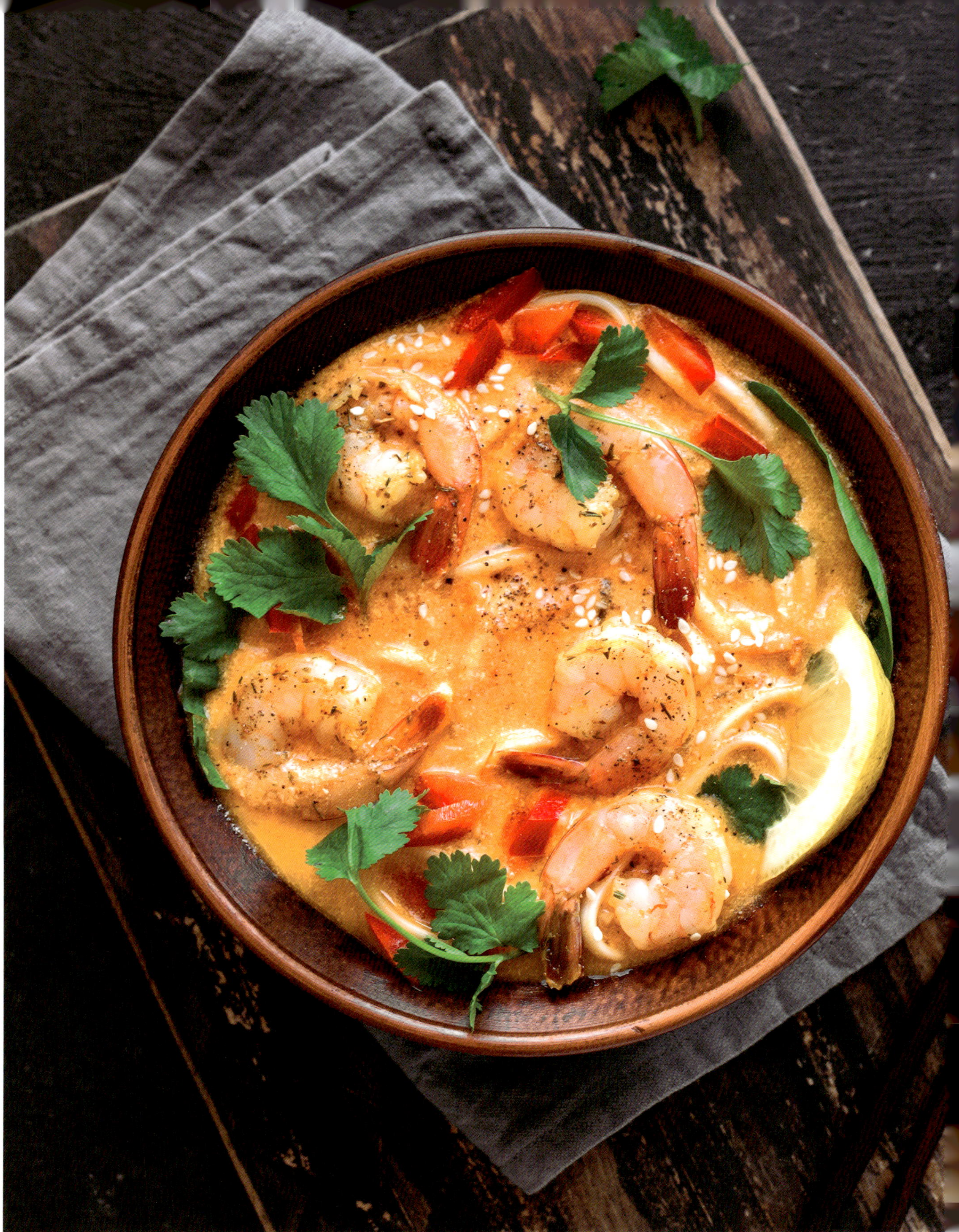

SERVES 4 | PREP + COOK TIME: 25 MINS | GLUTEN FREE | DAIRY FREE |

PRAWN LAKSA

2 tbsps coconut oil

2 red chillies, finely sliced

5 tbsps Thai red curry paste

4 cups (1L) vegetable or chicken stock

1 x 400ml can coconut milk

2 tbsps fish sauce

Pepper to taste

Juice of 1 lime

500g king prawns, tails intact, peeled and cooked

250g rice noodles, cooked according to packet instructions

Coriander leaves, to garnish

½ red capsicum, diced, to garnish

1 tsp sesame seeds

Lemon wedges to serve

STEPS

1. Heat the oil in a large pan over medium heat. Add the chilli and cook for 1 minute until fragrant. Add the curry paste, stir and cook for 1 minute more.
2. Pour in the stock and coconut milk and bring to the boil.
3. Add the fish sauce, a grind of pepper and a squeeze of lime juice.
4. Add the prawns and noodles and cook for 2-3 minutes until warm.
5. Spoon into four bowls. Top with coriander, diced capsicum, sesame seeds and a good grind of pepper. Serve with lemon wedges.

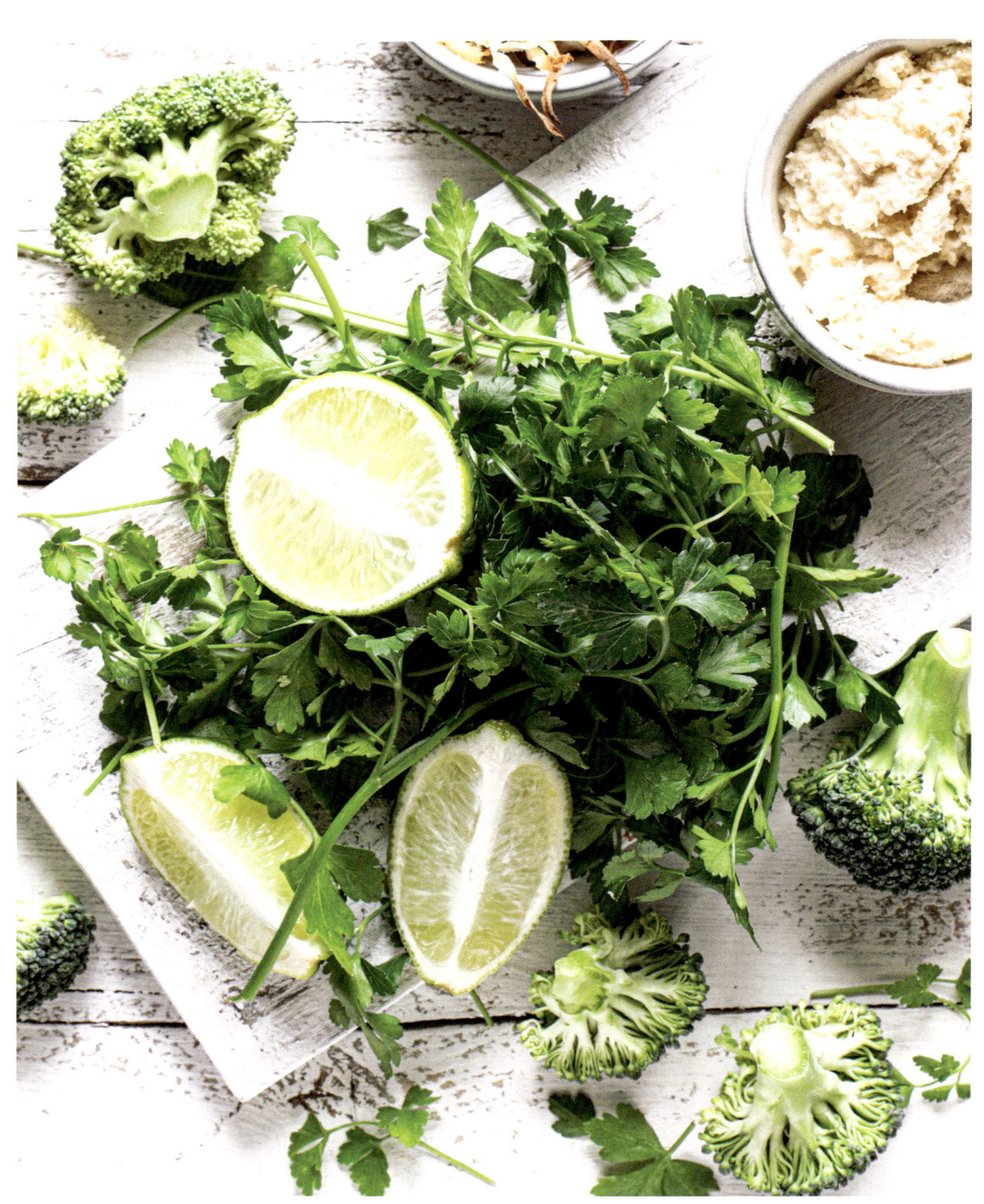

CHAPTER TWO

SIDES & SNACKS

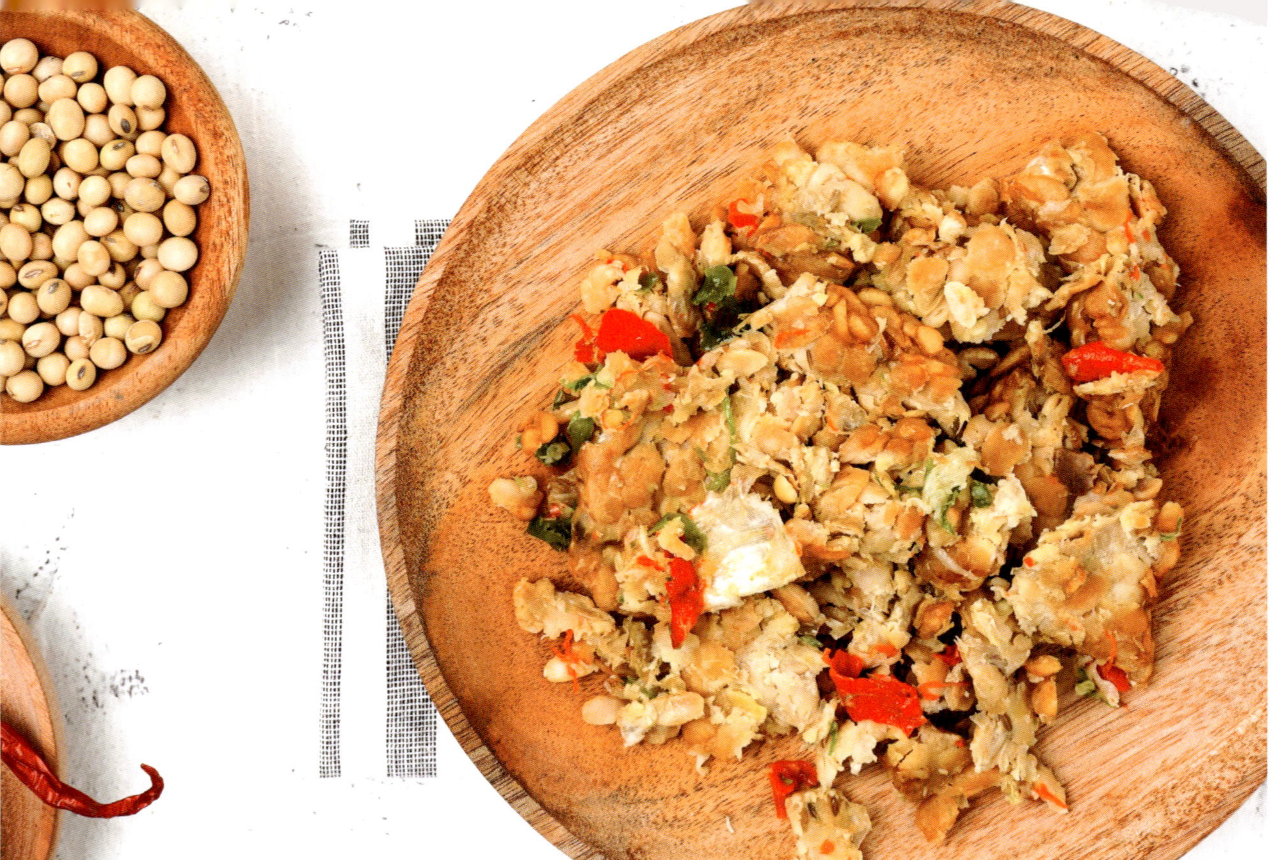

TEMPEH PENYET

4 cloves garlic, minced

2 tsps ground coriander

¾ cup (185ml) + 2 tbsps water

1¼ tsps salt

450g tempeh, cut into ½ cm-thick slices

¼ cup (60ml) canola oil + more as needed

Handful of Thai basil, roughly chopped

SAMBAL

¼ cup (60ml) canola oil

4 medium tomatoes, halved and thinly sliced

7 Asian shallots, sliced

10 long red chillies, deseeded and sliced

7 cloves garlic, sliced

¼ tsp salt

TO SERVE

1 tbsp lime juice

STEPS

1. In a large bowl combine the garlic, coriander, water and 1 teaspoon salt. Add tempeh and massage the marinade into all the pieces. Set aside.
2. Heat ¼ cup oil in a large frying pan over high heat. Add the tomatoes, shallots, chillies and garlic. Cook for 10 minutes, stirring. Reduce heat to medium and cook for a further 10 minutes, until reduced. Season with ¼ teaspoon salt. Set aside.
3. Drain tempeh in a colander.
4. Heat ¼ cup oil in a large frying pan over high heat. Add tempeh in a single layer. Fry for 2-3 minutes on each side, or until golden and crispy. Transfer to a paper towel–lined baking tray to drain; season with ¼ teaspoon salt.
5. Lay tempeh on top of sambal. Scatter with basil. Using a pestle, gently flatten each piece of tempeh into the sambal. Drizzle with lime juice to serve.

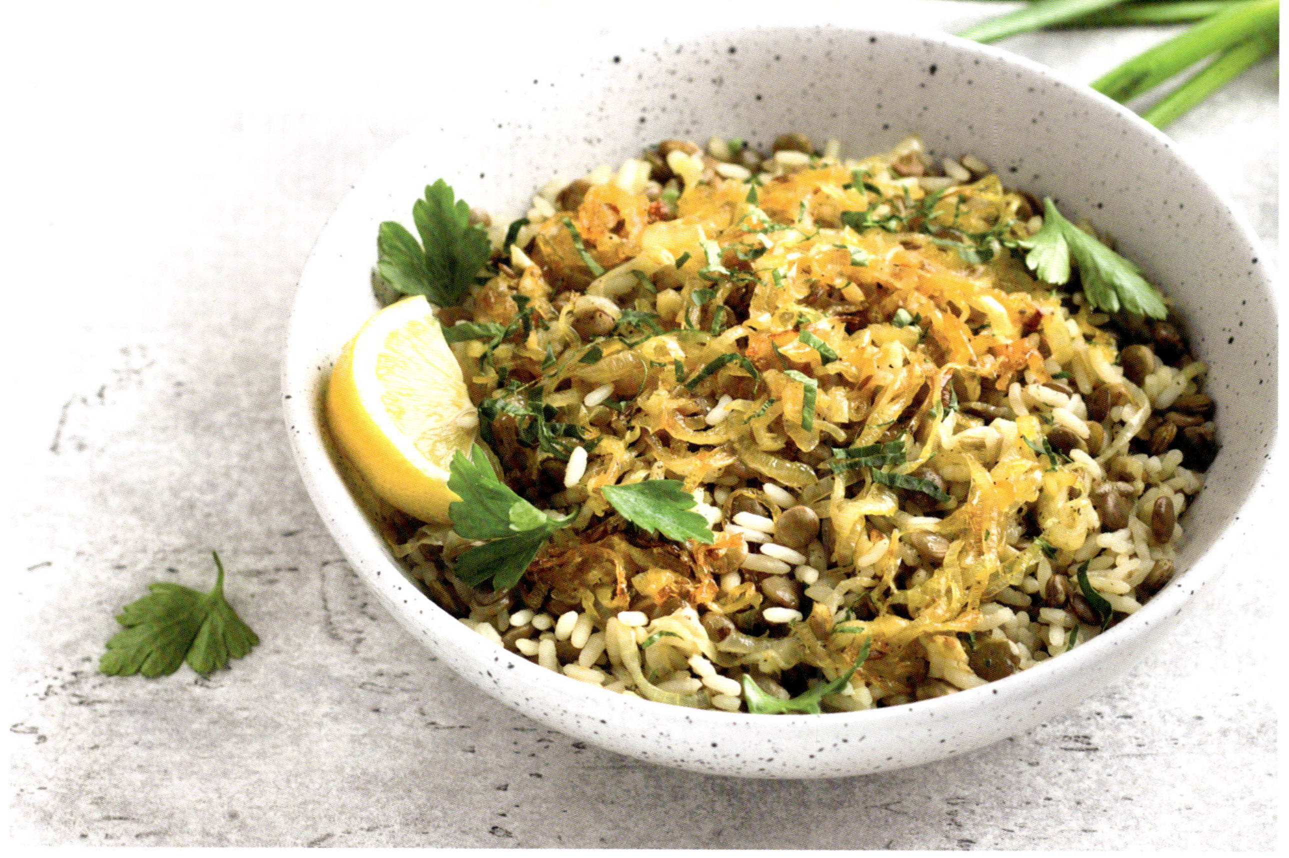

MUJADARA

¼ cup (60ml) + 1 tbsp olive oil
2 onions, sliced + ½ onion, diced
2 cloves garlic, minced
3½ cups (875ml) water
1 cup (185g) dried green lentils
1 tsp salt
1 cup (200g) long-grain rice
1 tsp cumin
½ tsp cinnamon
1 bay leaf
Juice of ½ lemon + lemon wedges to serve
2 tbsps chopped parsley

STEPS

1. Heat ¼ cup olive oil over high heat. Add 1 onion and cook, stirring constantly, for about 20 minutes, until the onions are browned and start to crisp around the edges. Transfer to a plate lined with paper towel and set aside.
2. Heat 1 tablespoon oil in a large saucepan over medium-high heat. Fry remaining onion and garlic, stirring regularly, for 5 minutes until soft and translucent.
3. Add water, lentils and salt to the pan. Bring to a boil. Cover with a lid and simmer for 10 minutes.
4. Add rice, cumin, cinnamon and bay leaf to the lentils. Stir to combine. Simmer covered for about 15 minutes, or until rice is cooked.
5. Squeeze over lemon juice and serve lentils and rice topped with caramelised onions, chopped parsley and lemon wedges.

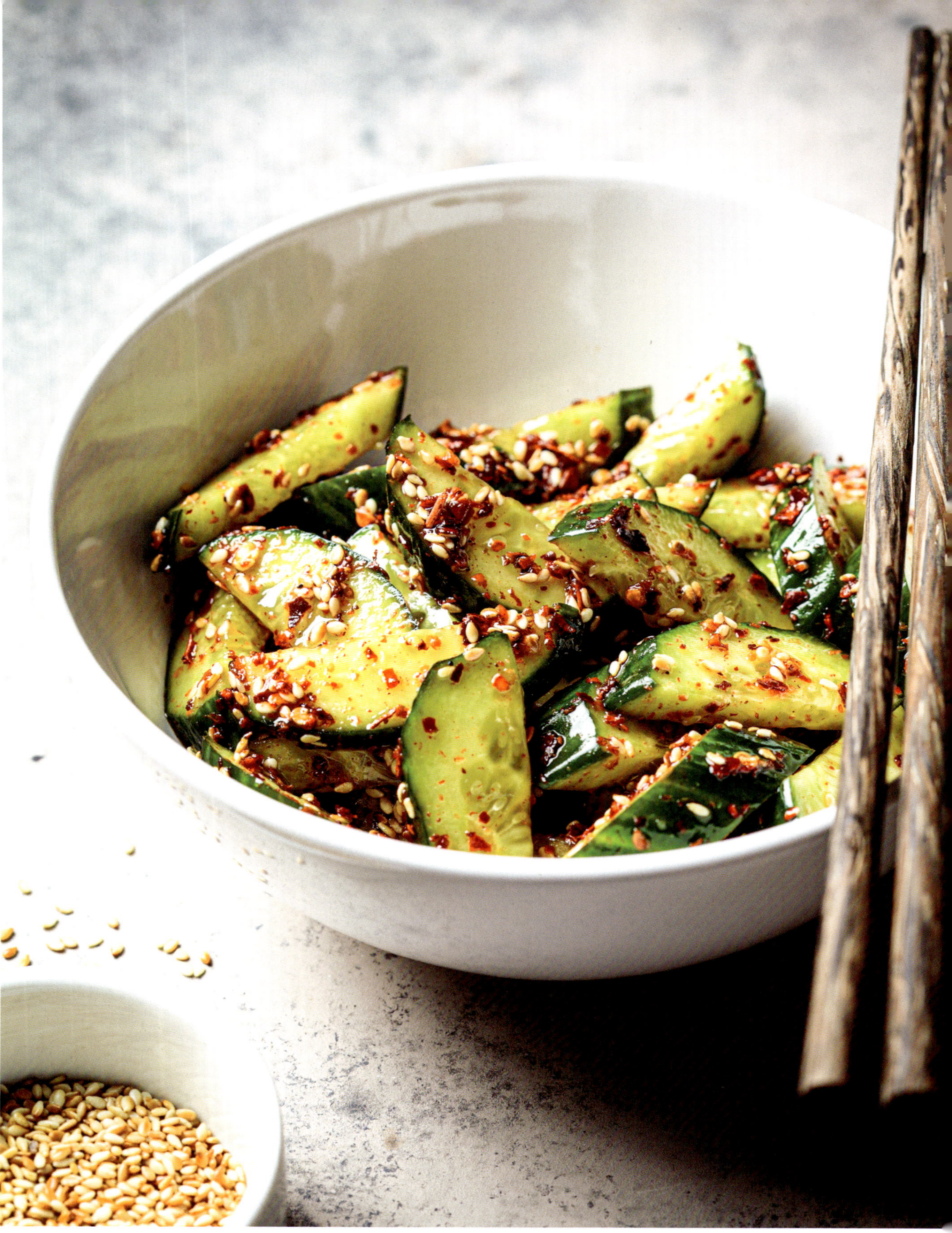

SPICY CUCUMBER SALAD

SERVES 4 | PREP + COOK TIME: 30 MINS + CHILLING | VEG | DAIRY FREE |

6 Lebanese cucumbers

½ tsp salt

2 cloves garlic, minced

1 tbsp soy sauce

1 tbsp rice wine vinegar

1 tsp sesame oil

1 tsp chilli oil

½ tsp sugar

½ tsp toasted sesame seeds

¼ tsp gochugaru (Korean chilli flakes)

STEPS

1. Cut the cucumbers in half lengthwise then slice diagonally into ½ cm-thick slices.
2. Add cucumbers and salt to a bowl and let them sit for 10 minutes. Drain away any liquid.
3. Add the remaining ingredients to the cucumbers and stir to combine. Serve immediately, or chill for up to 4 days until ready to serve.

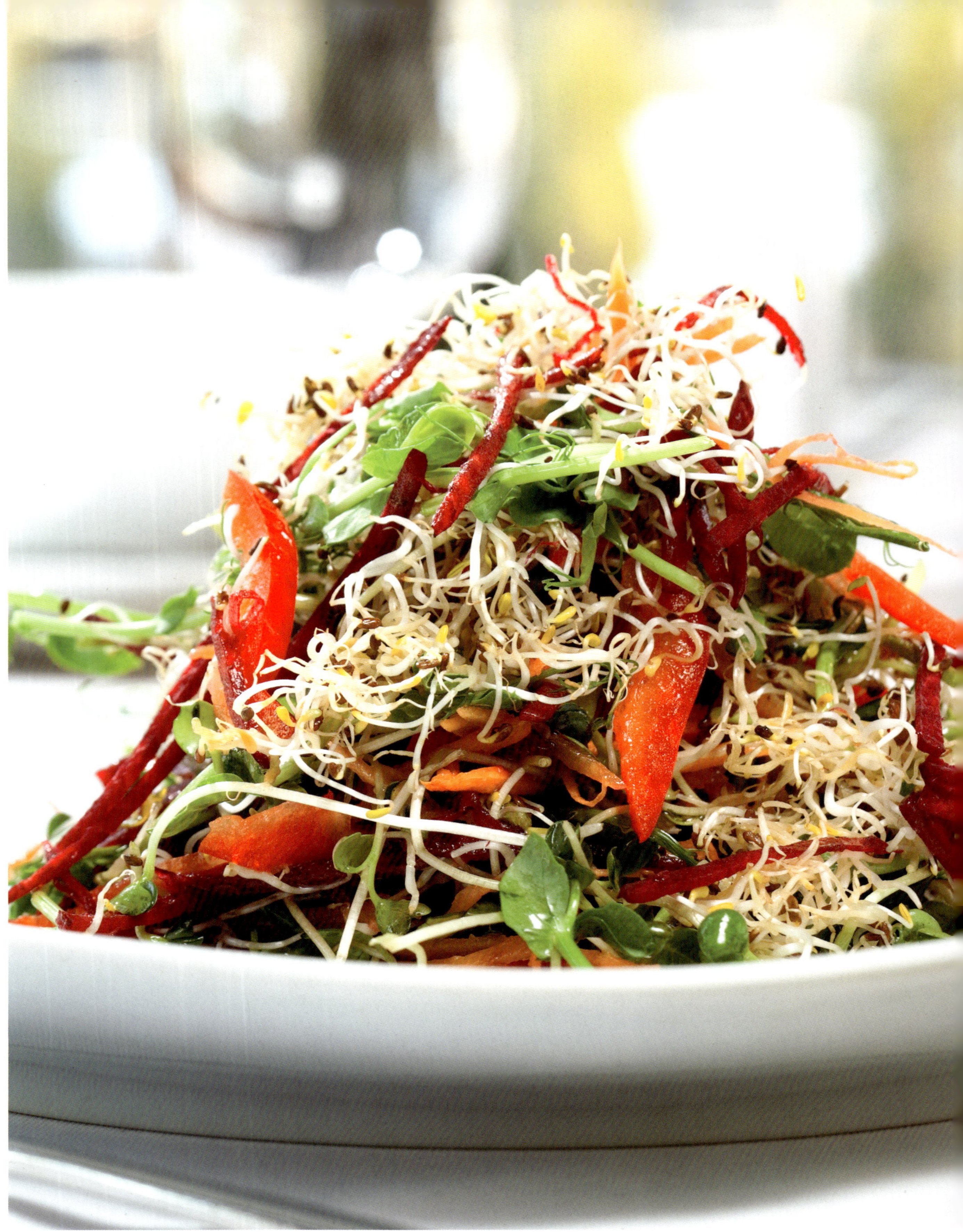

THAI SPROUT SALAD

SALAD

1 cup (35g) alfalfa sprouts

1 cup (35g) sunflower sprouts

1 red capsicum, sliced

1 carrot, julienned

1 large beetroot, julienned

MAPLE-SESAME DRESSING

1 clove garlic

¼ cup (55g) almond butter

2 tbsps fresh lime juice

2 tbsps tamari

2 tbsps water

2 tsps maple syrup

1 tbsp toasted sesame oil

1 tsp freshly grated ginger

STEPS

1. Place all dressing ingredients in a jar with a sealable lid and shake until thoroughly combined.
2. Place the salad ingredients in a large bowl and pour over dressing. Toss well to coat.
3. Arrange salad on individual plates and serve.

SERVES 2 | PREP + COOK TIME: 20 MINS | VEG | GLUTEN FREE | DAIRY FREE |

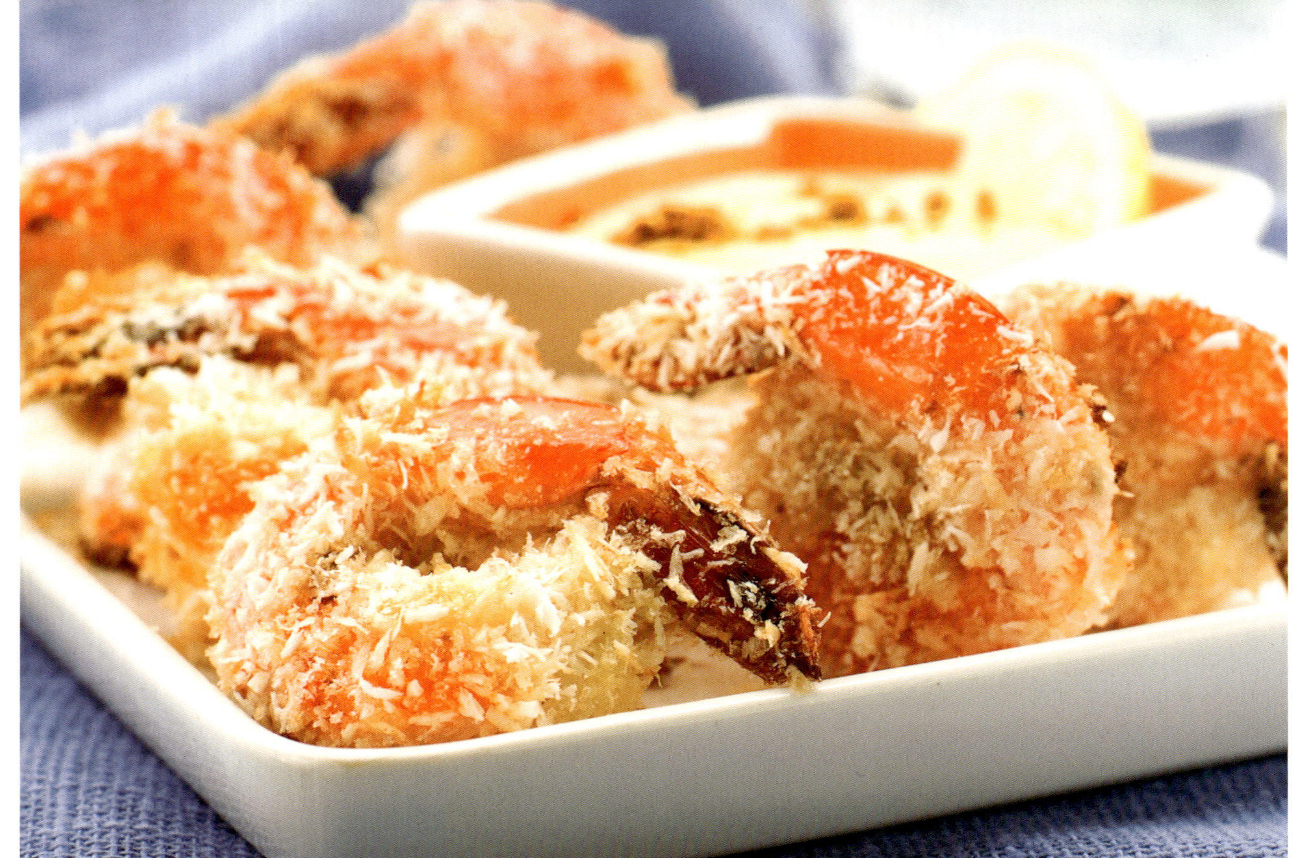

COCONUT PRAWNS

COCONUT PRAWNS

1 cup (120g) plain flour

3 eggs

2 cups (180g) desiccated coconut

⅔ cup (80g) panko breadcrumbs

Peanut oil for frying

900g green king prawns, peeled and deveined

MUSTARD YOGHURT DIP

⅓ cup (80ml) Greek yoghurt

2 tsps Dijon mustard

1 tsp cracked pepper

STEPS

1. Place the flour in a shallow bowl. Beat the eggs in a second shallow bowl. Combine the coconut and breadcrumbs in a third bowl.

2. Dip the prawns first into the flour, then into the eggs, shaking off any excess. Next press into the breadcrumbs, being sure to fully coat each prawn.

3. Pour 5cm peanut oil into wok or deep pan and place over medium heat. When the oil is hot and bubbles start to form fry prawns in batches for 2-3 minutes until risen to the top of the oil and golden brown in colour.

4. Remove prawns with a slotted spoon and drain on a plate lined with paper towel.

5. Stir together the ingredients for mustard yoghurt dip. Serve with cooked prawns.

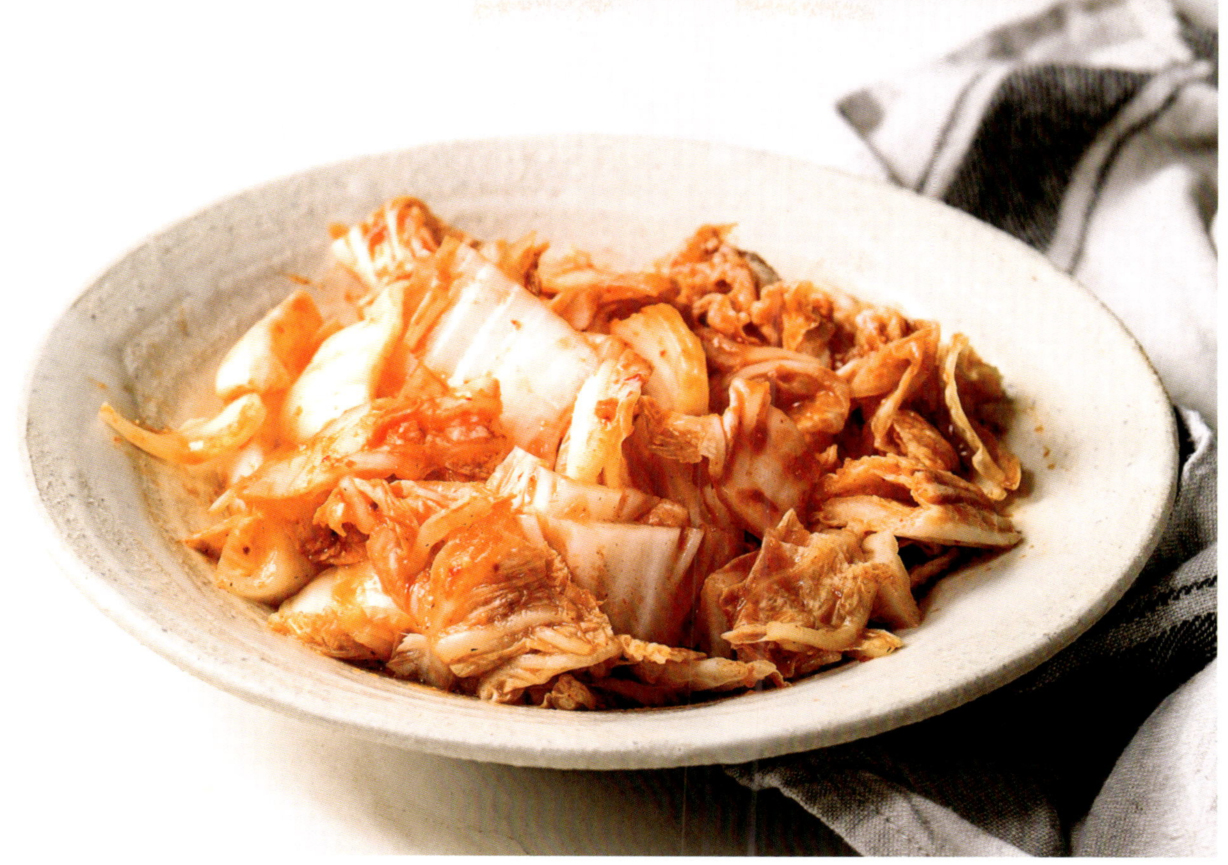

MAKES 6 CUPS | PREP + COOK TIME: 15 MINS + FERMENTING | VEG | DAIRY FREE |

KIMCHI

1 head Chinese cabbage (wombok), leaves removed and roughly chopped

1 daikon, chopped

2 tbsps coarse salt

8 spring onions, white parts only

8 cloves garlic

Medium piece ginger, peeled and roughly chopped

½ cup (50g) gochugaru (Korean chilli flakes)

2 tbsps white miso paste

1 tbsp sugar

1 cup (250ml) water

STEPS

1. Place cabbage leaves and daikon in a large bowl and sprinkle over salt. Toss to combine. Cover and allow to sit at room temperature for a minimum of 1 hour.
2. Meanwhile, combine spring onion, garlic, ginger, gochugaru, miso paste and sugar in a food processor and blend into a rough paste.
3. Pour chilli mixture over cabbage. Add water and toss to coat well.
4. Pack the mixture into glass jars, pressing down firmly to remove any trapped air. Pour in soaking liquid to completely cover cabbage. Seal the jars tightly.
5. Keep jars at room temperature for 24 hours then transfer to the fridge to ferment for 1 week before serving.

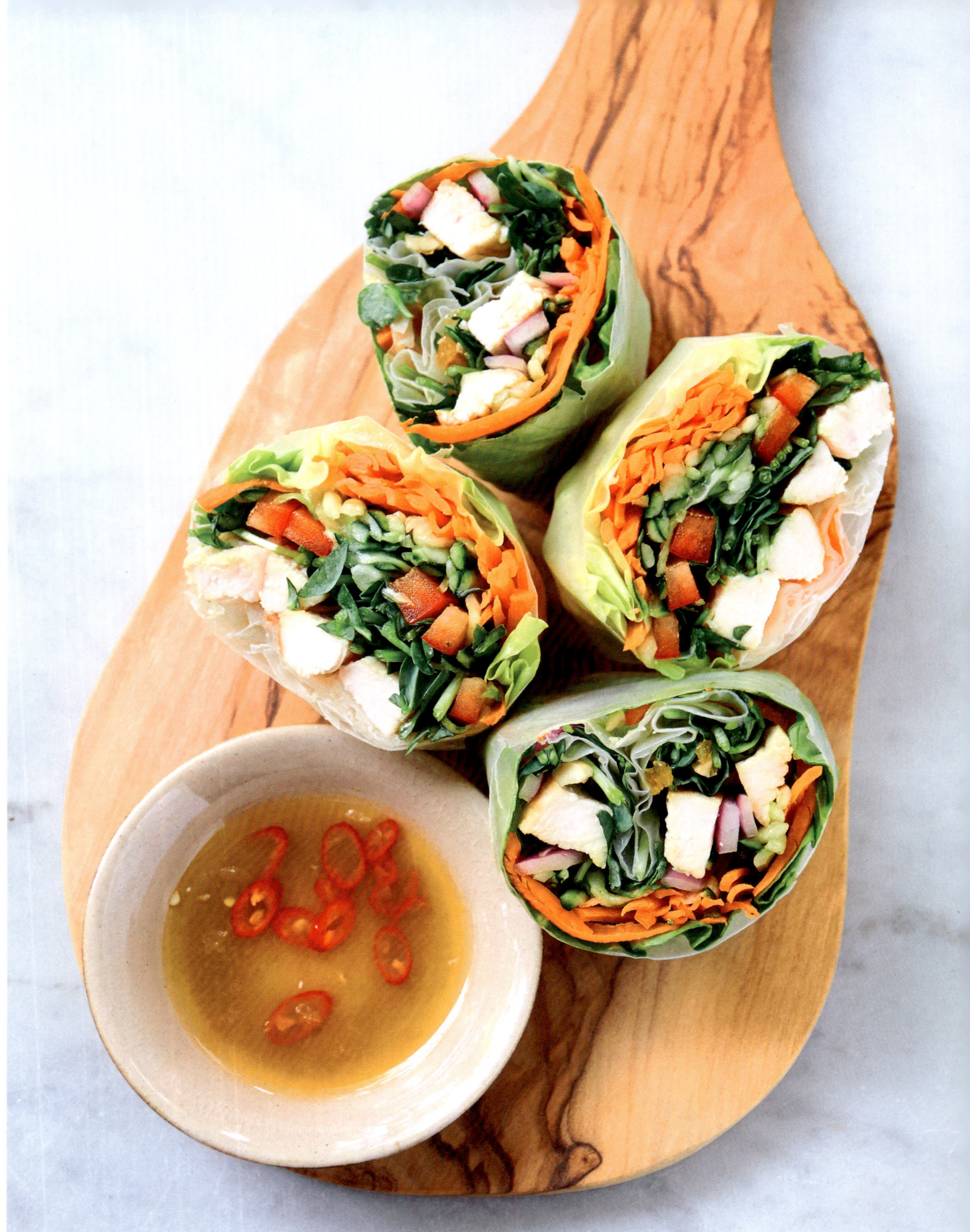

CHICKEN RICE PAPER ROLLS

2 small carrots, julienned or grated

1 medium Lebanese cucumber, cut into thin strips

1 red capsicum, cut into thin strips

½ red onion, cut into thin strips

1 cup (100g) pea shoots

350g cooked chicken breast, cut into strips

2 spring onions, cut into thin strips

6 butter lettuce leaves, cut in half

12 rice paper rounds

DIPPING SAUCE

6 tbsps warm water

2 tbsps sugar

2 tbsps lime juice

2 tbsps fish sauce

1 clove garlic, minced

2 Thai chillies, sliced

STEPS

1. Fill a large shallow bowl with lukewarm water. You need to make the rolls one at a time. Dip a rice paper sheet into the water for 10 seconds until transparent. Place on a clean, flat work surface.
2. Place small amounts of each vegetable along with some chicken in the middle of each sheet. Fold ends in and roll up firmly. Repeat with remaining rice paper sheets: dipping in water, filling and rolling.
3. Combine dipping sauce ingredients in a small bowl and stir to dissolve sugar.
4. Cut rolls in half with a very sharp knife and serve with dipping sauce.

SERVES 4 | PREP + COOK TIME: 20 MINS | GLUTEN FREE | DAIRY FREE |

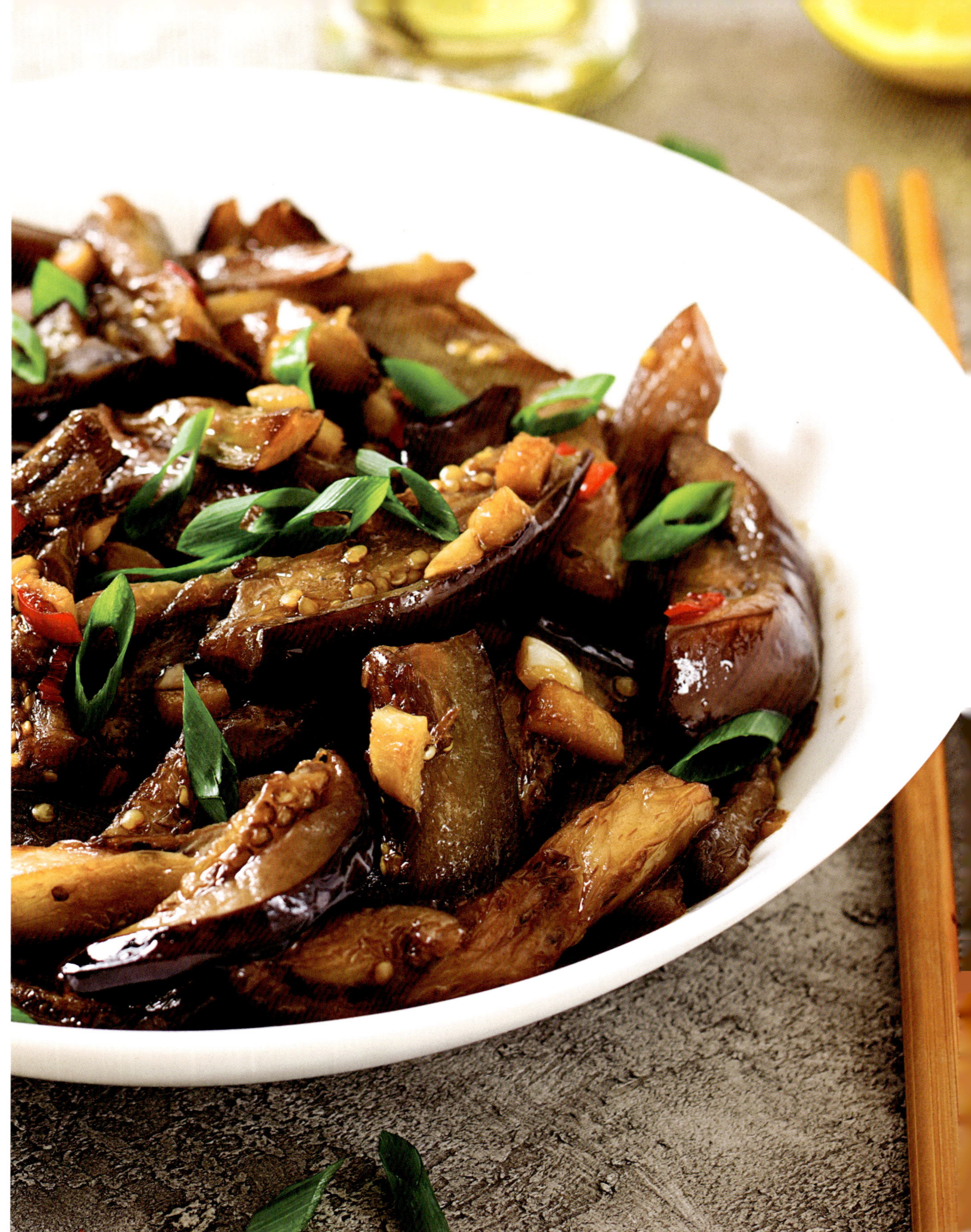

SPICY KOREAN EGGPLANT

2 large eggplants, cut into 5cm-long strips

3 cloves garlic, minced

1 red chilli, deseeded and chopped

Medium piece ginger, chopped

2 tbsps soy sauce or tamari

2 tsps toasted sesame oil

¼ tsp sugar

½ tsp gochugaru (Korean chilli flakes)

TO SERVE

1 spring onion, chopped

½ red chilli, chopped (optional)

STEPS

1. Place the eggplant in a steamer over a pan of boiling water on high heat. Cook, covered, for 15 minutes until soft.
2. Transfer to a bowl to cool.
3. Place the garlic, chilli, ginger, soy sauce or tamari, sesame oil, sugar and gochugaru in a small bowl. Whisk or stir to combine.
4. Pour over the eggplant and toss thoroughly to coat.
5. Sprinkle with chopped spring onion and chopped red chilli, if desired, to serve.

SERVES 4 | PREP + COOK TIME: 20 MINS | VEG | DAIRY FREE |

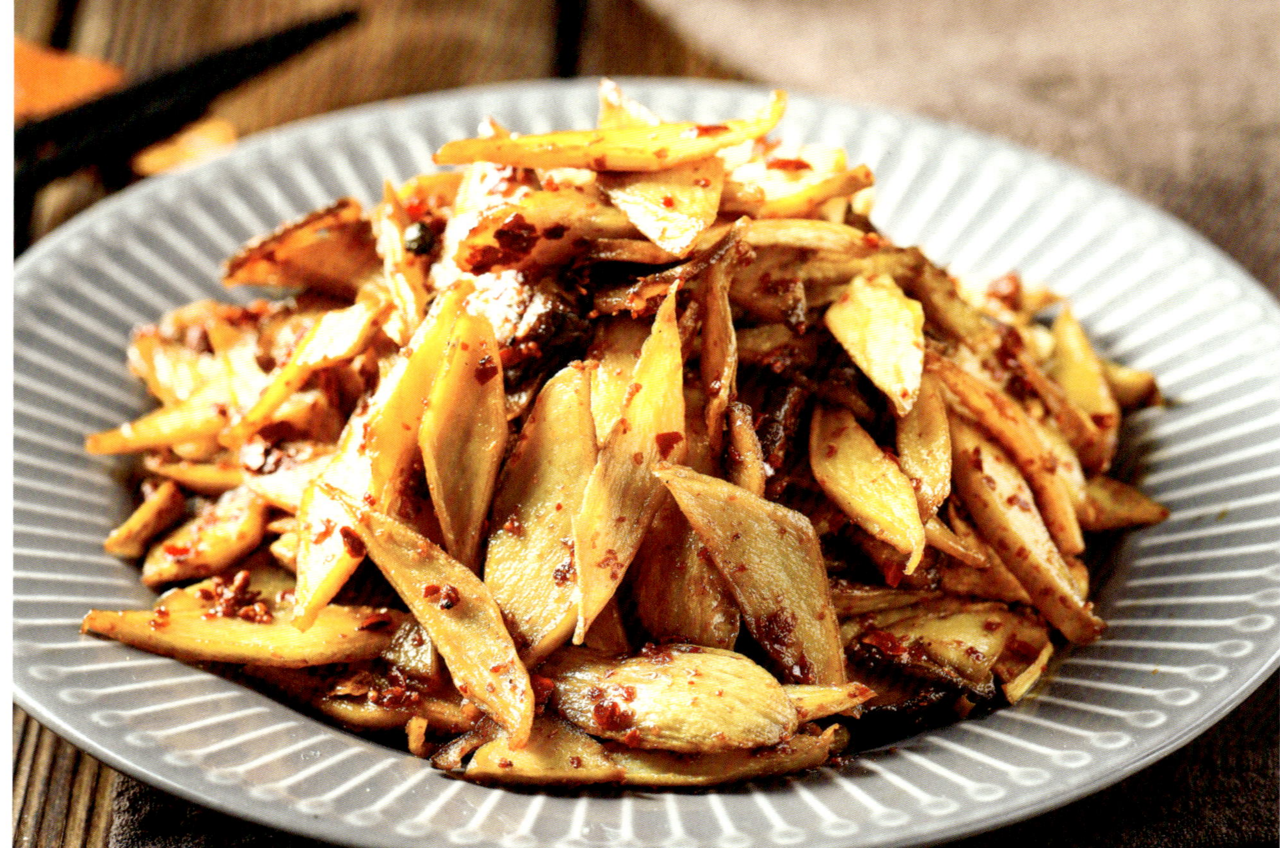

SPICY KING OYSTER MUSHROOMS

2 tbsps vegetable oil

2 cloves garlic, minced

Medium piece ginger, minced

350g king oyster mushrooms, cut into thin, 5cm-long strips

1 tbsp Chinese chilli bean sauce (toban jang)

2 tbsps soy sauce

1 tbsp oyster sauce

1 tbsp rice wine vinegar

1 tsp sugar

STEPS

1. Heat the vegetable oil in a large frying pan or wok over medium-high heat. Add garlic and ginger. Stir-fry for 30 seconds until fragrant.

2. Add the sliced mushrooms and stir-fry for 3-4 minutes until golden brown.

3. In a small bowl, whisk together Chinese chilli bean sauce, soy sauce, oyster sauce, rice wine vinegar, and sugar.

4. Pour the sauce over the mushrooms. Stir-fry for an additional 2-3 minutes, allowing the flavours to meld.

5. Serve immediately.

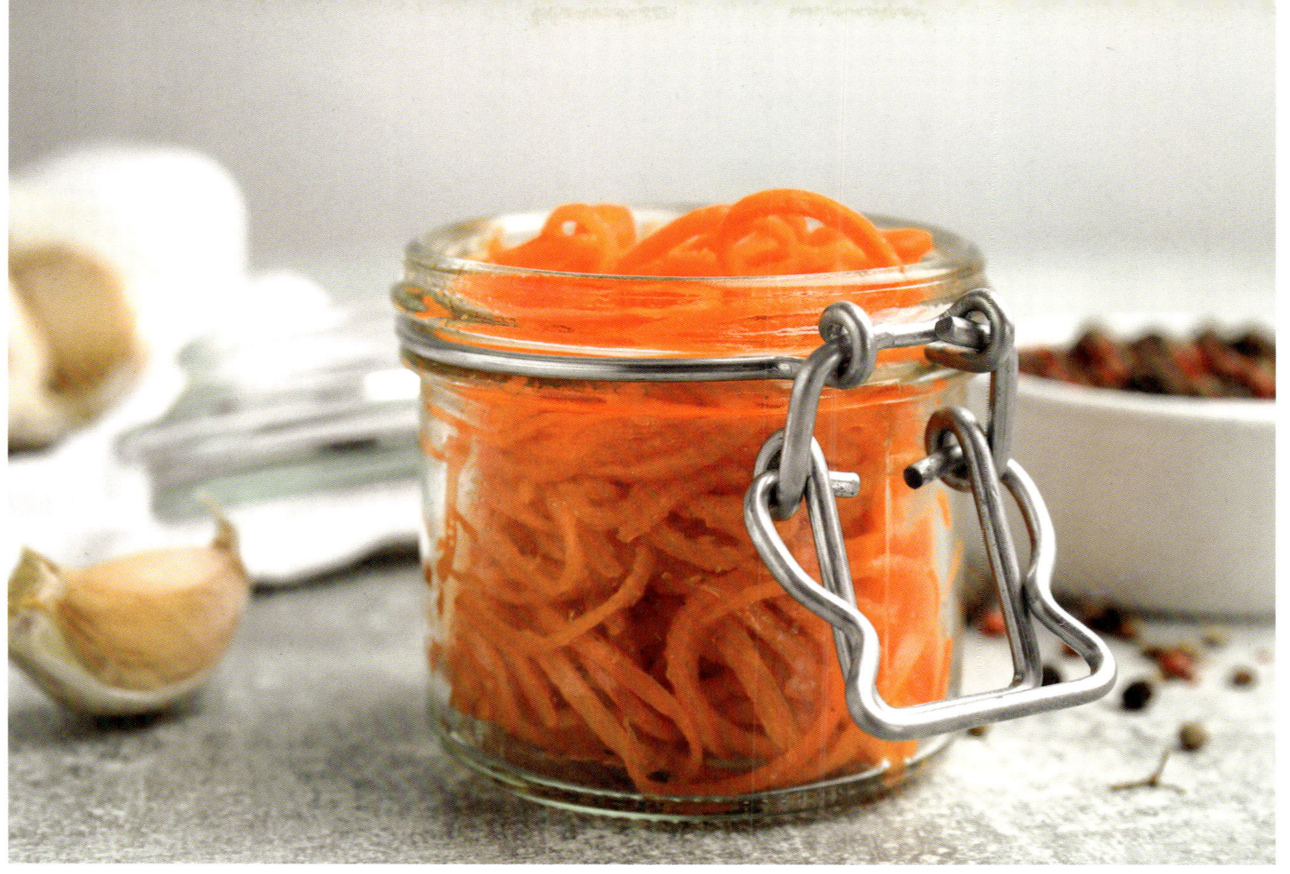

KOREAN CARROT SALAD

8 carrots, julienned or spiralised

1 tsp salt

⅓ cup (80ml) olive oil

1 large onion, finely chopped

6 cloves garlic, minced

¼ tsp cayenne pepper

½ tsp paprika

¼ tsp pepper

1 tbsp sugar

1 tbsp white wine vinegar

½ tsp ground coriander

STEPS

1. In a large bowl, combine carrots and half the salt. Set aside.
2. Heat the oil in a frying pan over medium heat. Cook the onion for 5 minutes until soft and translucent. Remove pan from heat and mix in minced garlic.
3. Once the onions are cool, add the remaining salt, cayenne pepper, paprika, pepper, sugar, vinegar and ground coriander. Mix well.
4. Spoon over the carrots and toss until completely combined. Cover and refrigerate for at least 2 hours.
5. Serve cold.

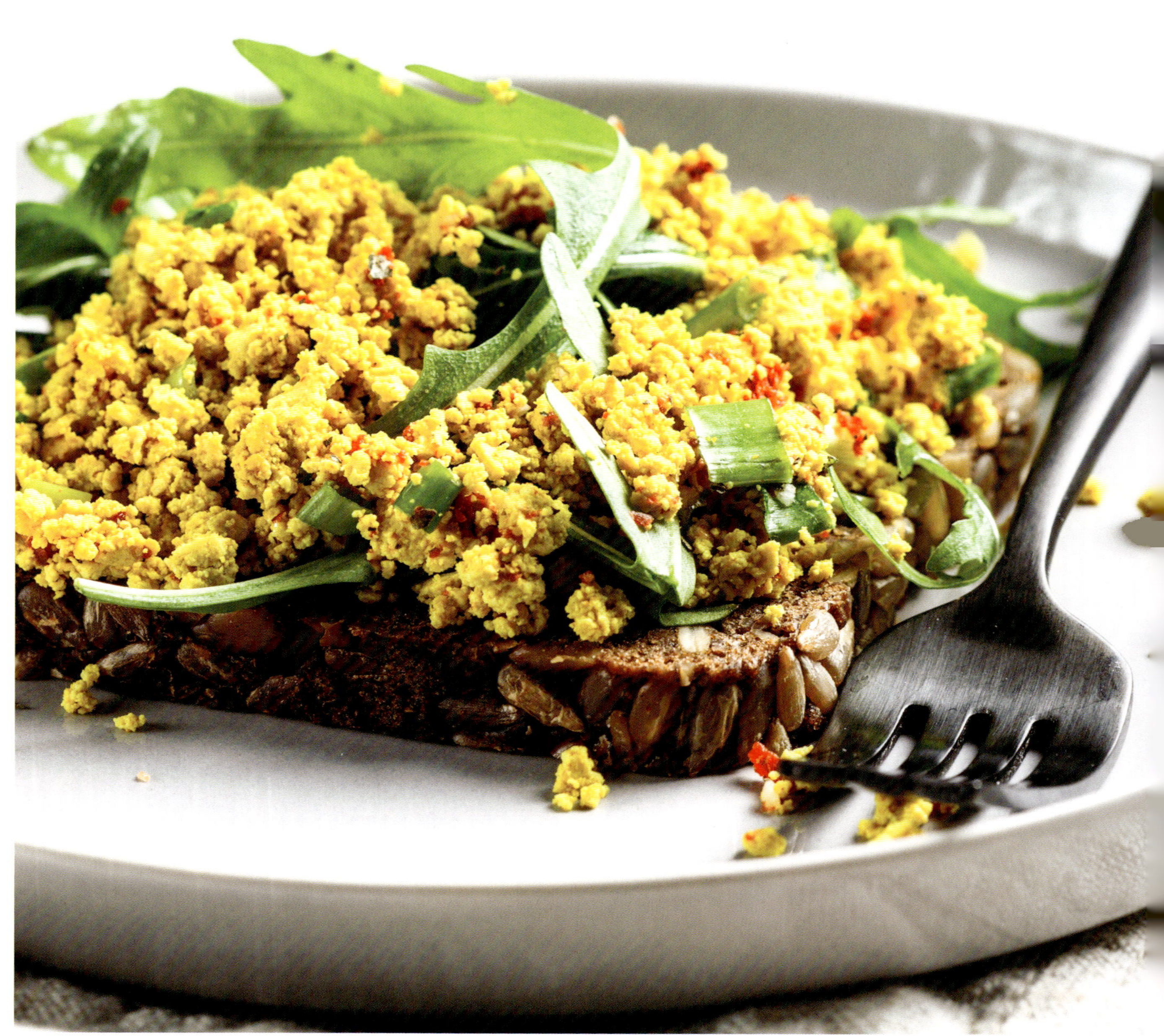

TURMERIC SCRAMBLED TOFU

1 tbsp olive oil

1 tsp grated fresh turmeric

2 spring onions, finely sliced, white and green parts separated

¼ red chilli, chopped

225g silken tofu

2 slices seeded bread, toasted

Handful of rocket

STEPS

1. Heat the oil and turmeric in a frying pan over a medium heat. Allow to cook for 2 minutes before adding the white part of the spring onions and the chilli. Saute for 2-3 minutes.
2. Add the tofu to the frying pan and stir well, leaving some larger chunks and breaking the rest of the tofu down to a 'scrambled egg' consistency. Continue to stir-fry the tofu mix for about 3 minutes until thoroughly heated through. Scatter with spring onion tops.
3. Top toasted seeded bread with scrambled tofu and rocket leaves to serve.

SERVES 2 | PREP + COOK TIME: 15 MINS | VEG | DAIRY FREE |

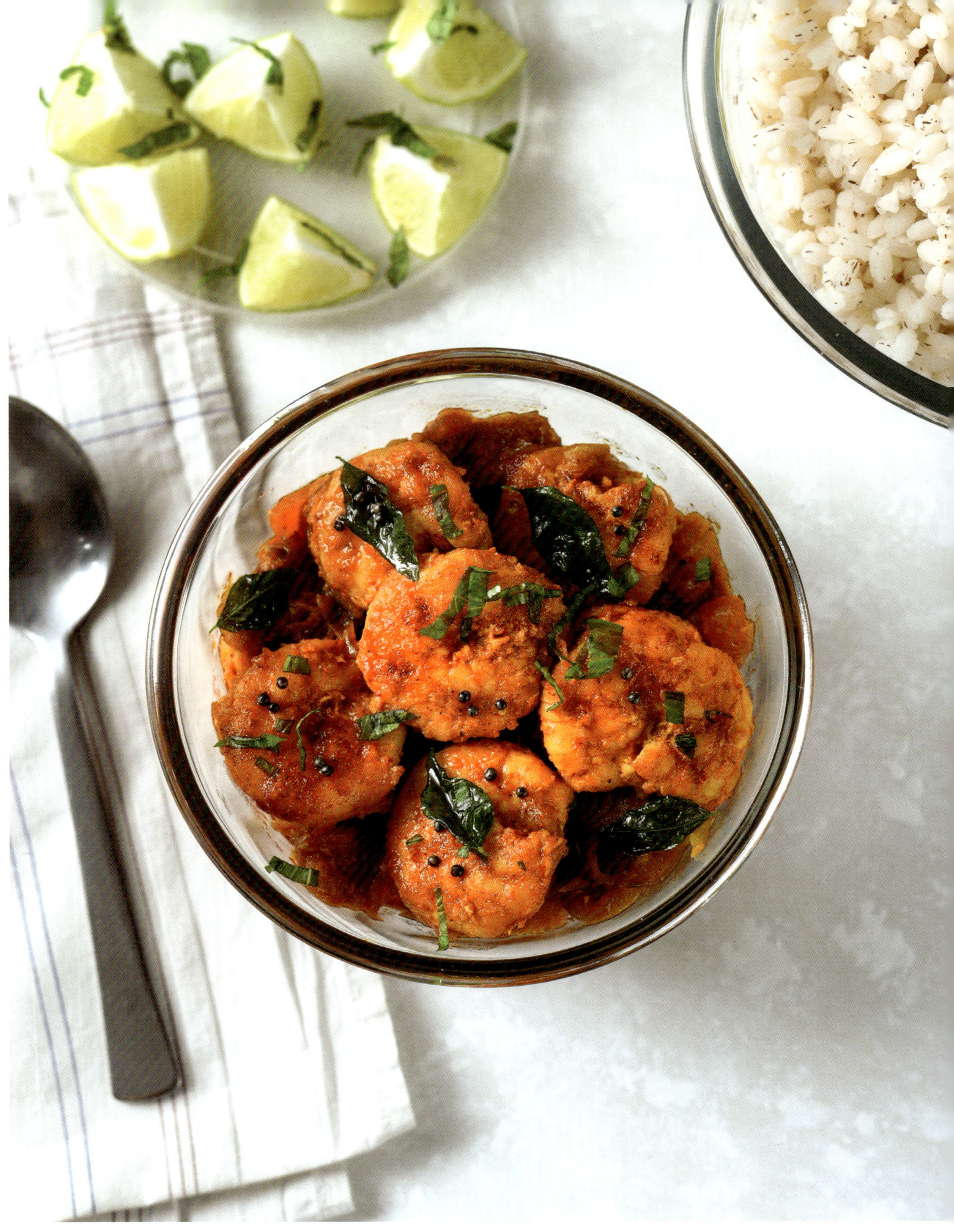

BENGALI SPICED PRAWNS

2 tbsps vegetable oil
600g raw prawns, peeled and deveined
1 tsp black mustard seeds
1 onion, finely chopped
3 cloves garlic, finely chopped
Small piece fresh ginger, grated
1 tsp ground turmeric
1 tsp chilli powder
1 tsp ground cumin
1 tsp ground coriander
1 tsp salt
1 tsp caster sugar
1 x 400g can chopped tomatoes
½ cup (125ml) coconut cream
10-12 curry leaves
1 tsp garam masala
2 tbsps chopped coriander leaves

STEPS

1. Heat 1 tablespoon oil in a large frying pan over medium heat. When hot, add the prawns and cook for 1-2 minutes on each side until they just turn pink. Transfer to a plate and set aside.
2. Add another tablespoon oil to the pan. When hot add the mustard seeds and cook 1 minute until they pop. Add the onion, garlic and ginger to the pan and gently cook, stirring occasionally, for 5 minutes or until they begin to turn golden. Stir in the turmeric, chilli, cumin and coriander, then season with the salt and sugar.
3. Stir in the chopped tomatoes, coconut cream and curry leaves. Bring to a boil, gently stirring. Simmer for 10 minutes.
4. Add the cooked prawns, gently spooning over the sauce to cover, then simmer for a few minutes to warm through. Taste and season if necessary.
5. Sprinkle over the garam masala and scatter with chopped coriander to serve.

SERVES 4 | PREP + COOK TIME: 45 MINS | GLUTEN FREE | DAIRY FREE |

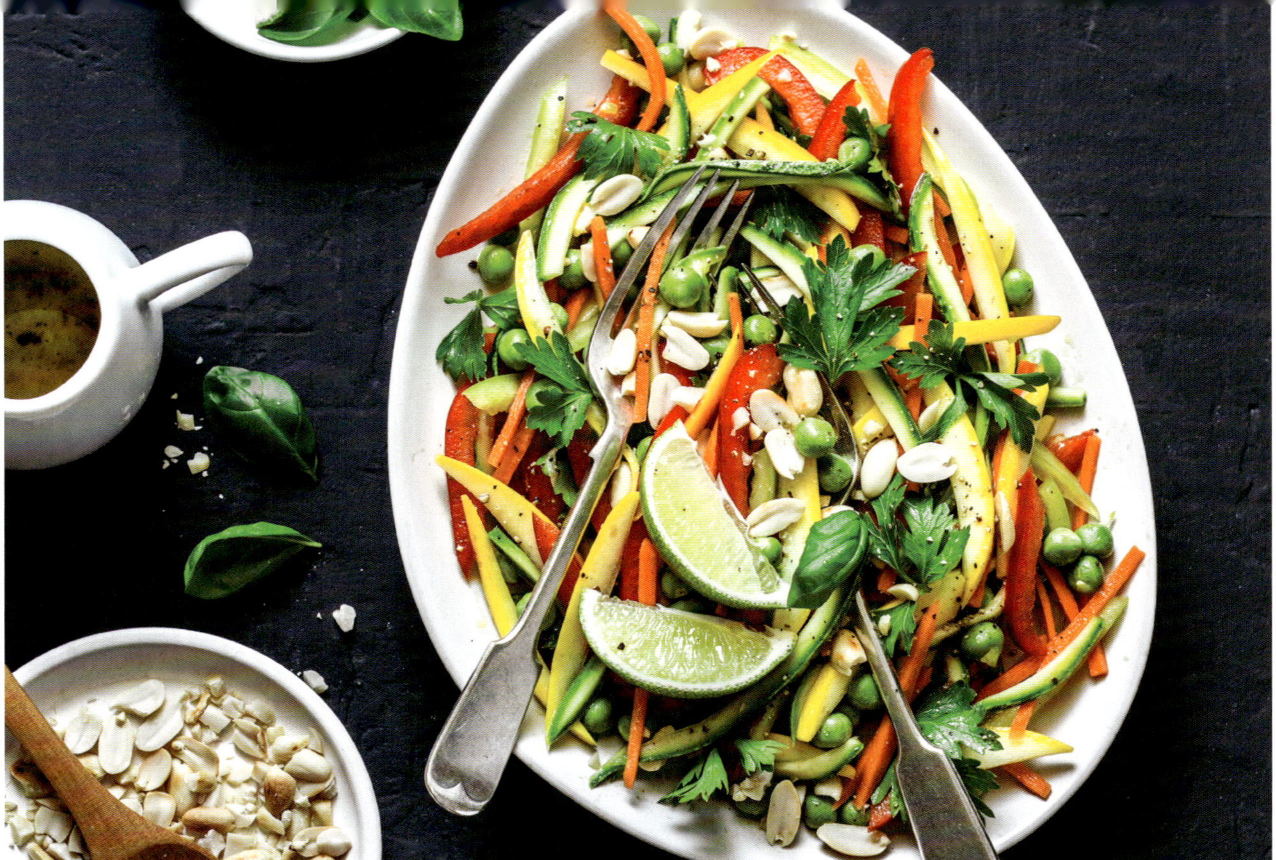

CRUNCHY THAI SALAD

2 green zucchinis, cut into long, thin batons

2 yellow zucchinis, cut into long, thin batons

2 carrots, cut into long, thin batons

1 red capsicum, cut into long, thin batons

½ cup (80g) peas

¼ cup (65g) smooth peanut butter

3 tbsps soy sauce or tamari

2 tbsps lime juice

1 tbsp honey

1 tsp Sriracha

1-2 tbsps water as needed

Pepper to taste

¼ cup (10g) parsley leaves, roughly torn

¼ cup (5g) Thai basil (or regular basil) leaves, roughly torn

¼ cup (30g) peanuts, coarsely chopped

Lime wedges to serve

STEPS

1. Place the vegetables in a large serving bowl or plate.
2. Place peanut butter in a small bowl and microwave for 15-30 seconds to soften, then add soy sauce or tamari, lime juice, honey and Sriracha. Whisk to combine. Add water as needed until a smooth, dressing-like consistency is reached.
3. Add dressing to vegetables and toss to combine. Season with pepper. Scatter with parsley, Thai basil and peanuts and serve with lime wedges.

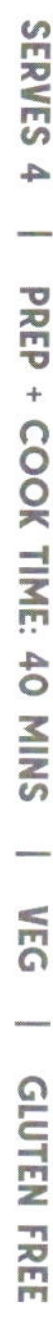

CURRY ROASTED CAULIFLOWER

1 tbsp coconut oil

3 cloves garlic, minced

Medium piece ginger, minced

1 small onion, finely chopped

2 tbsps melted butter or ghee

1 tsp curry powder

Pinch of salt

Pepper to taste

1 small cauliflower, broken into florets

Chopped coriander leaves to serve

YOGHURT SAUCE

¾ cup (185ml) Greek yoghurt

¼ cup (5g) mint leaves, chopped

3 tbsps lemon juice

2 cloves garlic, minced

Salt and pepper to taste

STEPS

Preheat the oven to 200°C.

1. Heat a small frying pan over medium-high heat. Add coconut oil, garlic, ginger and onion and fry, stirring, for 10 minutes until sticky and soft.
2. Mix the melted butter or ghee, curry powder, salt and pepper together in a mixing bowl. Add the cauliflower and garlic-ginger mix.
3. Transfer to a lined baking tray arranging in one single layer. Roast for 20 minutes then toss with chopped coriander.
4. Mix together the yoghurt sauce ingredients. Serve with the roasted cauliflower.

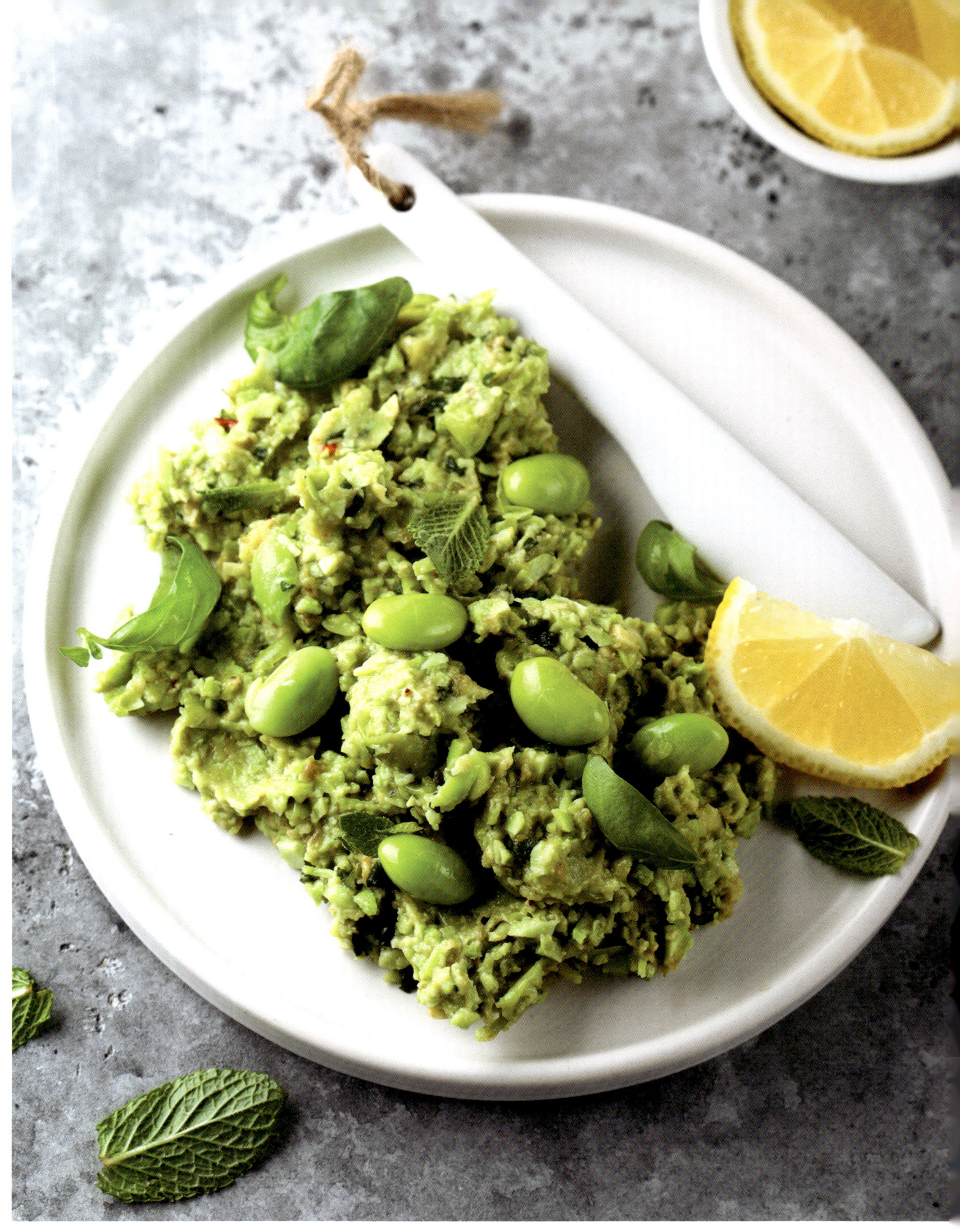

EDAMAME DIP

¾ cup (100g) walnuts

450g frozen edamame, thawed
+ ¼ cup (50g) extra to garnish

2 tsps white miso paste

½ tsp salt

2 tbsps fresh lemon juice

2 tbsps fresh chives, minced

2 cloves garlic, minced

¼ red chilli, chopped (or to taste)

½ cup (125ml) olive oil

Basil and mint leaves to garnish (optional)

STEPS

Preheat oven to 180°C.

1. Arrange the walnuts on a baking tray and bake for 10-15 minutes or until fragrant. Remove from the oven and set aside to cool slightly.
2. Combine edamame, toasted walnuts, miso paste, salt, lemon juice, chives, garlic and chilli in a food processor and process until ingredients become a rough paste. Keeping the food processor running, drizzle in olive oil until all incorporated.
3. Spoon into a bowl and garnish with extra edamame and mint and basil leaves, if desired.

SERVES 4 | PREP + COOK TIME: 20 MINS | VEG | DAIRY FREE |

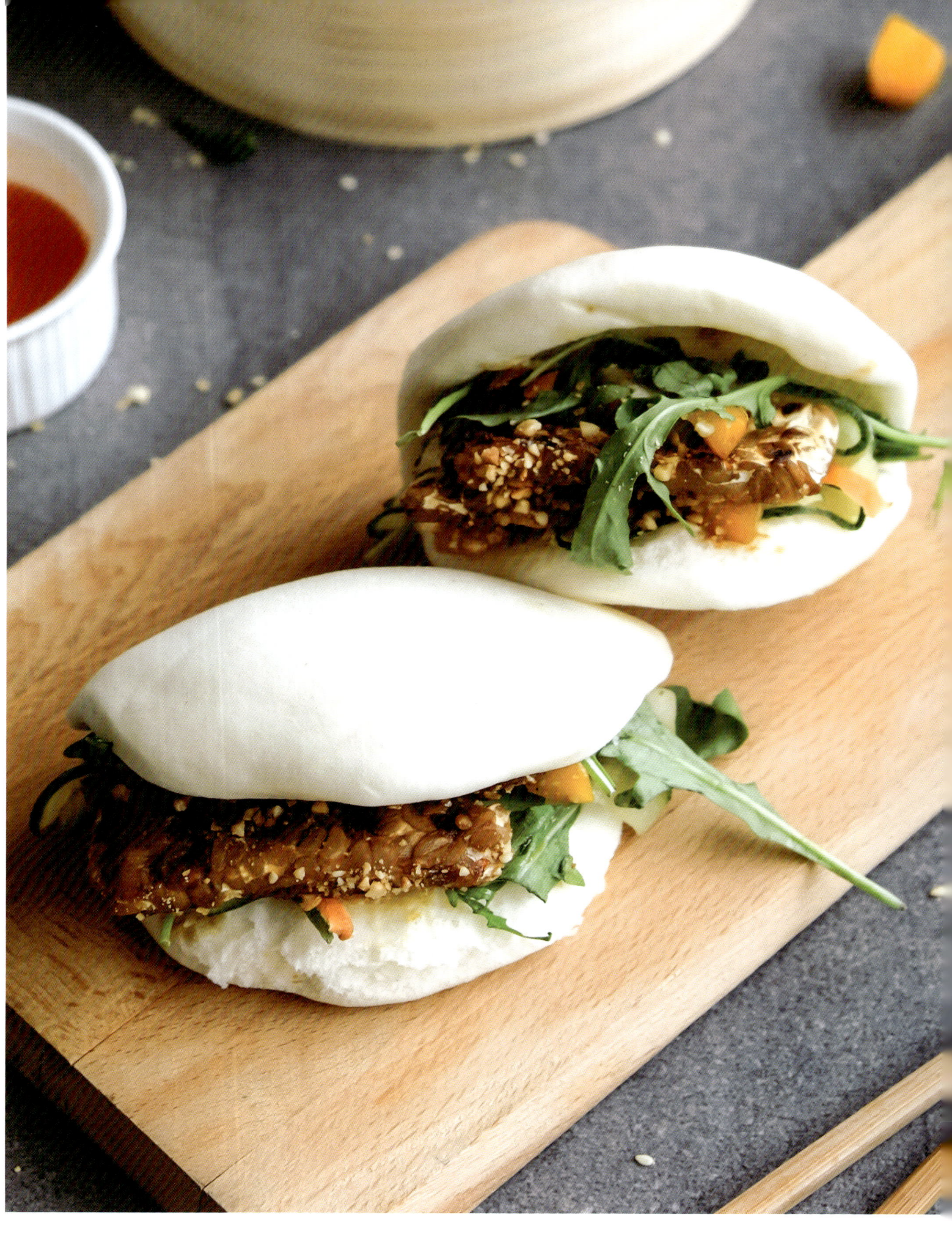

TEMPEH GUA BAO

1 x 300g package tempeh

½ cup (125ml) + 1½ tsps water

2 tsps vegetable oil

2 tsps gochujang (Korean chilli paste)

1 tbsp maple syrup

1½ tsp soy sauce

¼ tsp garlic powder

12 bao buns

2 cups (60g) rocket leaves

1 carrot, peeled into ribbons or julienned

1 Lebanese cucumber, cut into thin ribbons, using a vegetable peeler

1 yellow capsicum, diced

1 tbsp sesame seeds

STEPS

1. Place the tempeh in a large nonstick frying pan with ½ cup of water. Cover with a lid and steam for 15 minutes over medium-high heat, or until all the water is absorbed. Reduce the heat to medium and pour the oil into the pan. Fry 2-3 minutes on each side until golden and crispy.

2. In a small bowl, mix together the gochujang, maple syrup, soy sauce, garlic powder and 1½ teaspoons of water to form a thick sauce. Pour it over the tempeh and cook for 1 minute, tossing to coat all the pieces evenly with the sauce.

3. Place bao buns in steamer baskets lined with greaseproof paper. Steam for 7-8 minutes until piping hot.

4. Open the buns and fill with rocket, carrot, cucumber, capsicum and tempeh. Sprinkle with sesame seeds to serve.

SERVES 4 | PREP + COOK TIME: 35 MINS | VEG | DAIRY FREE |

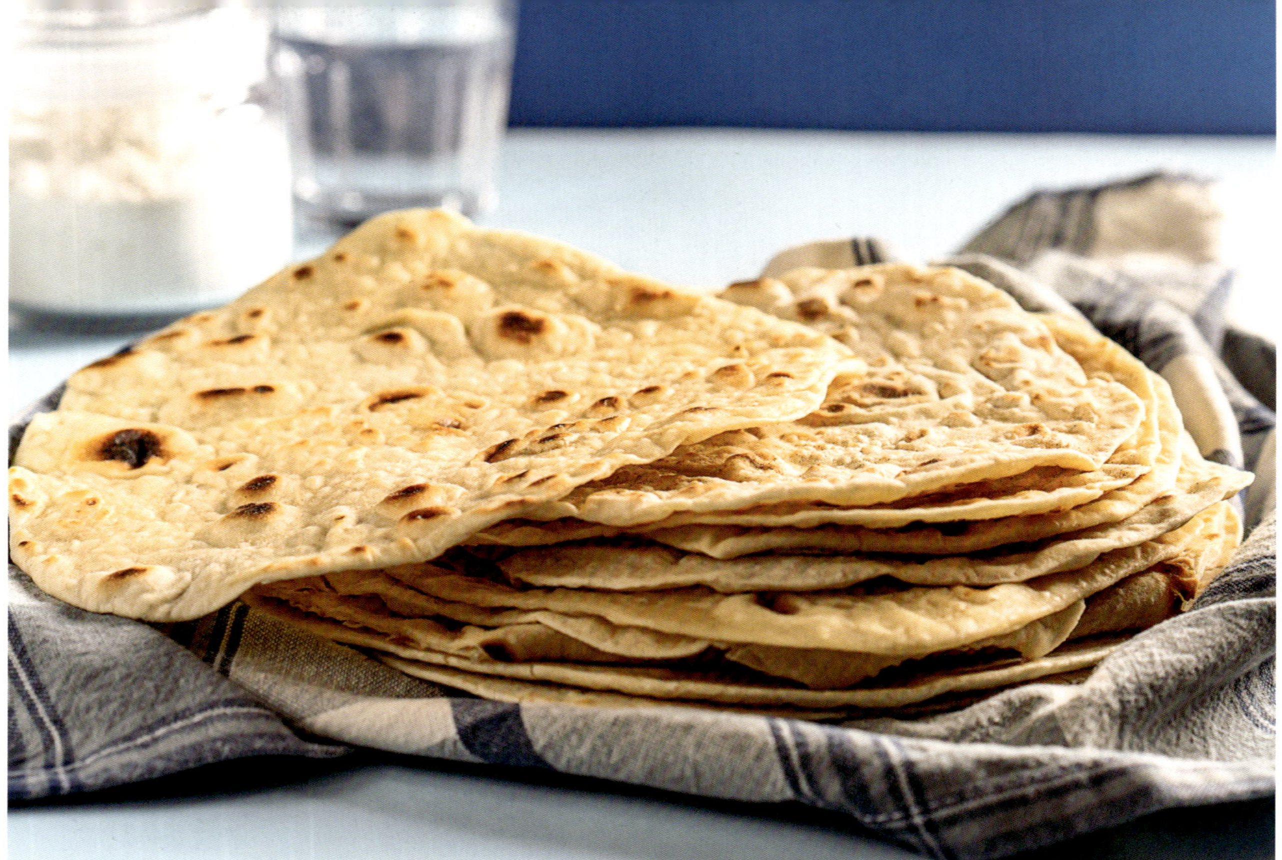

CHAPATIS

1 cup (125g) whole wheat flour

1 cup (125g) plain flour

1 tsp salt

¾ cup (185ml) hot water or as needed

2 tbsps ghee or butter

STEPS

1. Mix flours and salt in a large bowl. Use a wooden spoon to stir in water. Mix until a soft, elastic dough forms, adding more water if needed. Knead dough on a lightly floured surface until smooth.
2. Divide dough into 10 equal portions. Roll each piece into a ball and let rest for a few minutes.
3. Lightly grease a frying pan with ghee or butter and place over medium heat.
4. Working on one dough ball at a time, use a rolling pin to roll out on a lightly floured surface until very thin.
5. Place a chapati in the hot pan. Cook for about 30 seconds until bottom has brown spots, then flip and cook 30 seconds more. Repeat with remaining chapatis.

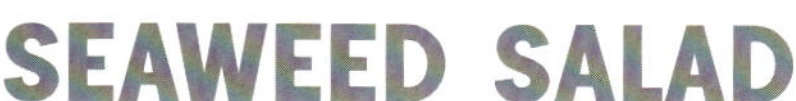

SEAWEED SALAD

SERVES 2 | PREP + COOK TIME: 20 MINS | VEG | DAIRY FREE

60g dried green seaweed (wakame, arame or hijiki)

2 tbsps rice wine vinegar

2 tsps sugar

2 tsps ginger, grated

½ tsp wasabi powder

⅛ red chilli, very finely chopped

2 tsps soy sauce

1 tbsp roasted sesame oil

1 lime, juiced

1 tsp toasted black and white sesame seeds

Salt to taste

STEPS

1. Cover the seaweed with cold water in a large bowl. Soak for 10 minutes, until soft. Drain and pat dry with paper towel. Use scissors to snip into bite-size pieces. Transfer to a serving bowl.

2. Whisk together the rice wine vinegar, sugar, ginger, wasabi powder, chilli, soy sauce and sesame oil. Transfer to a serving jug.

3. Pour half of the dressing over the soft seaweed. Pour on the lime juice.

4. Add the sesame seeds and toss gently.

5. Season with salt to taste. Serve accompanied with the extra dressing in the jug.

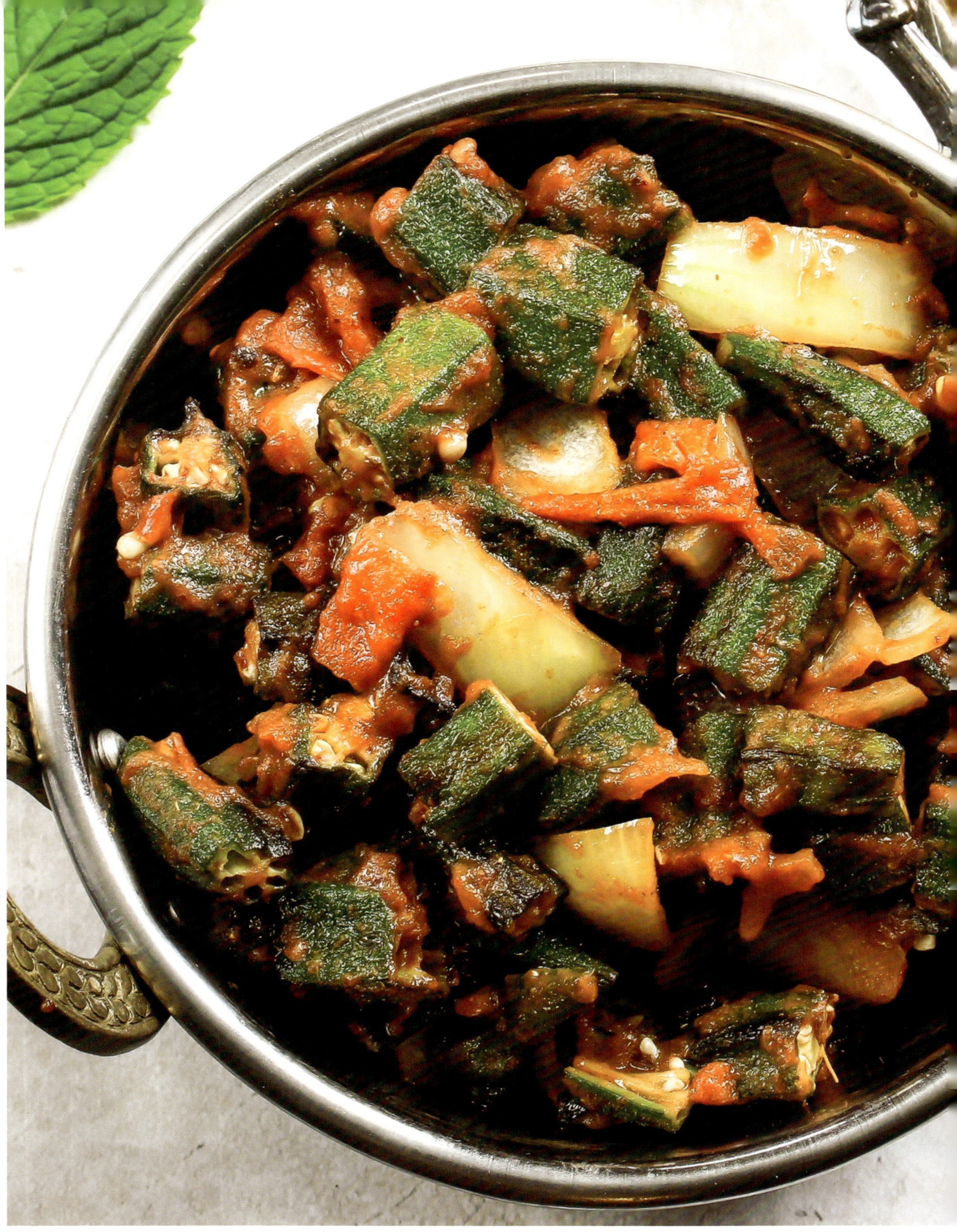

BHINDI MASALA

500g okra

3 tbsps oil

1 tsp cumin seeds

1 large onion, thickly sliced

Small piece ginger, grated

2 cloves garlic, minced

1 large tomato, diced

1½ tsps salt

¼ tsp ground turmeric

1 tsp Kashmiri red chilli powder

1 tsp ground coriander

¼ tsp garam masala

STEPS

1. Rinse and completely dry okra with paper towels. Cut into 2cm pieces.
2. Heat half of the oil in a large frying pan over medium heat. Add okra and cook, stirring occasionally, for 8 minutes, until the okra is tender-crisp. Do not over-stir. Transfer the okra to a plate and set aside.
3. Add the remaining oil to the same pan. Add cumin seeds and allow them to sizzle. Add sliced onion and cook for 5 minutes, stirring frequently. Add ginger, garlic and tomatoes. Stir to combine. Add salt, turmeric, red chilli powder, ground coriander and garam masala and mix well. Cook for 2 minutes or just until the onions start to soften.
4. Return the okra to the pan and cook, stirring, for 2-3 minutes until the okra is tender.

SERVES 4 | PREP + COOK TIME: 45 MINS | VEG | GLUTEN FREE | DAIRY FREE |

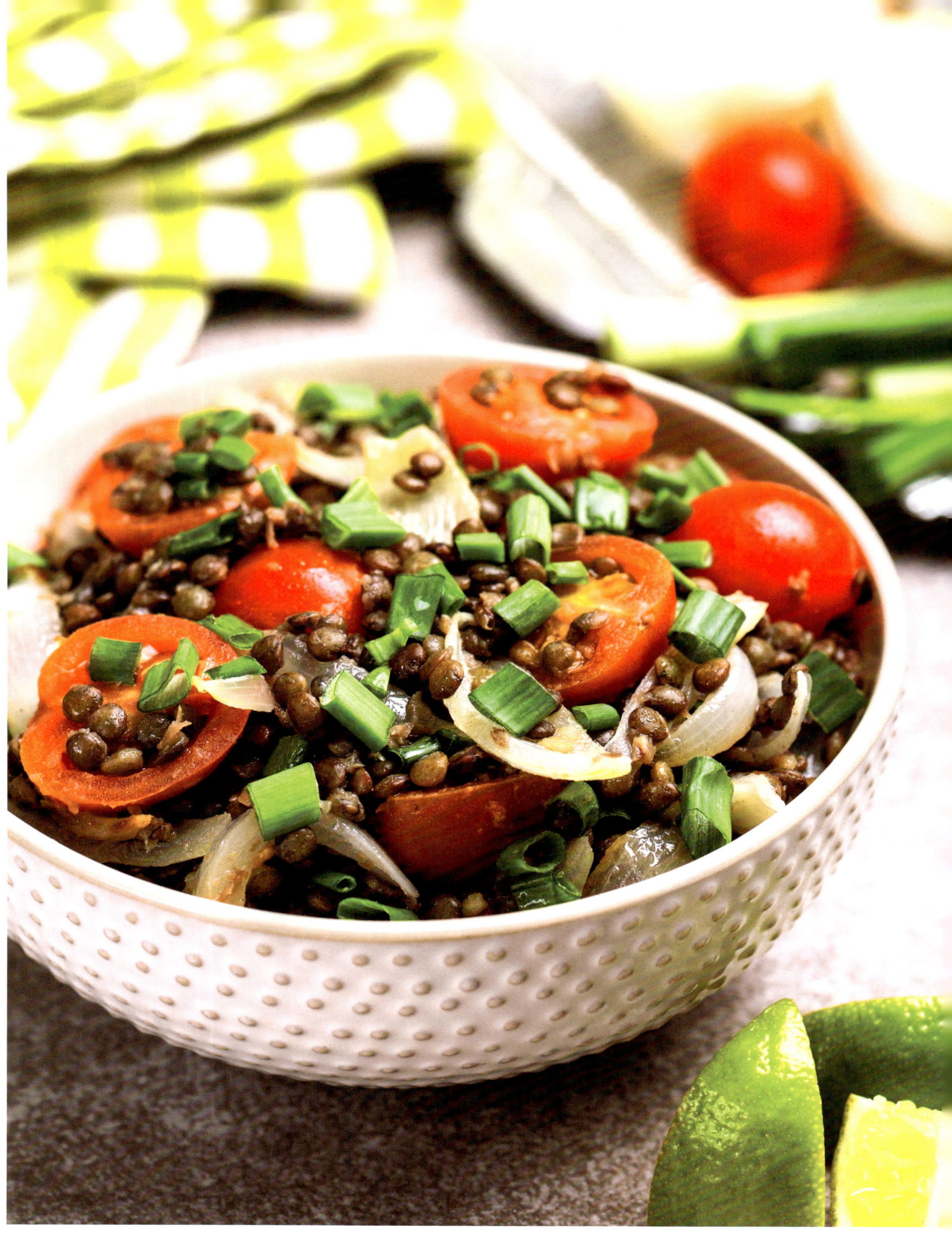

WARM LENTIL SALAD

2 tbsps olive oil
1 onion, thickly sliced
1 tbsp fresh ginger, minced
2 cloves garlic, minced
1 red chilli, finely diced
1 tsp ground cumin
1 tbsp curry powder
1 tsp salt
2½ cups (625ml) water
1 cup (185g) dried green lentils
1 tsp ground cinnamon
⅔ cup (150g) cherry tomatoes, halved
2 spring onions, green parts only, chopped
Lime wedges to serve

STEPS

1. Heat oil in a large saucepan over medium-high heat. Add onion and cook for 5 minutes, stirring, until soft and golden. Add ginger, garlic and chilli and cook for a further 1 minute.
2. Add cumin, curry powder and salt and cook for 1 minute.
3. Stir in water and lentils and bring the mixture to a boil. Reduce to a simmer and cook uncovered for 15 minutes, allowing most of the moisture to evaporate.
4. Add cinnamon and simmer covered for 5 more minutes until the lentils are tender.
5. Toss with cherry tomatoes and scatter with spring onion tops. Squeeze over lime wedges to serve.

SERVES 2 | PREP + COOK TIME: 40 MINS | VEG | GLUTEN FREE | DAIRY FREE |

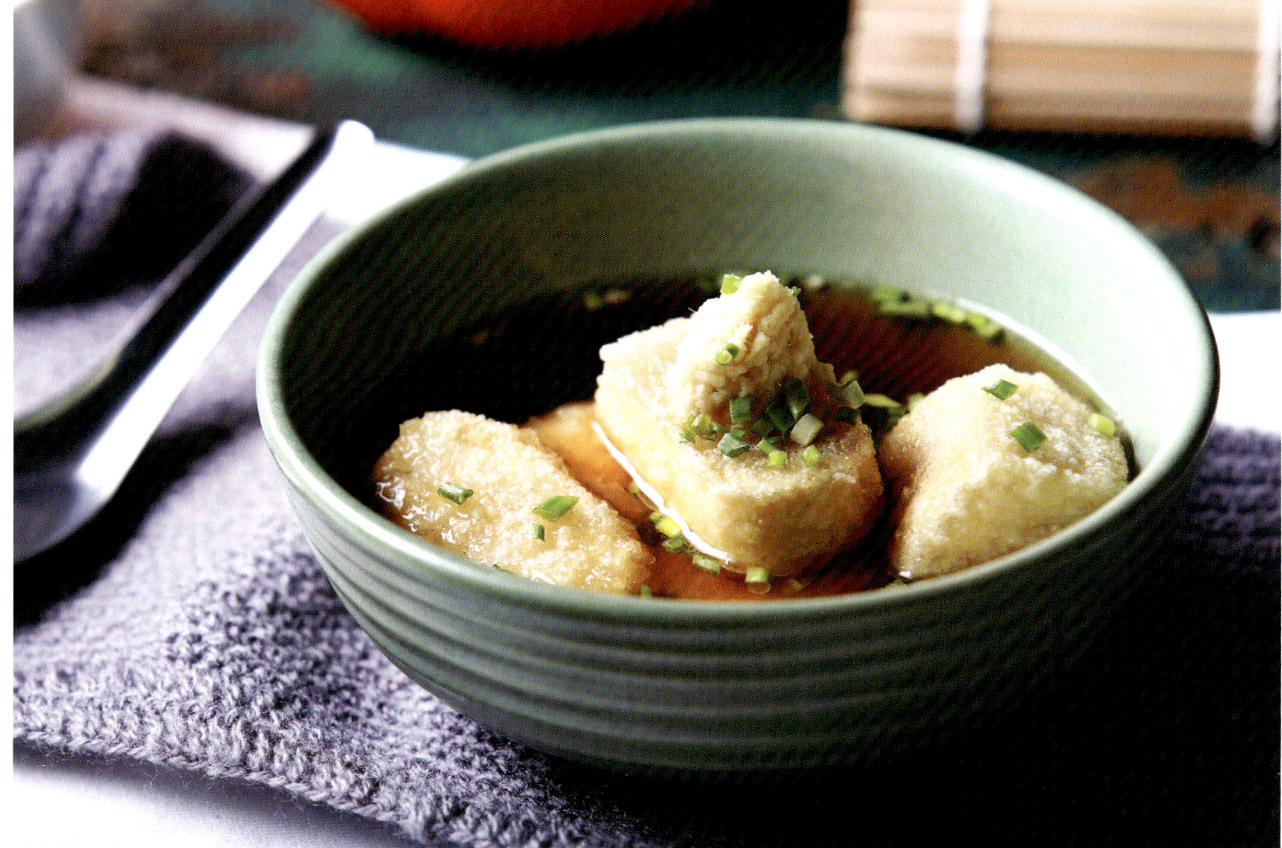

AGEDASHI TOFU

400g silken tofu
4 tbsps potato starch
Vegetable oil for deep-frying
1 spring onion, finely chopped

SAUCE
1 cup (250ml) kombu dashi
2 tbsps tamari (or soy sauce)
2 tbsps mirin

STEPS

1. Wrap the tofu in three or four layers of paper towel and place on a plate. Place another flat plate on top of the tofu and leave for 15 minutes. Drain off any excess liquid and discard paper towels.
2. Cut tofu into eight pieces and roll in potato starch to coat well.
3. Put kombu dashi, tamari and mirin in a saucepan and bring to a boil. Turn off heat and set aside.
4. Heat 5cm oil in a large, heavy-bottomed pan. When hot deep-fry tofu until light brown and crispy. Remove the tofu and drain on a plate lined with paper towels.
5. To serve, place tofu in two bowls. Pour the sauce around the tofu. Scatter with spring onion.

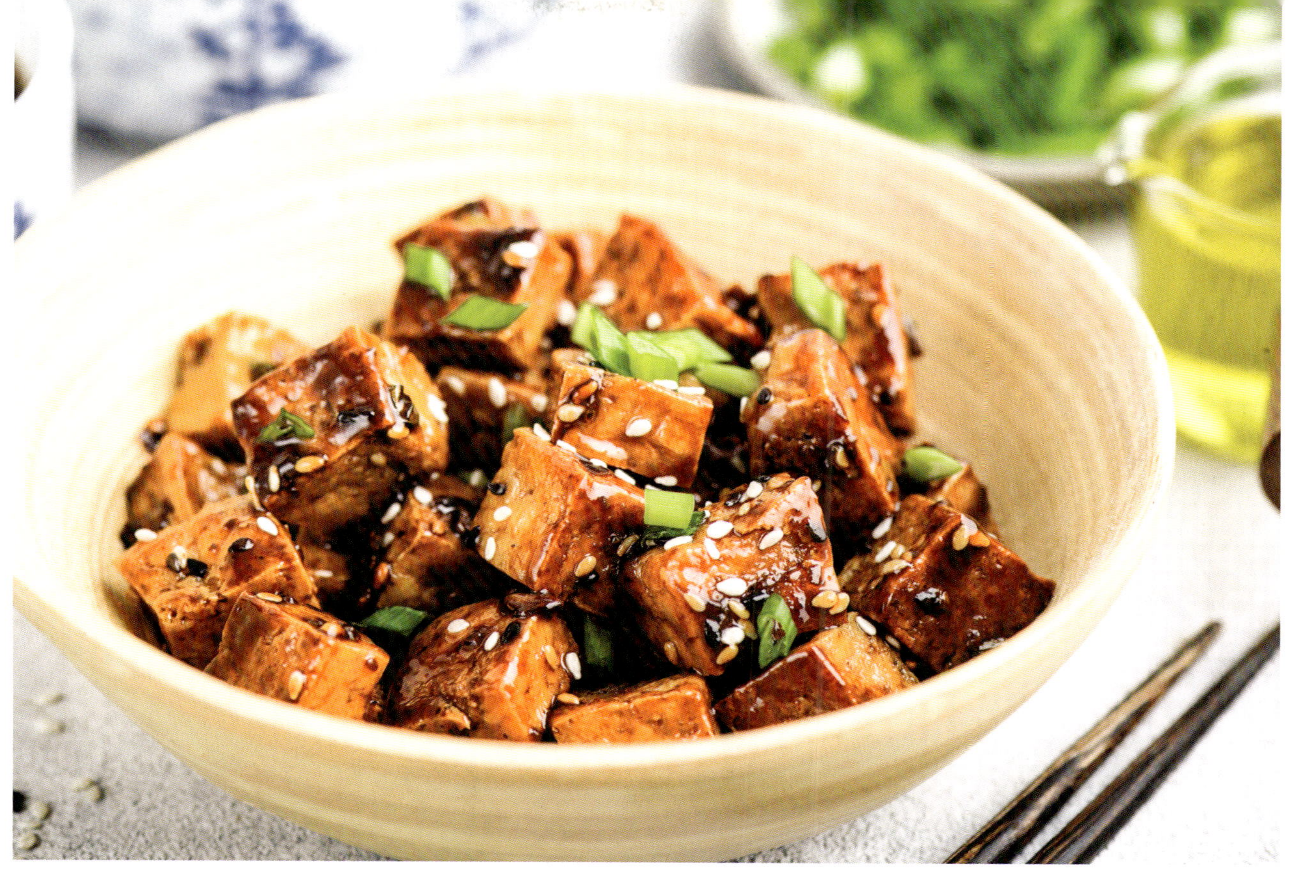

CHILLI-SOY-GLAZED TOFU

350g firm tofu, diced
⅓ cup (80ml) water
3 tbsps tamari
1 tbsp apple cider vinegar
1 tbsp maple syrup
1 clove garlic, minced
Pinch of cayenne pepper
½ tsp chilli flakes
1 tbsp neutral-flavoured oil
2 tsps tapioca flour
1 spring onion, chopped, to garnish
1 tbsp sesame seeds, to garnish

STEPS

1. Mix tofu, water, tamari, vinegar, syrup, garlic, cayenne and chilli flakes in a large bowl until well combined. Refrigerate, covered, for 30 minutes. Strain the tofu, retaining the liquid.
2. Heat oil in a frying pan over medium-high heat. Add tofu and saute for 5 minutes. Mix the tapioca flour into the remaining marinade. Pour the sauce into the frying pan and cook, stirring, for 3 minutes until it thickens.
3. Spoon the tofu into bowls. Top with sauce, spring onions and sesame seeds.

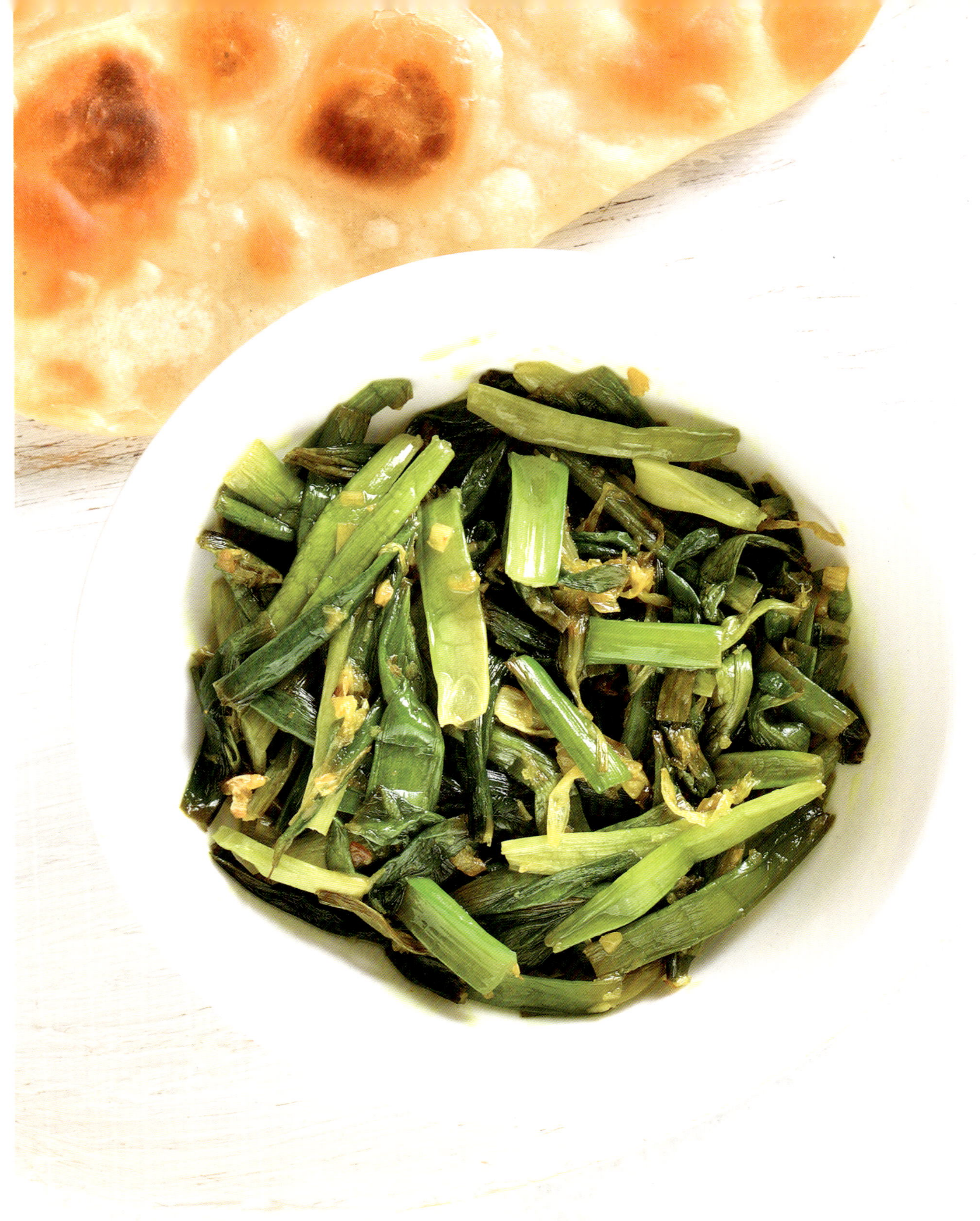

SPRING ONION SABZI

SERVES 4 | PREP + COOK TIME: 15 MINS | VEG | GLUTEN FREE |

3 tbsps ghee

2 pinches asafoetida

8 cloves garlic, finely chopped

2 bunches spring onions, white part finely chopped, green part chopped into 5cm pieces

4 green chillies, finely chopped

Salt to taste

STEPS

1. Heat ghee in a large frying pan, add asafoetida and saute for 30 seconds until it turns light brown. Add garlic and cook for a further 30 seconds until fragrant.
2. Add white part of the spring onion and green chillies and saute for 1 minute.
3. Add green parts of spring onion. Stir-fry for 5 minutes over medium-high heat, then reduce heat to low and season with salt. Cook for a further 5 minutes.
4. Serve with chapatis or rice.

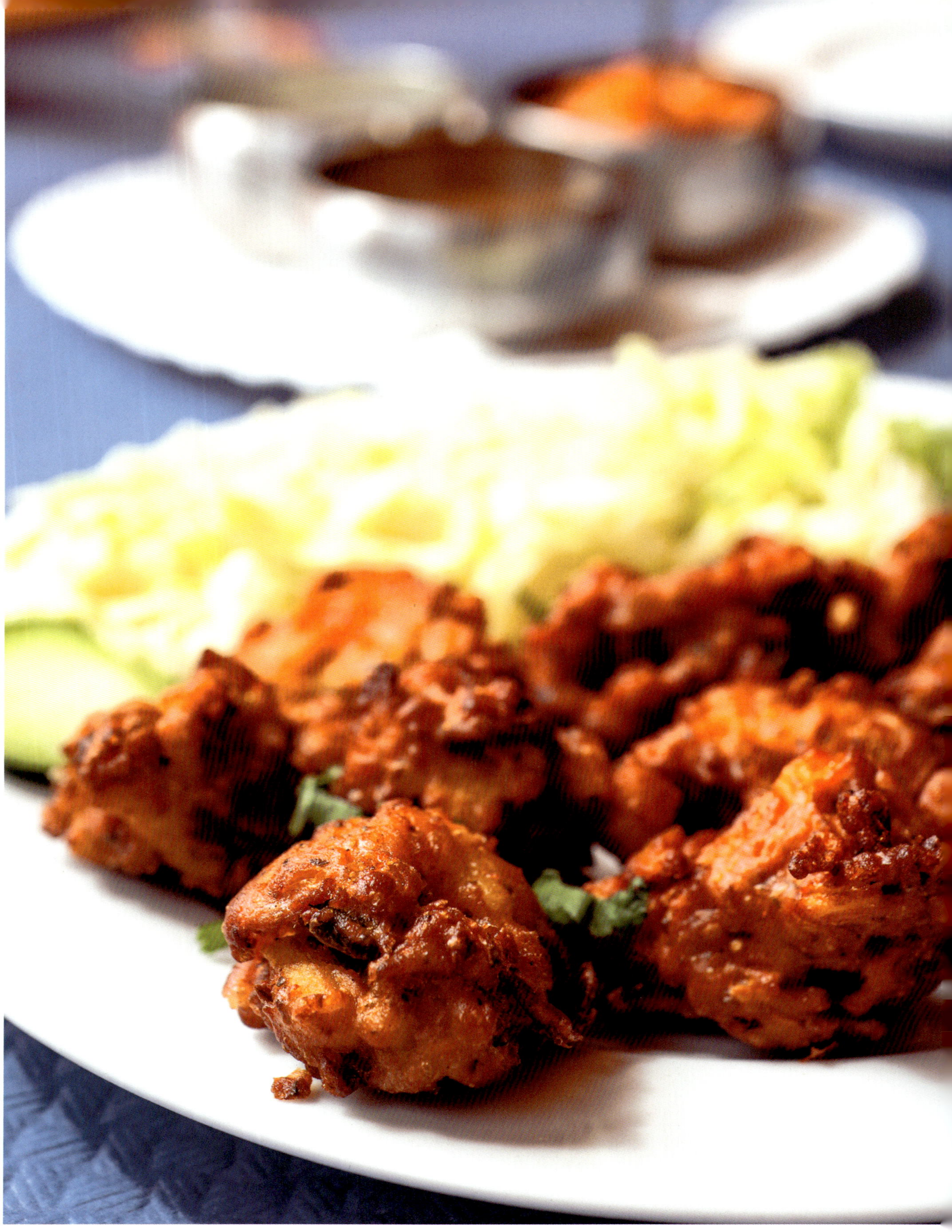

ONION PAKORAS

SERVES 4 | PREP + COOK TIME: 30 MINS | VEG | DAIRY FREE

3 onions, thinly sliced

2 eggs, beaten

¾ cup (90g) plain flour

1 tsp ground coriander

1 tsp ground cumin

½ tsp ground turmeric

Vegetable oil for deep-frying

Salt to taste

Handful of fresh coriander leaves to serve

STEPS

1. Combine onion and egg in a bowl. Stir in flour and spices.
2. Heat 10cm oil in a deep-fryer or large saucepan to 180°C.
3. Carefully drop tablespoons of onion mixture into the oil in batches (the hot oil will spit). Cook for 2 minutes or until golden and crisp, turning occasionally.
4. Remove with a slotted spoon and set aside in a warm place on paper towels. Repeat with remaining mixture.
5. Scatter with salt and fresh coriander leaves. Serve warm.

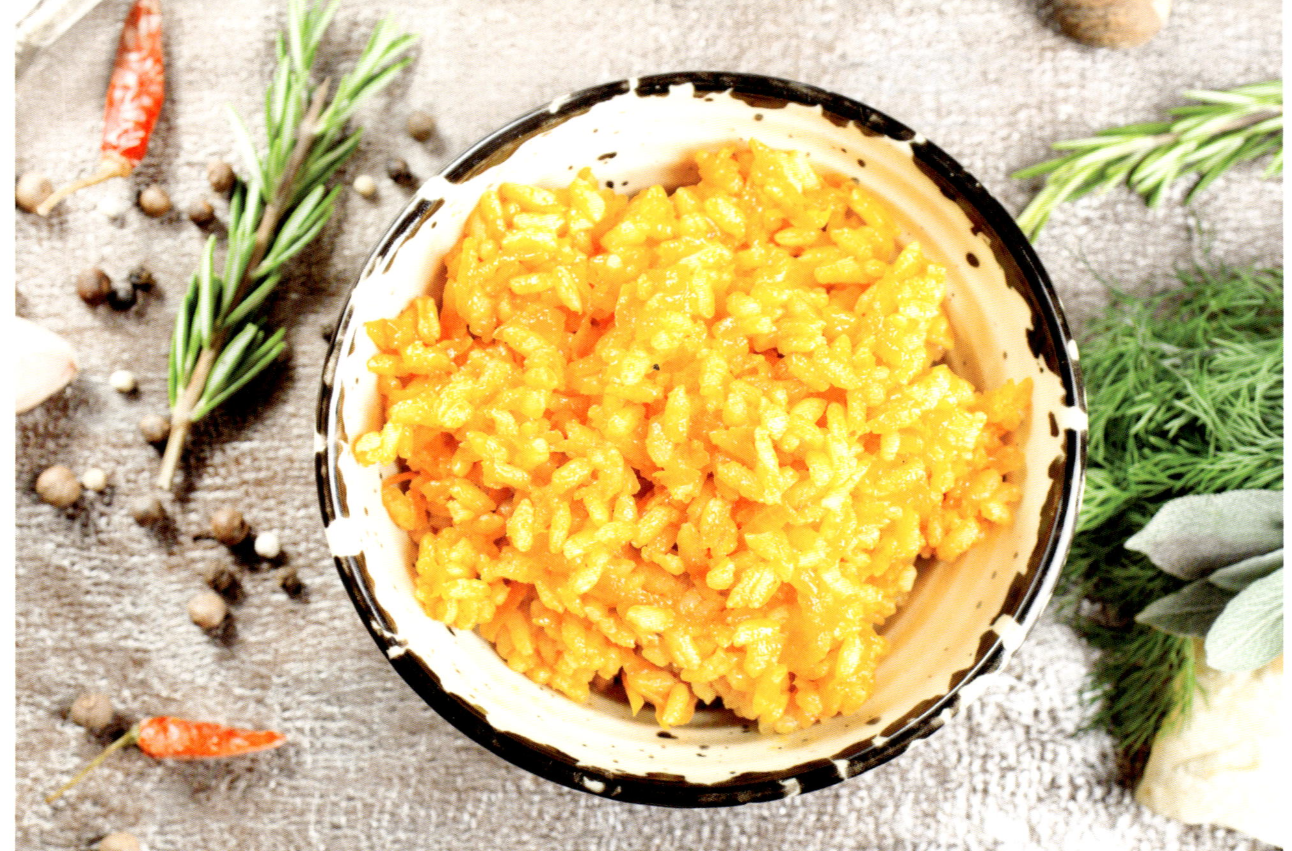

INDIAN SPICED RICE

8 cups (2L) water

2 tsps salt

2 cups (310g) long-grain basmati rice

2 cloves

2 green cardamon pods

1 cinnamon stick

3 tbsps ghee or vegetable oil

¼ tsp dried chilli flakes

1 onion, chopped

½ tsp ground cumin

3 cloves garlic, chopped

¼ tsp ground turmeric

STEPS

1. Bring the water and the salt to a boil in a large pot. Add the rice, cloves, cardamon and cinnamon and simmer for 8-10 minutes until the rice is tender and cooked. Drain rice and discard whole spices.
2. Heat oil in a large frying pan over medium heat. Add chilli flakes and cook for 30 seconds then add onion and cumin. Cook for 5 minutes until onion is soft.
3. Add garlic and cook for 2 minutes, then add rice and sprinkle with turmeric. Continue to cook for 3-4 minutes, stirring regularly.
4. Remove from the heat and serve.

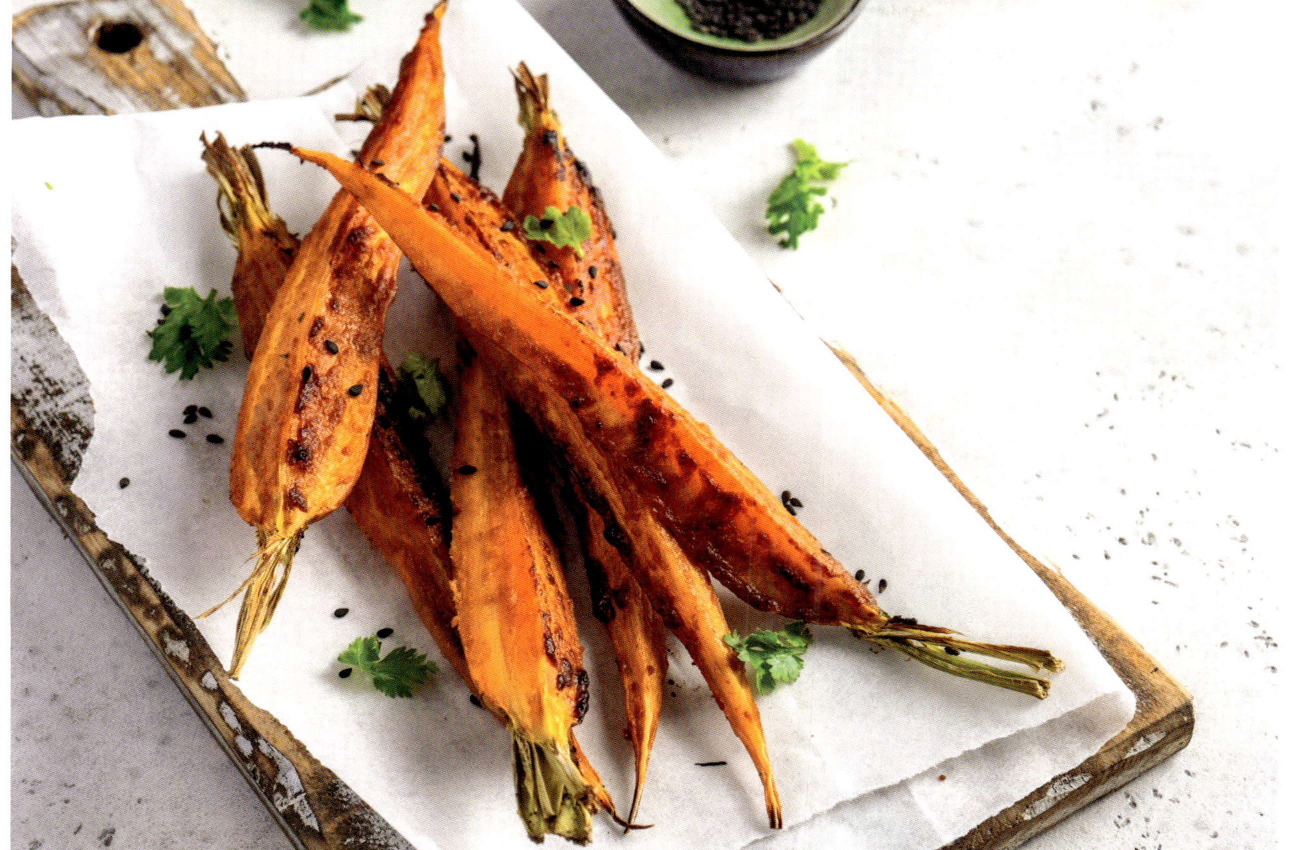

SERVES 4 | PREP + COOK TIME: 35 MINS | VEG | DAIRY FREE |

MISO-GLAZED CARROTS

¼ cup (60ml) olive oil
4 cloves garlic, minced
1 tbsp white miso paste
3 tbsps maple syrup
1kg carrots, cut into quarters lengthwise
Salt and pepper to taste
1 tbsp black sesame seeds
Handful of fresh coriander leaves to serve

STEPS

Preheat oven to 200°C.

1. Heat oil in a large ovenproof frying pan on medium heat. Add garlic, miso paste and maple syrup. Saute for a few seconds until garlic is fragrant.
2. Add carrots and season with salt and pepper. Toss and mix well to coat carrots evenly.
3. Cover with foil and bake in the oven for approximately 20 minutes until carrots are tender and starting to turn golden. Remove foil and bake for a further 5 minutes until carrots start to caramelise.
4. Remove from oven. Sprinkle with sesame seeds and coriander leaves to serve.

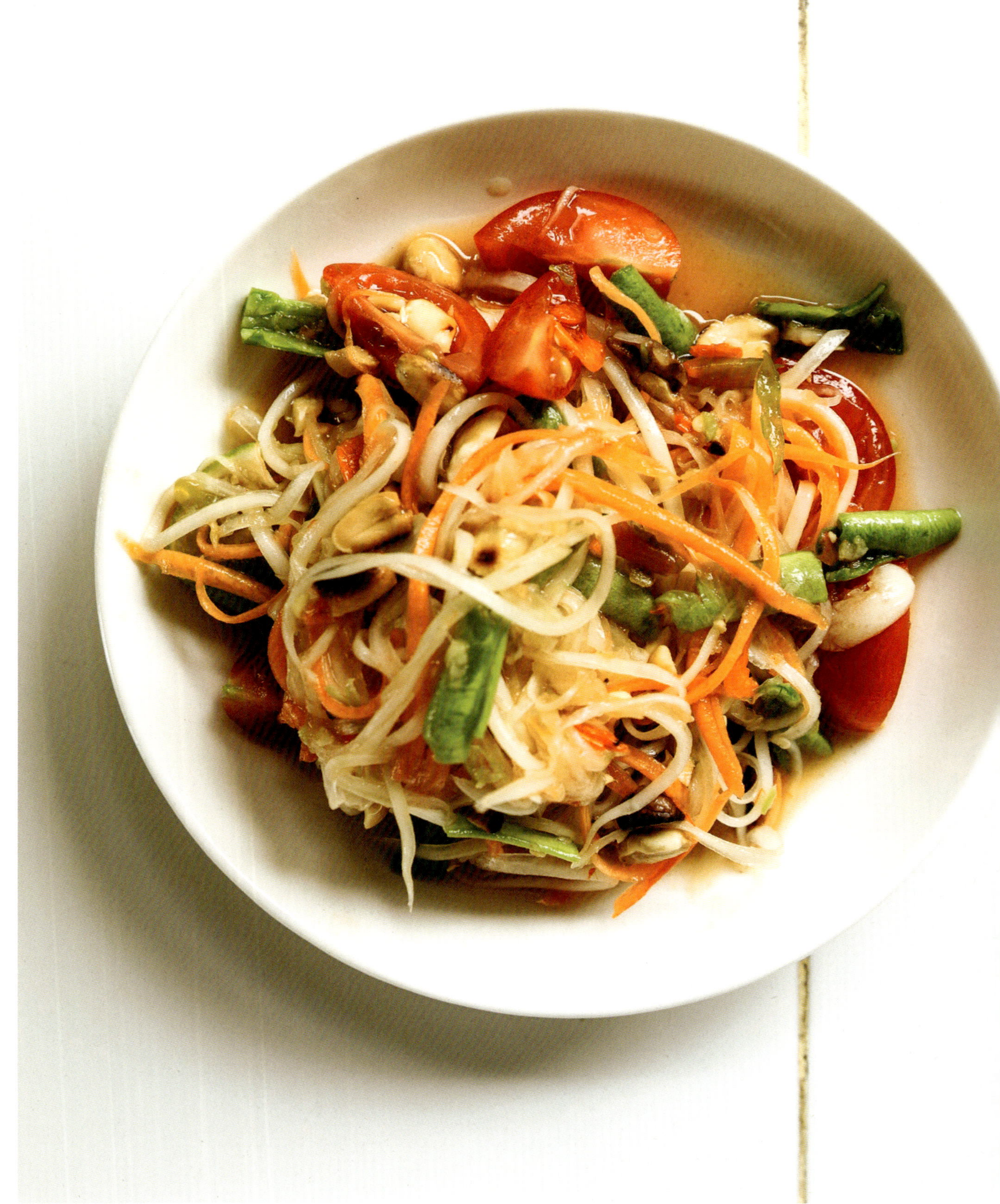

GREEN PAPAYA SALAD

SERVES 4 | PREP + COOK TIME: 20 MINS | GLUTEN FREE | DAIRY FREE |

DRESSING

10 cloves garlic, roughly chopped

6 bird's-eye chillies, roughly chopped

6 tbsps dried shrimp (available in Asian supermarkets)

1 cup (200g) loosely packed grated palm sugar or brown sugar

½ cup (125ml) lime juice

½ cup (125ml) fish sauce

SALAD

20 snake beans or green beans, cut in 5cm pieces

500g green papaya

2 carrots

3 cups (675g) cherry tomatoes, quartered

1 cup (125g) roasted unsalted peanuts, roughly chopped

½ cup (10g) Thai basil leaves

STEPS

1. Place garlic and chilli in a blender and process into a paste. Add dried shrimp and pulse a few times to incorporate. Add sugar, lime juice and fish sauce and pulse to combine. Pour dressing into a large bowl.
2. Add beans to a mortar (in batches if needed), and pound with a pestle to bruise and split. Alternatively bash the beans with a rolling pin. Add beans to dressing.
3. Shred papaya and carrot with a mandoline or vegetable peeler.
4. Add tomatoes, papaya, carrot, peanuts and basil to bowl. Toss well to combine. Serve immediately.

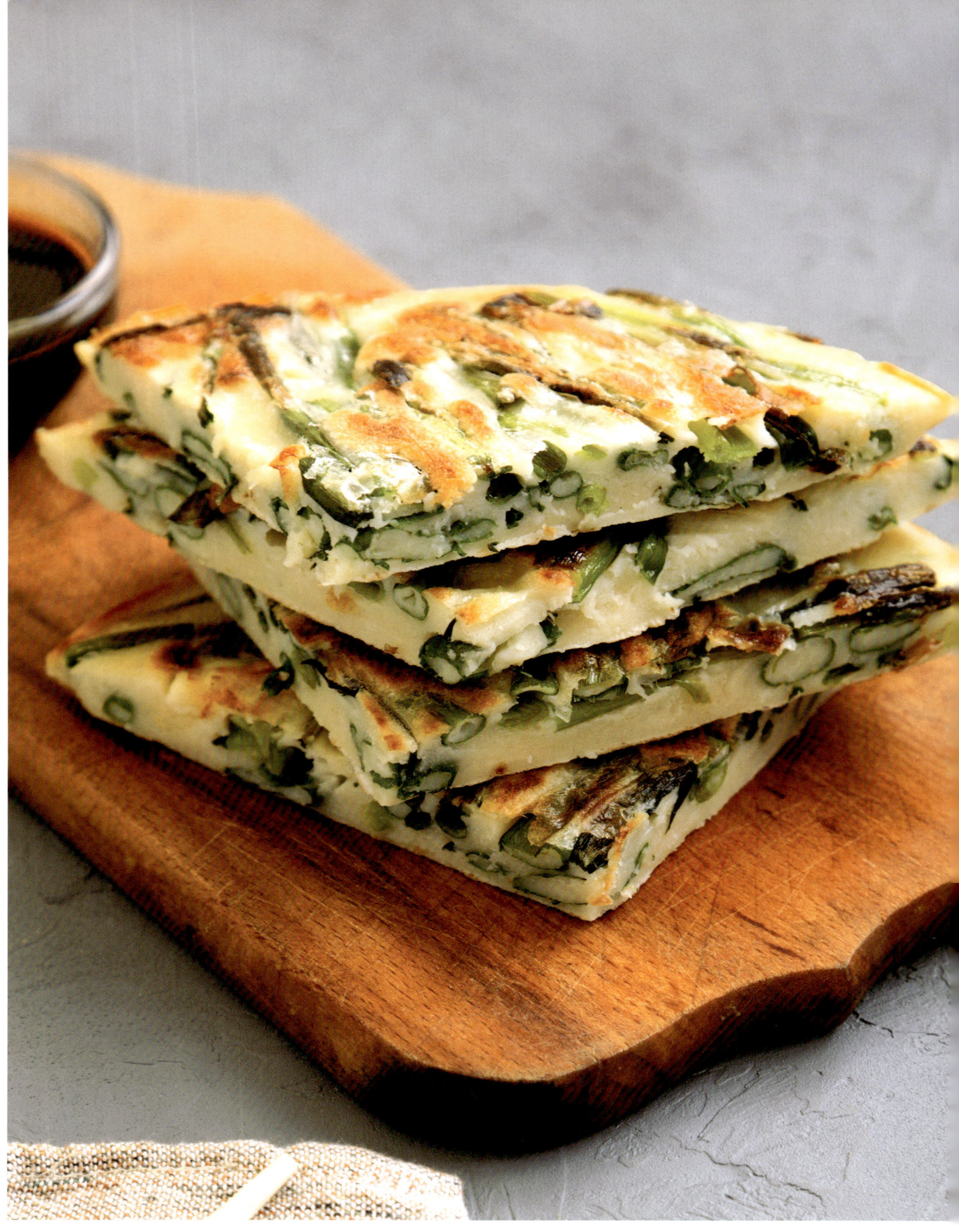

PAJEON (SPRING ONION PANCAKE)

1½ tsps soy bean paste (or miso)

¾ cup (185ml) water

12 medium spring onions, white parts finely chopped, green parts cut into 3cm lengths

⅓ cup (50g) rice flour

½ tsp caster sugar

1 cup (125g) plain flour

Salt and pepper to taste

1½ tbsps vegetable oil

STEPS

1. Whisk together the soy bean paste and 2 tablespoons of the water in a large bowl. Add the white parts of the onions, rice flour, sugar, remaining water, plain flour and a couple of grinds of salt and pepper.
2. Heat the oil in a large nonstick frying pan over medium-high heat. Add the green spring onion sections and fry for 1 minute.
3. Pour the batter mixture over the top. Reduce heat to medium and let the batter cook for 3 minutes until it has mostly set.
4. Gently flip the pancake over and cook for 2 more minutes or until it is golden brown on the bottom and cooked through.
5. Serve cut into wedges.

SERVES 2 | PREP + COOK TIME: 45 MINS | VEG | DAIRY FREE |

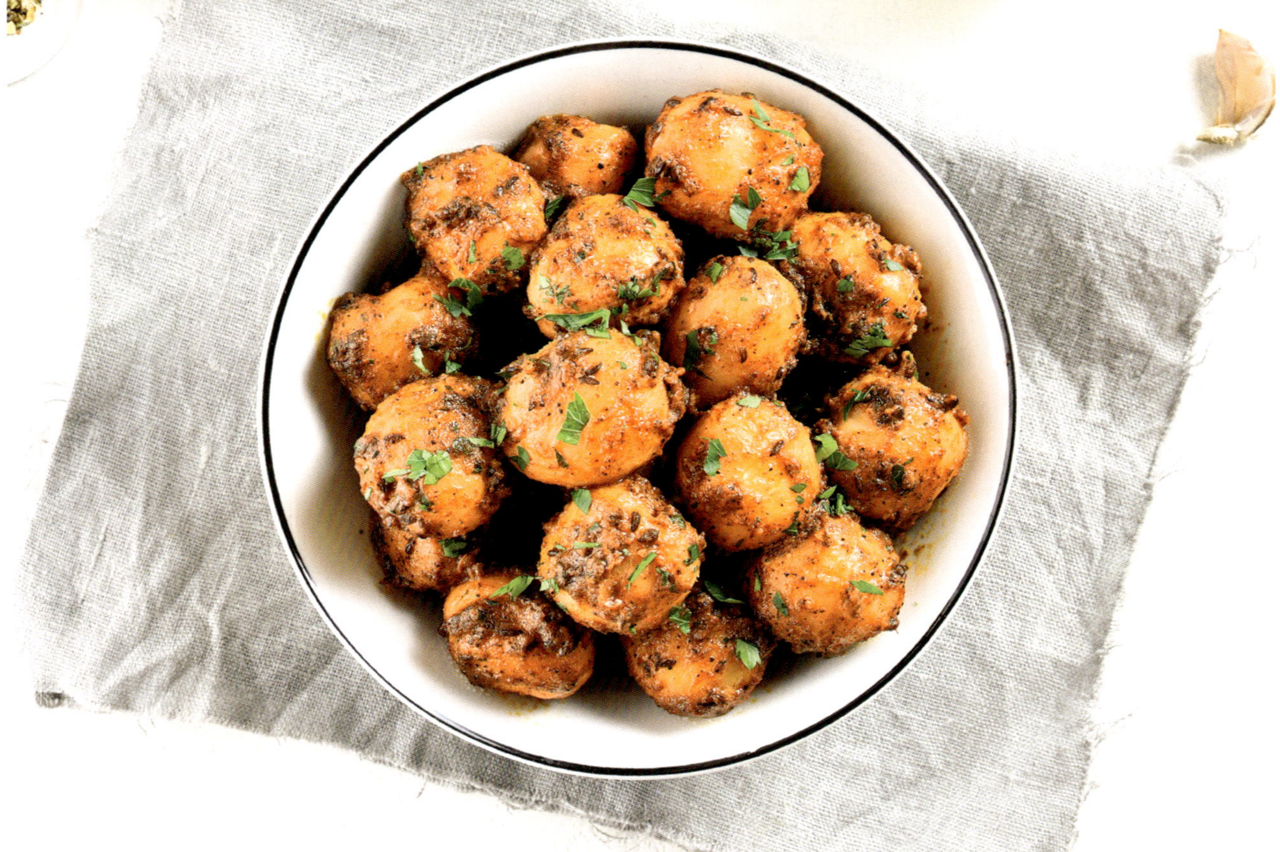

BOMBAY POTATOES

- 1kg small potatoes, peeled
- 1 tsp salt
- 3 tbsps vegetable oil
- 1 tsp mustard seeds
- 2 onions, finely chopped
- 2 bay leaves
- 1 tsp ground turmeric
- 1 tsp chilli powder
- 2 tsps garam masala
- 3 tbsps chopped fresh coriander

STEPS

1. Place the potatoes and salt in a large saucepan of boiling water and cook for 10 minutes. Drain.
2. In a large, deep frying pan or wok, heat oil over medium heat. Add mustard seeds and fry until they start to pop, then add onions and cook for 2 minutes. Add bay leaves, turmeric, chilli powder and garam masala and stir to combine. Add the potatoes to the pan and toss them to coat thoroughly.
3. Stir gently for another 5 minutes, until the potatoes are cooked through. Season to taste and serve sprinkled with fresh coriander.

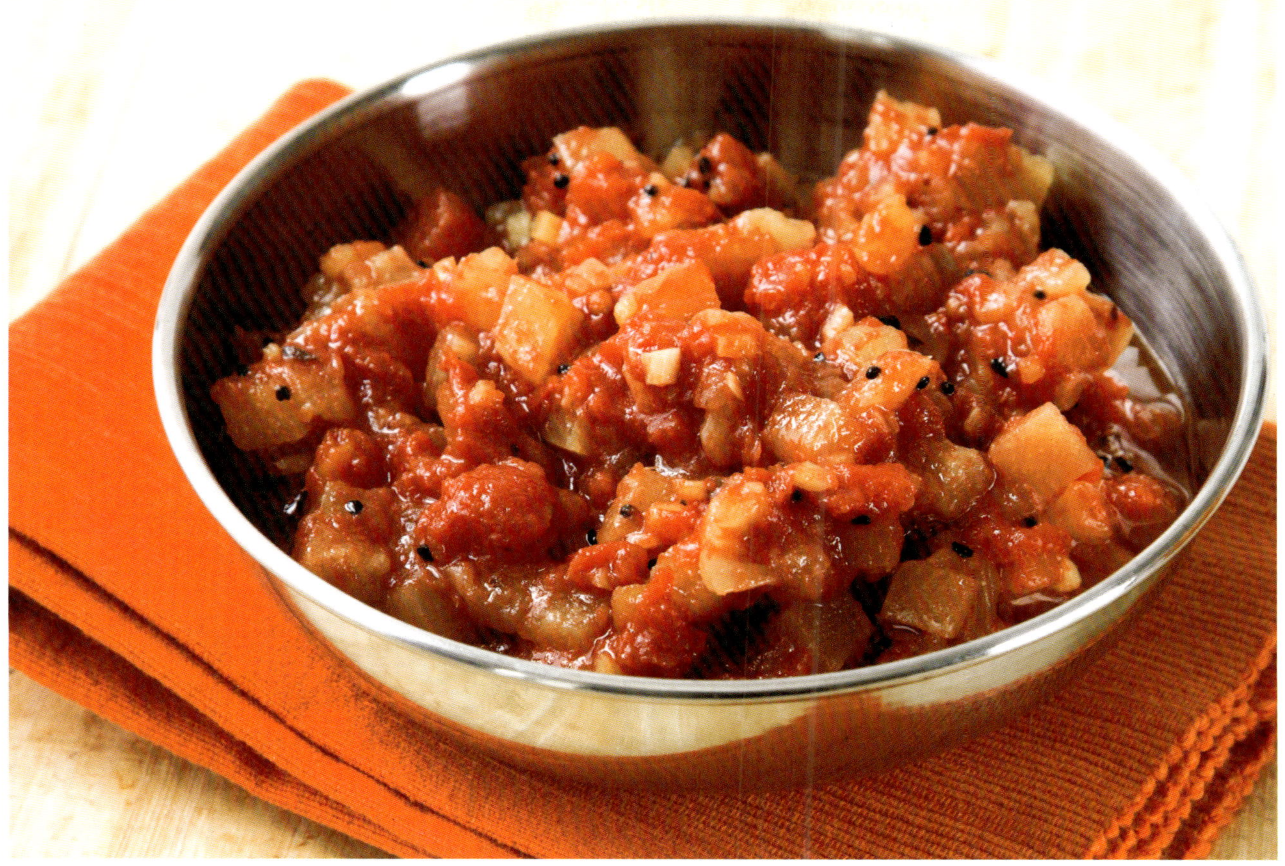

PINEAPPLE CHUTNEY

1 tbsp olive oil

1 tsp brown mustard seeds

1 small red onion, chopped

1 cup (250ml) water

1 cup (225g) diced fresh pineapple

1 clove garlic, finely chopped

8 dates, chopped

⅔ cup (160ml) apple cider vinegar

2 tsps brown sugar

1 tsp salt

½ tsp black peppercorns

¼ tsp ground cardamon

½ tsp chilli flakes

¼ tsp ground coriander

2 tsps sultanas

1 tsp currants

STEPS

1. Heat oil in a saucepan over medium-high heat. Add mustard seeds and cook for 30 seconds until the mustard seeds begin to pop. Add onion and cook for 3-5 minutes until soft and translucent. Reduce heat to low.

2. Add water, pineapple, garlic and dates and cook for 20 minutes until water is absorbed. Add vinegar, sugar, salt, peppercorns, cardamon, chilli flakes and coriander.

3. Cook, covered, for 1 hour until thick and dark. Stir in the sultanas and currants. To store, pour into dry, clean jars and seal.

MAKES 1.5 CUPS | PREP + COOK TIME: 1 HOUR 30 MINS | VEG | GLUTEN FREE | DAIRY FREE |

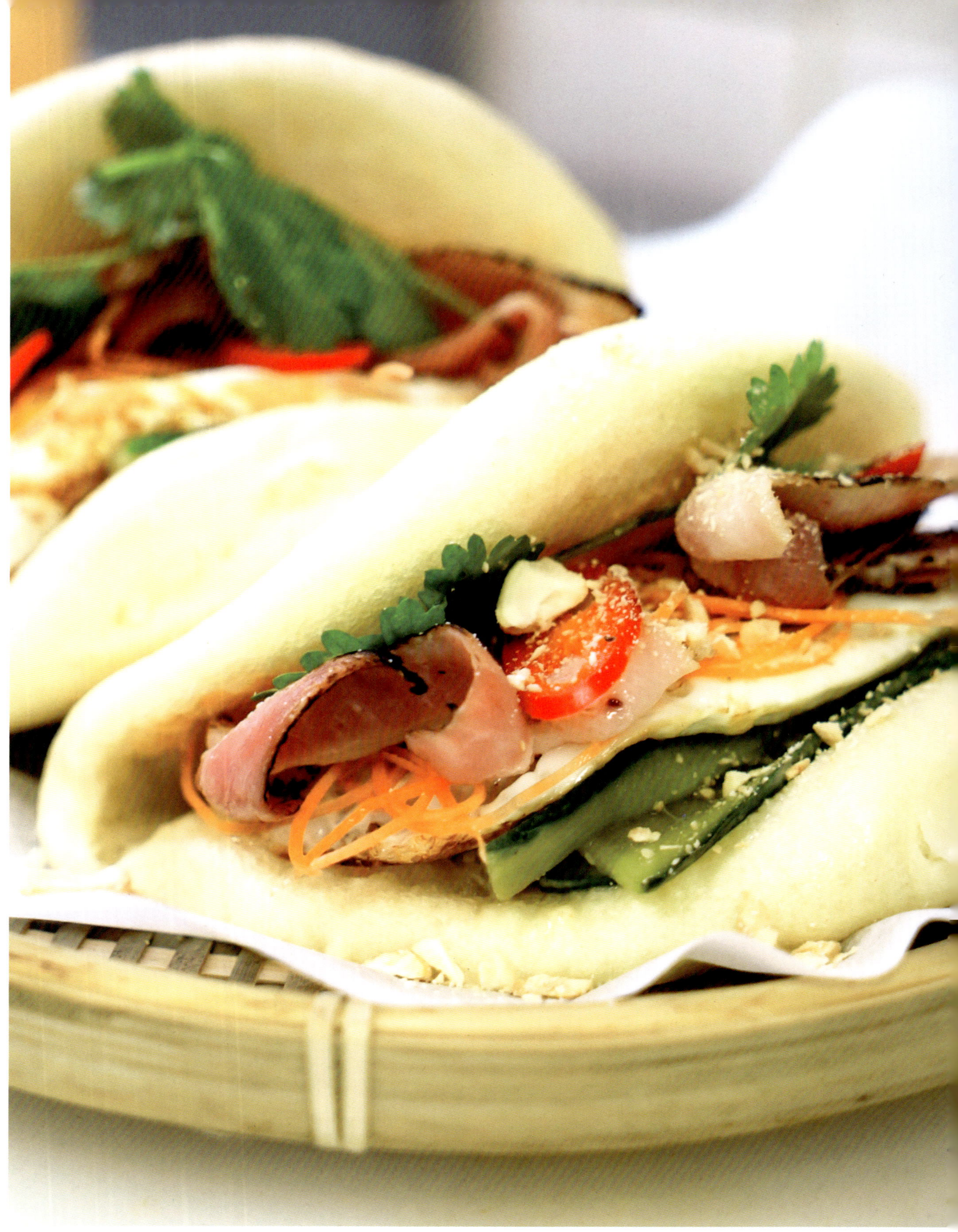

EGG & BACON BAO

8 rashers bacon

2 tbsps oil + more as needed

8 eggs

8 bao buns

¼ cup (60ml) hoisin sauce, or to taste

1 carrot, shredded

1 Lebanese cucumber, cut into ribbons with a vegetable peeler

1 cup (15g) coriander leaves

1 red chilli, sliced

80g goat's cheese, crumbled

STEPS

1. Place the bacon under a hot grill and cook for 2-3 minutes on each side until cooked to your liking.

2. Heat 1 tablespoon oil in a large frying pan over medium-high heat. Crack the eggs a few at a time into the pan and cook for 3-4 minutes until the white is cooked through and the yolk is still soft. Using a spatula transfer cooked eggs to a plate and keep warm while you cook the remaining eggs. Add more oil as needed.

3. Steam the bao buns in a steamer basket over a pan of simmering water for 7-8 minutes until piping hot.

4. Open the bao buns and spread with hoisin sauce. Fill with shredded carrot, cucumber, bacon, egg, coriander leaves and sliced chilli. Crumble over goat's cheese to serve.

SABUDANA VADA (TAPIOCA FRITTERS)

1 cup (150g) sago or tapioca pearls
2 potatoes, boiled and mashed
½ cup (60g) peanuts, roasted and crushed
1 tsp grated ginger
1 tsp ground cumin
1 green chilli, finely chopped
2 tbsps coriander leaves, finely chopped
1 tsp lemon juice
½ tsp salt
Oil for frying
Lime wedges to serve

STEPS

1. Soak tapioca or sago in a large bowl of water for 3 hours until soft. Then strain in a fine mesh sieve and allow to sit in the sieve, draining, for 30 minutes.
2. Transfer to a large bowl. Add potato and peanuts, ginger, cumin, chilli, coriander, lemon juice and salt. Mix and mash well with your hands. Shape into small patties.
3. Heat 5cm oil in a large, wide frying pan over medium heat to 180°C (it's ready if the oil sizzles when a small amount of batter is dropped in).
4. Cook the patties in batches for 4-5 minutes, turning with a slotted spoon, until golden brown on both sides.
5. Remove from the pan with a slotted spoon and drain on a plate lined with paper towel before serving, hot, with lime wedges.

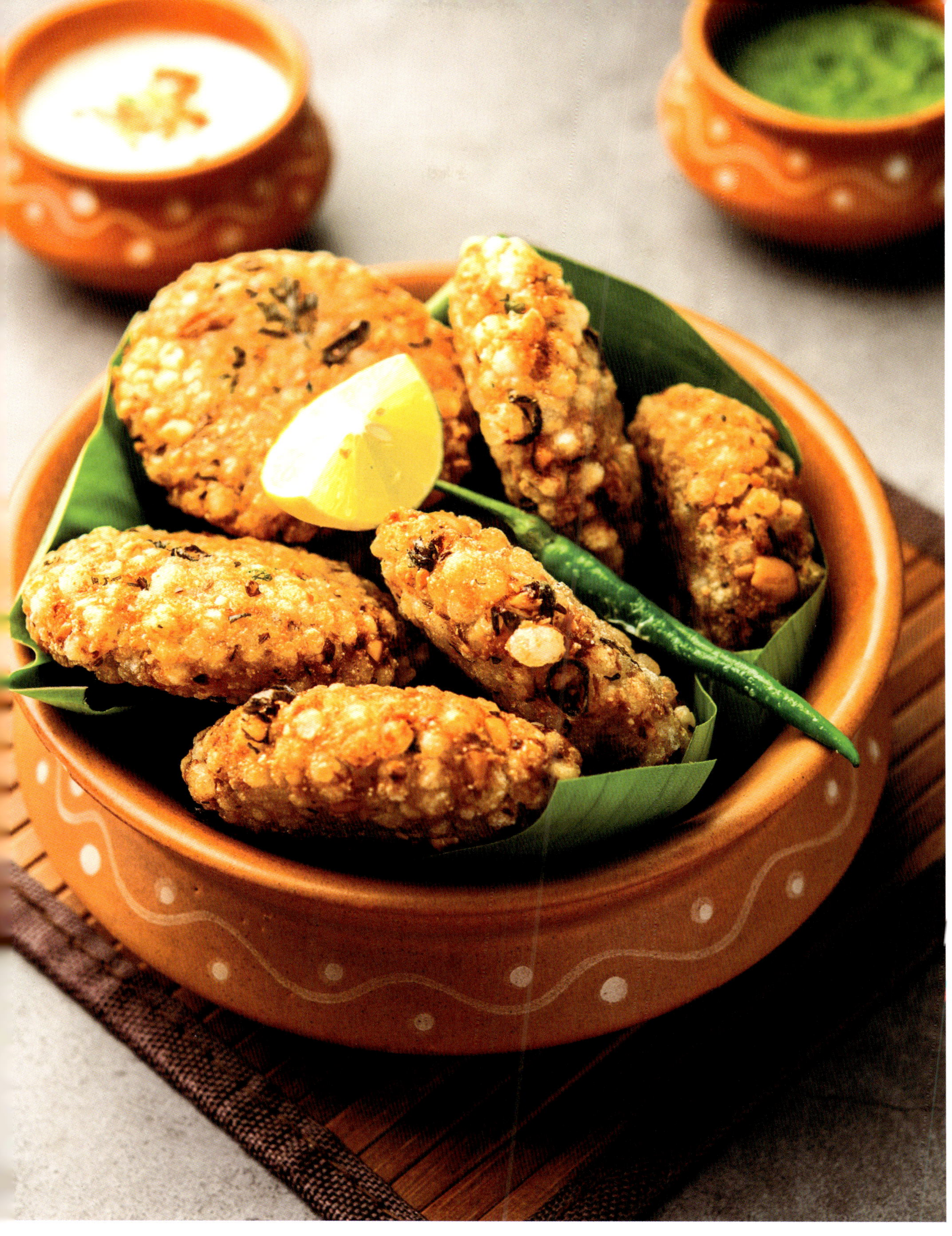

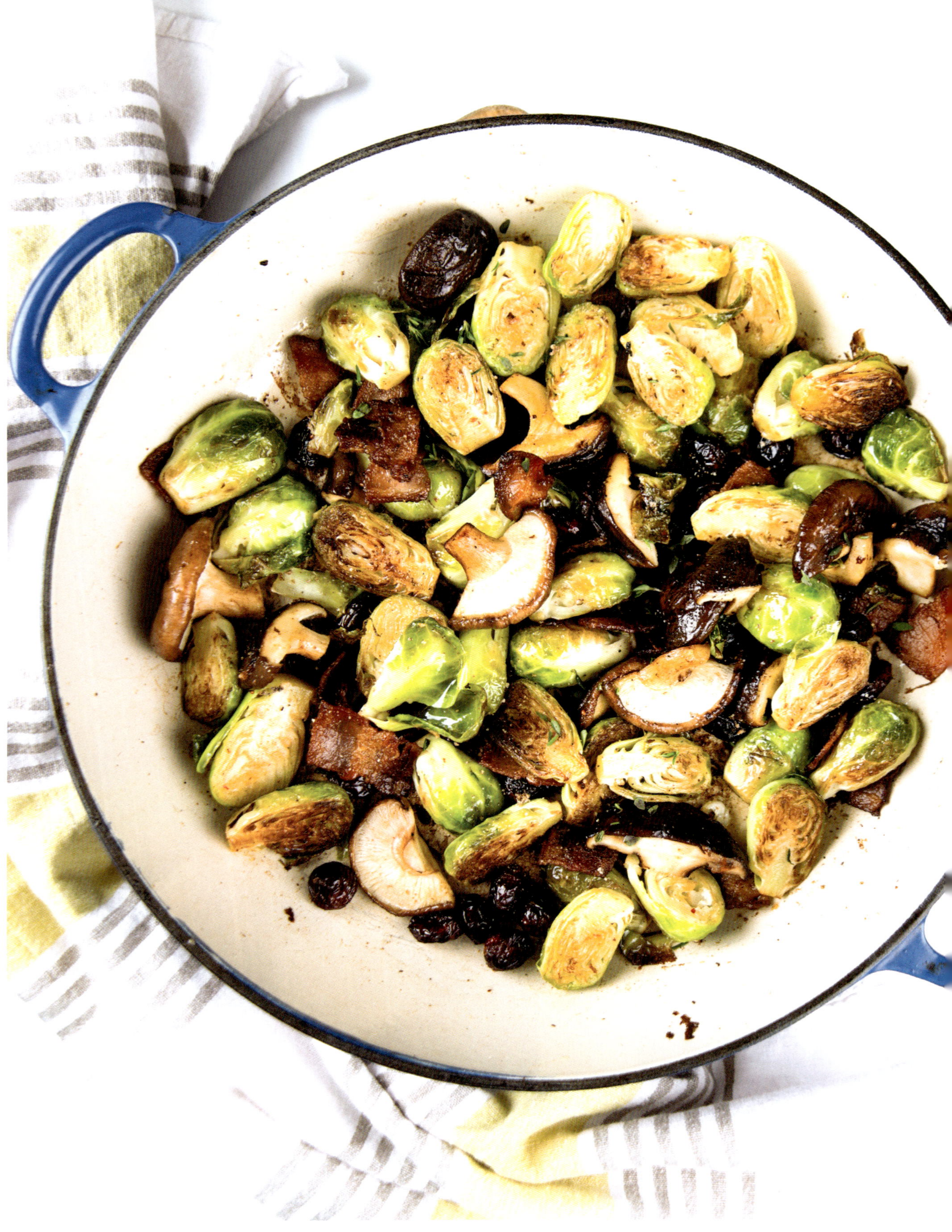

SHIITAKE MUSHROOM & SPROUTS

500g Brussels sprouts
2 tbsps olive oil
200g bacon (optional)
500g shiitake mushrooms, sliced
½ cup (125ml) vegetable stock
2 tbsps soy sauce
2 tsps balsamic vinegar
1 tsp Dijon mustard
¼ cup (30g) dried cranberries
Salt and pepper to taste

STEPS

1. Wash the Brussels sprouts. Trim the ends and remove any discoloured leaves and cut in half lengthways.

2. Heat 1 tablespoon oil in a large frying pan over medium-high heat. Add the bacon and fry for 4 minutes, until the bacon begins to crisp. Omit this step if not using the bacon.

3. Add the rest of the oil and then the Brussels sprouts. Cook for 5 minutes until the sprouts begin to brown. Add the mushrooms and fry for 1 minute.

4. Pour in the stock, soy sauce, vinegar and mustard. Cook until most of the liquid has evaporated, then remove from heat.

5. To serve, stir through the cranberries and season to taste.

SERVES 4 | PREP + COOK TIME: 25 MINS | DAIRY FREE |

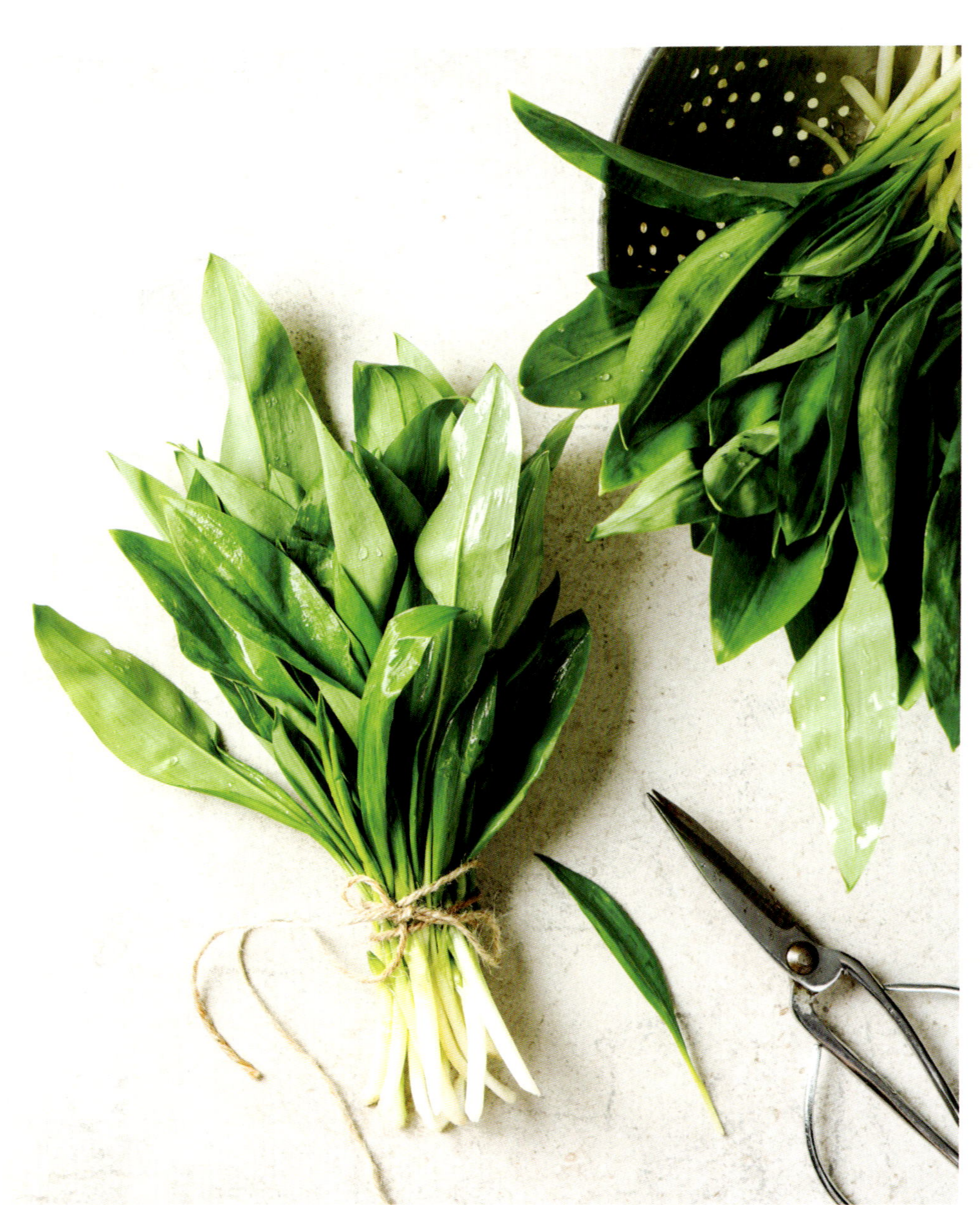

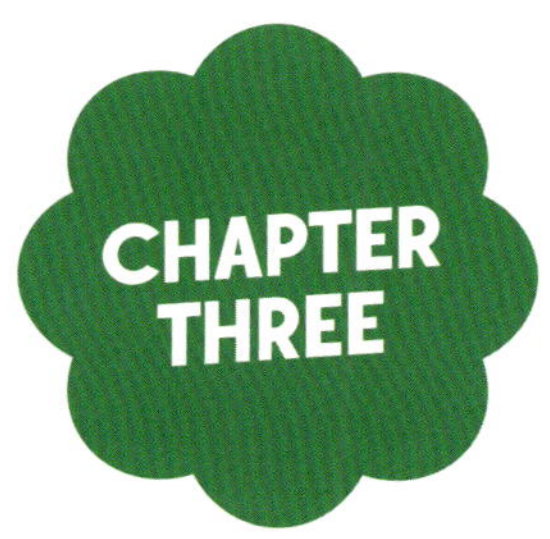

EVERYDAY DINNERS

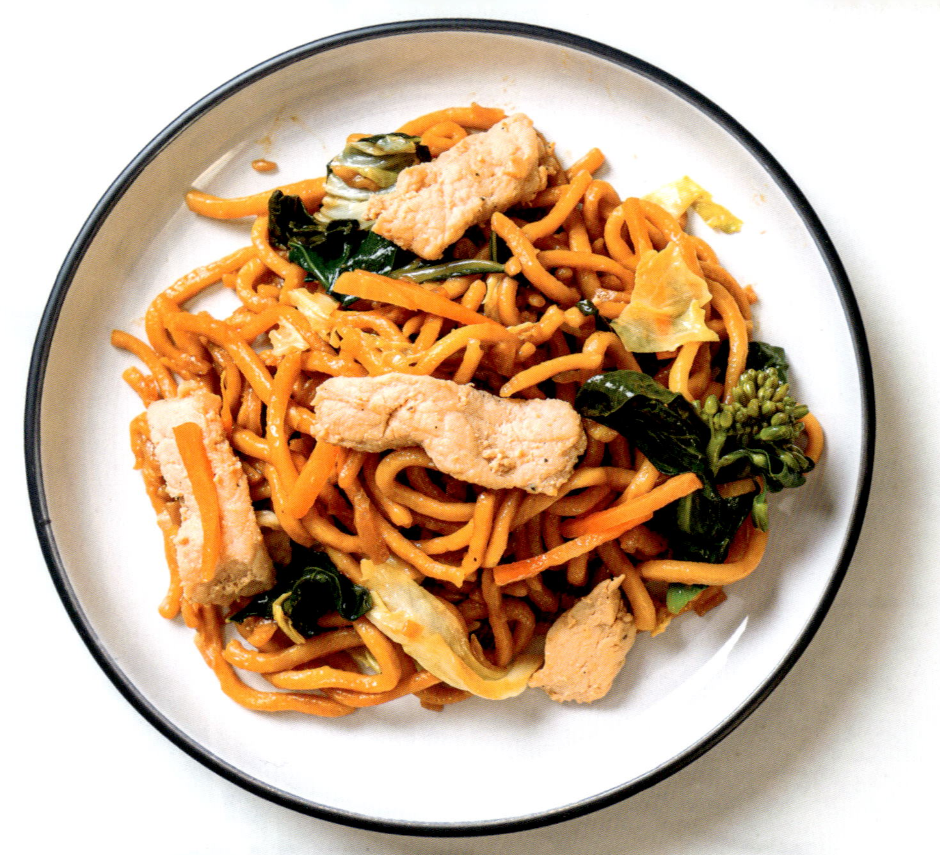

JAPANESE CHICKEN STIR-FRY

450g Hokkien noodles
2 tbsps sesame oil
1 clove garlic, minced
1 tbsp ginger, minced
350g chicken breast, sliced
2 carrots, julienned
Small bunch broccolini, stems trimmed
¼ green cabbage, roughly chopped

SAUCE

¼ cup (60ml) tamari
2 tbsps Worcestershire sauce
1½ tbsps Japanese rice wine vinegar
1 tbsp mirin
1 tsp tomato paste
3 tsps brown sugar
1 tbsp oyster sauce

STEPS

1. Cook noodles according to packet directions. Drain and set aside.
2. In a wok, heat the sesame oil over medium-high heat. Stir-fry the garlic and ginger for 1 minute. Add the chicken and cook for 4 minutes, until browned. Set chicken aside.
3. Add the vegetables to the wok and cook for 3-4 minutes until just softened. Return the chicken to the wok with all the sauce ingredients.
4. Stir-fry for 4 minutes then add the noodles and toss to combine. Cook gently on low heat for 2 minutes. Serve immediately.

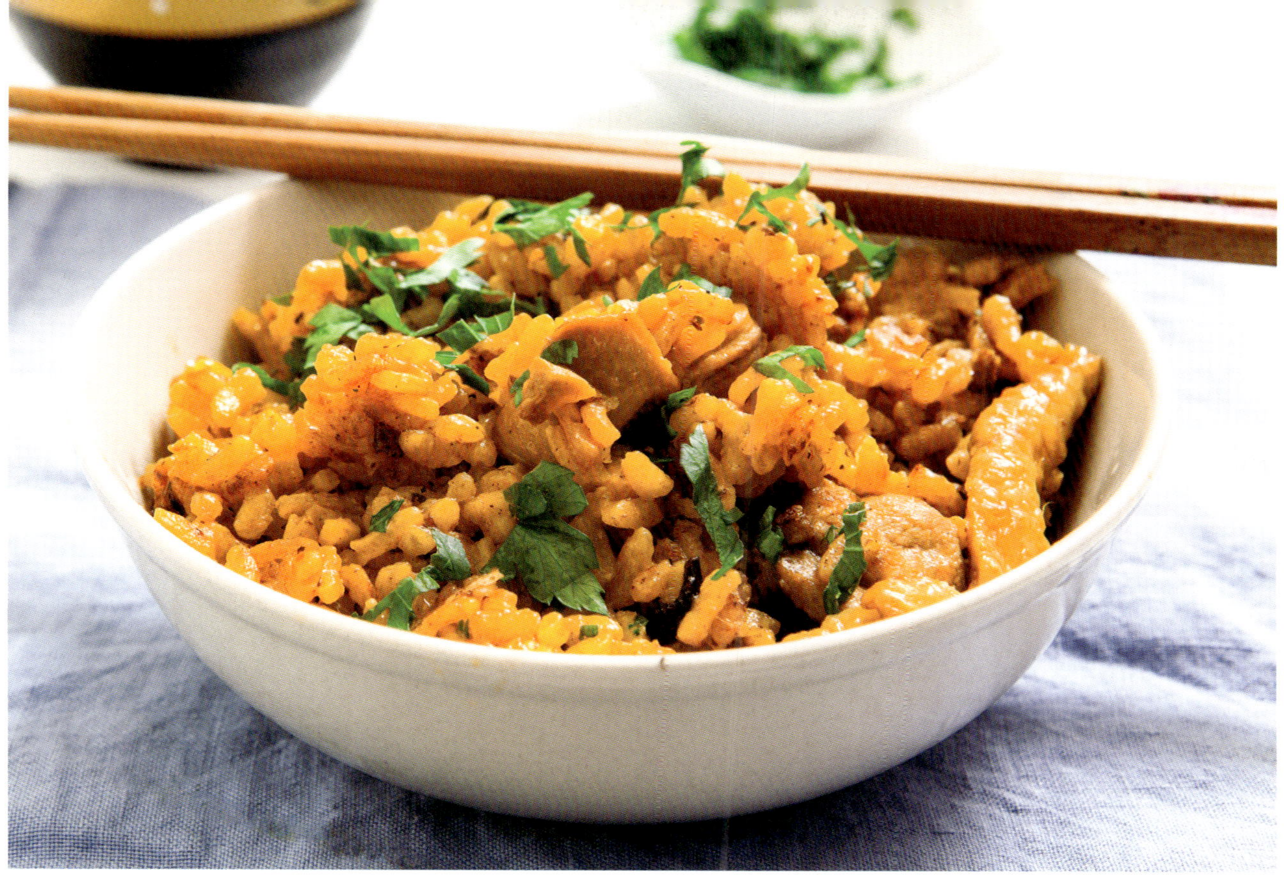

SERVES 4 | PREP + COOK TIME: 45 MINS | GLUTEN FREE |

CHICKEN BIRYANI

25g butter or ghee

1 onion, finely sliced

1 bay leaf

3 cardamon pods

1 cinnamon stick

1 tsp ground turmeric

4 skinless chicken breasts, cut into bite-size pieces

2 cups (300g) basmati rice, rinsed

3½ cups (875ml) chicken stock

2 tbsps chopped coriander

STEPS

1. Heat the butter or ghee in a saucepan and fry the onion with the bay leaf and other whole spices for 10 minutes. Sprinkle in the turmeric, then add chicken and pan-fry until aromatic.
2. Add the rice to the pan and stir for 1 minute before pouring in the stock. Cover and bring to a boil. Reduce heat to low and cook for another 5 minutes.
3. Remove from the heat and leave to stand with the lid on for 10 minutes.
4. Scatter over coriander to serve.

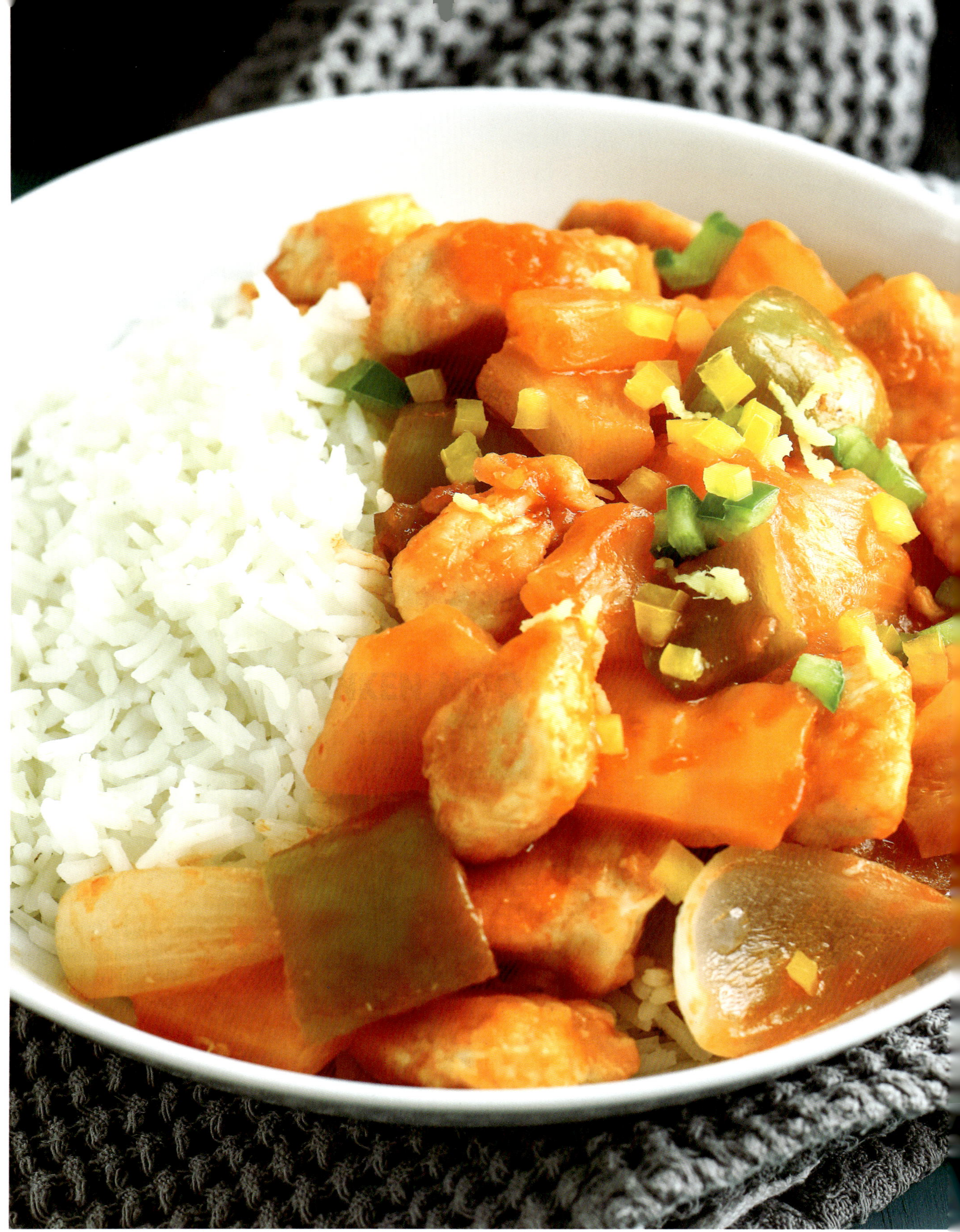

SWEET & SOUR CHICKEN

1½ cups (235g) rice

3 cups (750ml) water

2 tbsps peanut oil

700g chicken fillets, cut into bite-size strips

2 tsps cornflour

1 onion, thickly sliced

Small piece ginger, grated

1 red capsicum, cut into 2cm pieces

1 green capsicum, cut into 2cm pieces

1 yellow capsicum, cut into 2cm pieces

1 long red chilli, sliced

1 x 225g can diced pineapple in juice, drained, juice reserved

¼ cup (60ml) apple cider vinegar

¼ cup (60g) tomato ketchup

3 tbsps light brown sugar

2 tsps light soy sauce

TO SERVE

2 tbsps finely chopped green and yellow capsicum

1 tsp grated ginger

STEPS

1. Combine the rice with the water in a large saucepan over a medium-high heat and bring to the boil. Cover the pan and reduce the heat to low. Cook for 20 minutes, then remove from the heat and let the pan stand for a further 5 minutes.
2. Heat half the oil in a wok or frying pan over high heat. Toss chicken in cornflour then add to the pan and stir-fry for 2 minutes to brown. Remove from pan and set aside.
3. Reduce heat to medium and add remaining oil. Add onion; stir-fry for 3 minutes. Add ginger, capsicums and chilli; stir-fry for 2 minutes.
4. In a small bowl stir together pineapple juice, vinegar, ketchup, sugar and soy sauce. Add to wok with the pineapple. Bring to a simmer. Return chicken to the pan and simmer for a further 2 minutes until cooked through.
5. Serve over rice and scatter with chopped capsicum and grated ginger, if desired.

SERVES 4 | PREP + COOK TIME 45 MINS | DAIRY FREE |

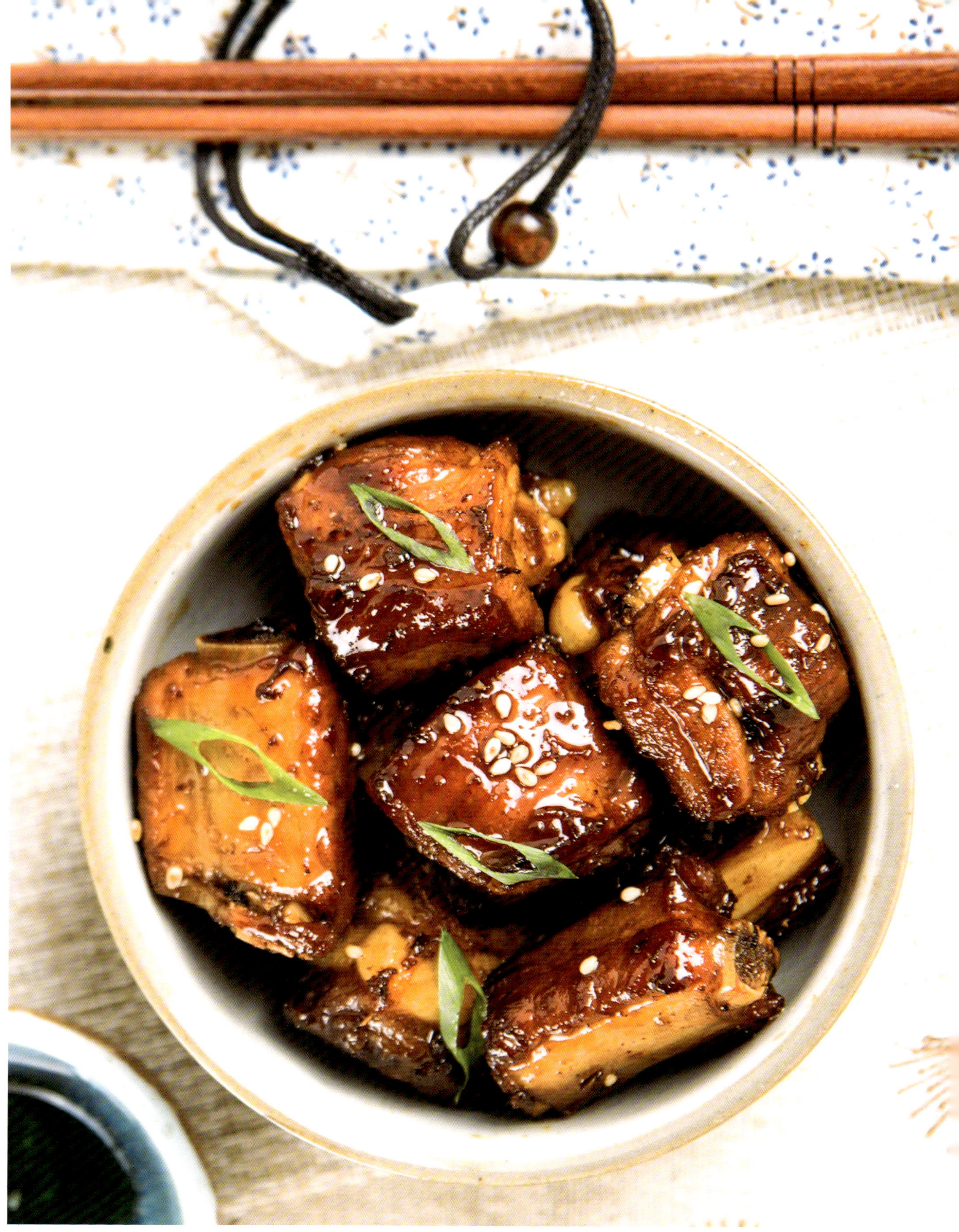

CHINESE SPARE RIBS

⅓ cup (115g) honey
¼ cup (60ml) soy sauce
¼ cup (60ml) tomato ketchup
¼ cup (40g) brown sugar
2 tbsps rice wine vinegar
2 tbsps lemon juice
2 tsps sesame oil
4 cloves garlic, minced
1kg pork ribs
1 tbsp sesame seeds
2 spring onions, chopped

STEPS

1. In a medium-size bowl, mix together honey, soy sauce, tomato ketchup, brown sugar, vinegar, lemon juice, sesame oil and garlic.
2. Pour about two-thirds of the marinade into a shallow baking dish along with the ribs. Toss to coat, then cover and refrigerate for at least 1 hour (or overnight if you can). Reserve the rest of the marinade.
3. Remove the ribs from the fridge 30 minutes prior to cooking. Preheat the oven to 175°C and line a shallow baking dish with foil.
4. Place the ribs in the prepared dish and bake for 45 minutes, basting with the remaining marinade every 20 minutes. Reduce heat to 160°C. Roast for a further 15 minutes.
5. Scatter with sesame seeds and spring onions to serve.

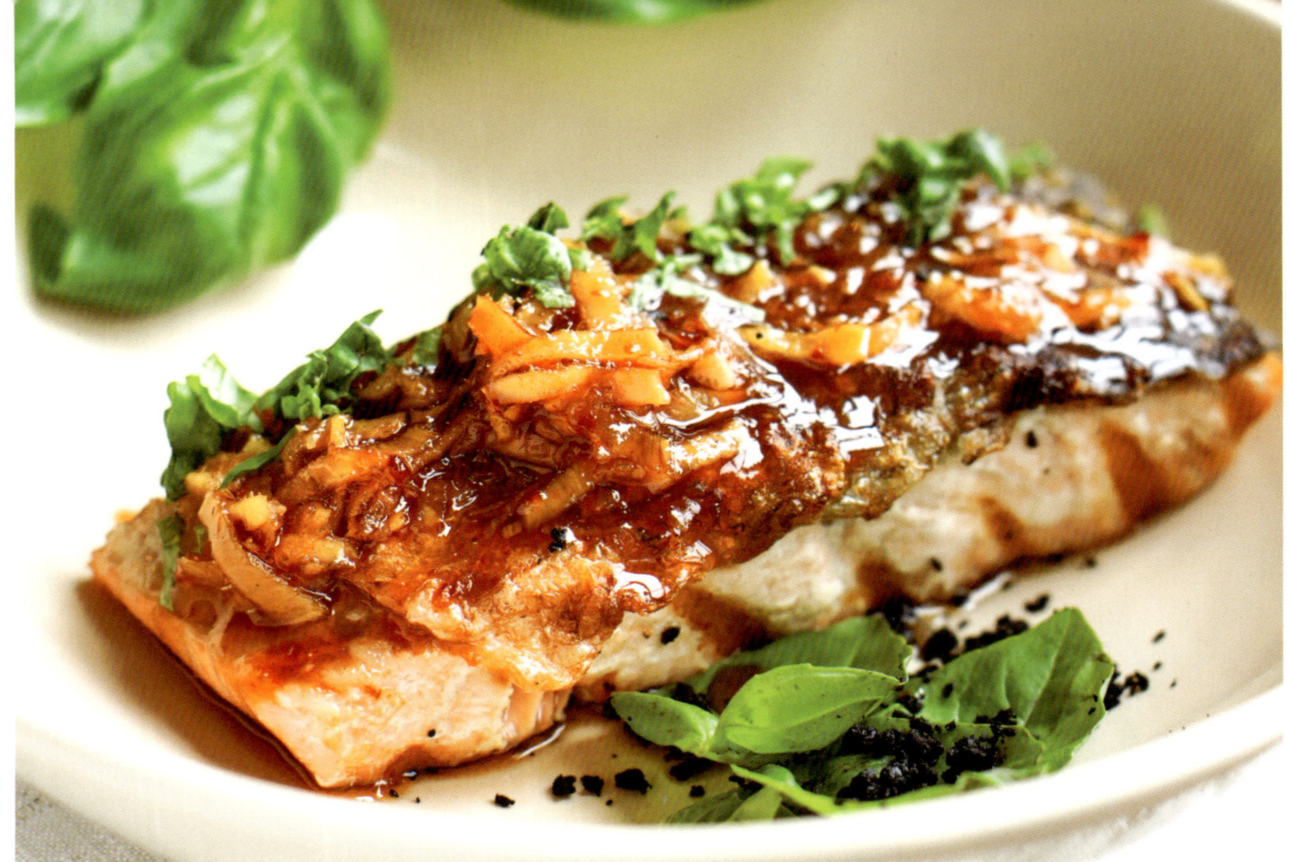

SALMON WITH HONEY GINGER GLAZE

4 tbsps unsalted butter

¼ cup (60ml) soy sauce

2 tbsps honey

1 tsp mirin

Large piece ginger, julienned

2 cloves garlic, minced

¼ chilli, finely chopped (optional)

4 x 175g salmon fillets

Salt and pepper to taste

STEPS

Preheat the oven to 200°C.

1. Melt the butter in a small saucepan over low heat. Add the soy sauce, honey, mirin, ginger, garlic and chilli, if using. Stir to combine and simmer for about 3 minutes. Remove from the heat and set aside to cool for a few minutes.
2. Place the salmon in a lined baking dish and season with salt and pepper.
3. Pour the honey ginger glaze over the salmon, making sure both sides are coated with the glaze.
4. Bake for 10-15 minutes or until the salmon is cooked through and flakes easily with a fork.

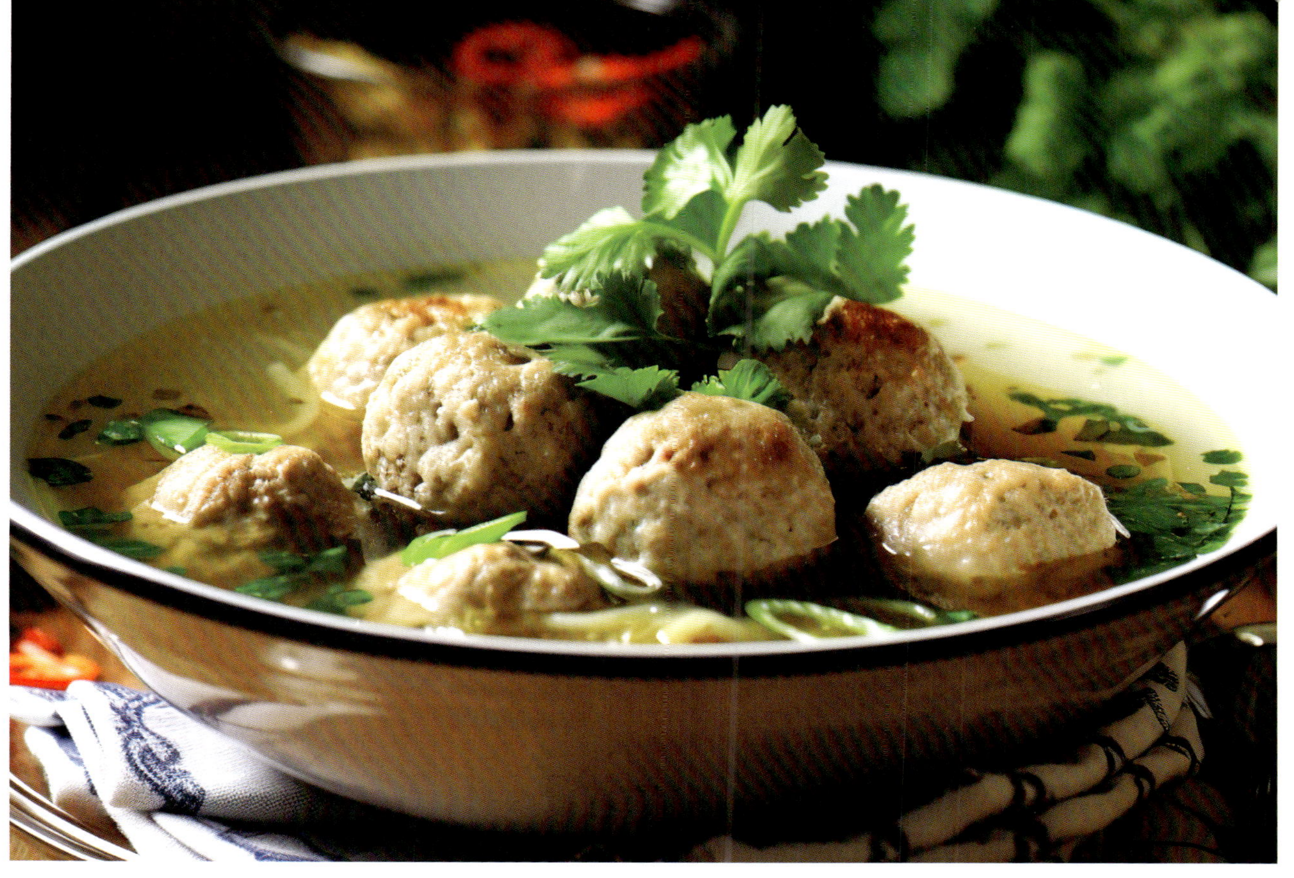

SERVES 4 | PREP + COOK TIME: 40 MINS | GLUTEN FREE | DAIRY FREE |

INDONESIAN MEATBALL SOUP

400g beef mince

3 tsps garlic

1 tbsp fried shallots

½ tsp baking powder

1 egg

¾ cup (100g) cornflour

⅓ cup (80ml) ice water

BROTH

3 cups (750ml) beef stock

1 spring onion, chopped

3 cloves garlic, chopped

Small piece ginger, grated

½ stalk celery, chopped

1 stalk lemongrass, crushed

½ tsp sugar

Salt and pepper to taste

350g rice noodles

2 tbsps chopped fresh coriander leaves

STEPS

1. Place beef mince, garlic, fried shallots, baking powder and egg into a large mixing bowl. Stir well. Add the cornflour and ice water and mix to combine using your hands. Roll mixture into balls.
2. Bring a large pan of water to a boil. Add the meatballs and cook for 15-20 minutes until the meatballs rise to the surface.
3. Meanwhile place stock, spring onion, garlic, ginger, celery, crushed lemongrass and sugar into a medium saucepan and bring to a boil. Continue to cook for 5 minutes before switching off the heat. Season with salt and pepper to taste.
4. Cook noodles according to packet directions.
5. Divide noodles between bowls. Top with meatballs and broth. Scatter with coriander to serve.

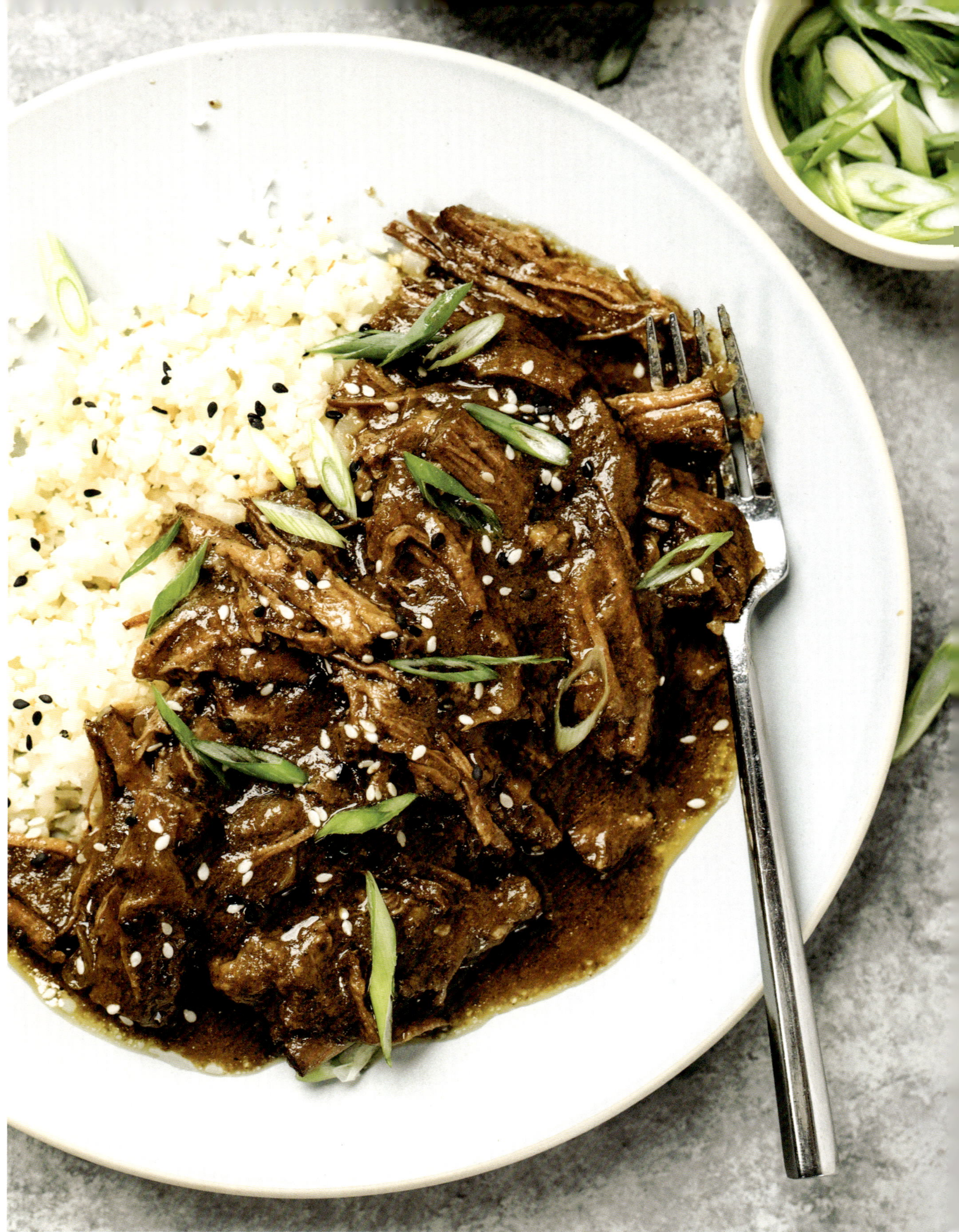

SLOW-COOKED KOREAN BEEF

2½ tbsps gochujang (Korean chilli paste)
4 cloves garlic, minced
Medium piece ginger, grated
3 tbsps soy sauce
2 tbsps red wine vinegar
1 tbsp sesame oil
3 tsps soft brown sugar
¼ tsp chilli flakes (optional)
Pepper to taste
700g beef flank steak, cut into 3cm-thick strips
1 onion, peeled and sliced
1 pear, peeled and diced
1½ tbsps cornflour
⅔ cup (150ml) apple juice
Cooked rice to serve
2 tsps black and white sesame seeds
2 spring onions, chopped

STEPS

1. In a large bowl combine the gochujang, garlic, ginger, soy sauce, vinegar, sesame oil, sugar and chilli flakes, if using. Season with a few grinds of pepper. Mix well.
2. Add the beef to the marinade. Stir well to ensure all of the beef is coated. Cover and refrigerate for 2 hours.
3. Place onion and pear into a slow cooker. Sprinkle with cornflour and stir to coat. Add the marinated beef, then pour in the apple juice and stir.
4. Cook on low for 6 hours or high for 4 hours.
5. Serve with rice and scatter with sesame seeds and spring onions.

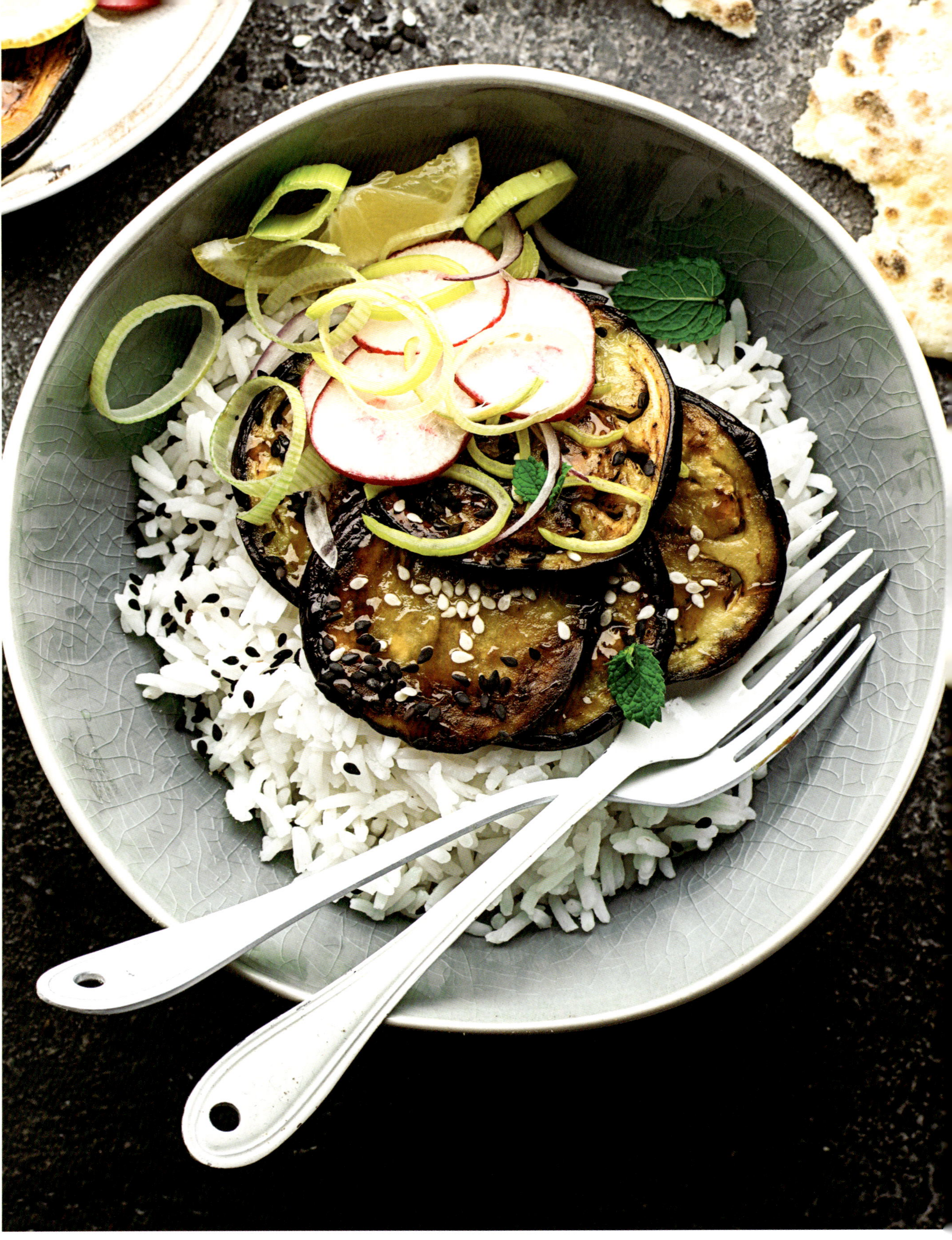

MISO-GLAZED EGGPLANT

SERVES 2 | PREP + COOK TIME: 40 MINS | GLUTEN FREE | DAIRY FREE |

1 medium eggplant
Oil for brushing
¼ cup (60ml) dashi
1 tbsp mirin
1 tbsp sake
2 tsps sugar
1 tbsp miso
Sesame seeds to garnish
Cooked rice to serve (optional)

STEPS

Preheat oven to 220°C.

1. Slice the eggplant into 1½ cm-thick rounds. Place eggplant slices on a lined baking tray and brush both sides of each round with olive oil. Bake for about 15 minutes, until tender, flipping halfway. Let cool on baking tray for 10 minutes.
2. Meanwhile bring dashi, mirin, sake and sugar to a gentle boil in a saucepan over a medium heat. Add miso and stir to combine. Remove from heat.
3. Spread about 2 teaspoons of miso mixture on each eggplant round. Place eggplant under a grill preheated to medium for 3-4 minutes until caramelised.
4. Scatter with sesame seeds and serve with rice, if desired.

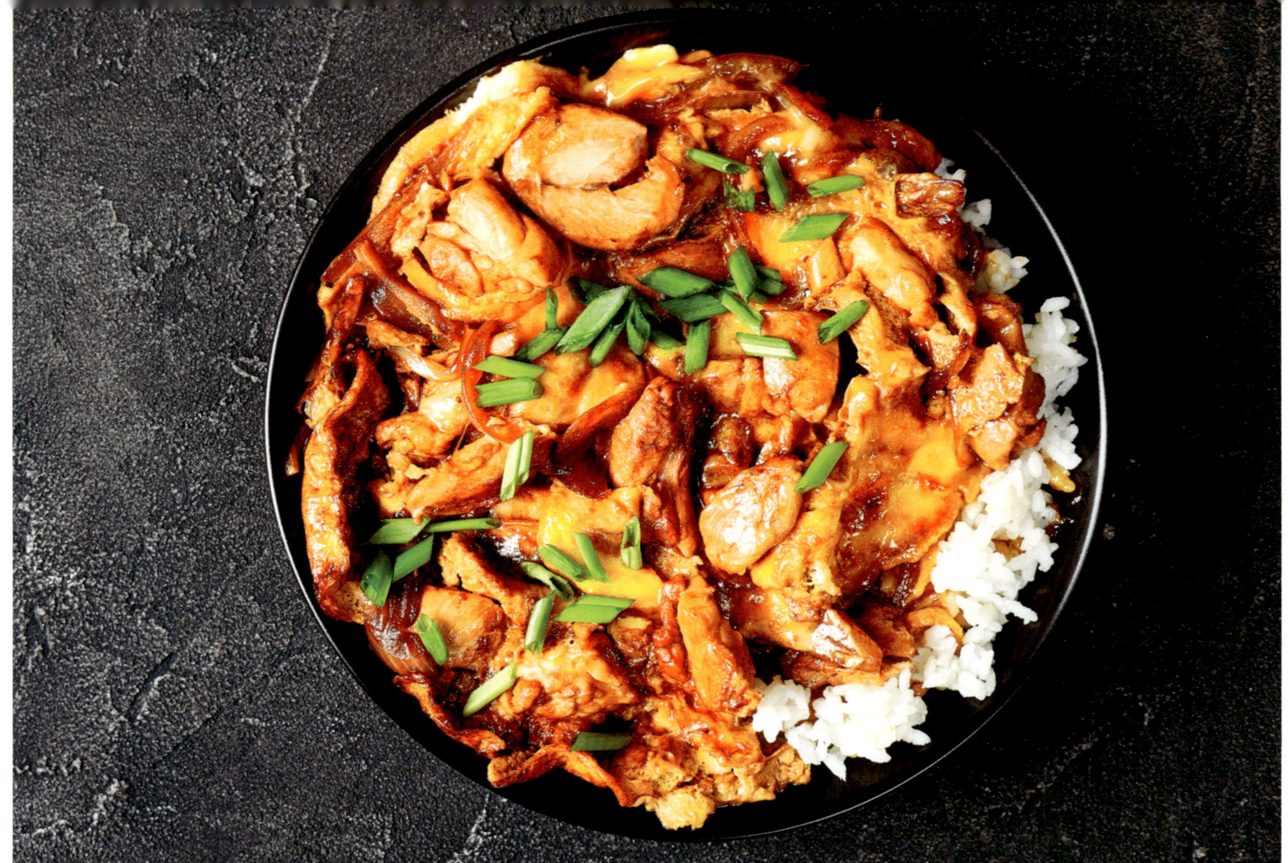

OYAKODON (CHICKEN, EGG, RICE BOWL)

2 cups (310g) Japanese short-grain rice

1 tbsp peanut or other neutral-flavoured oil

1 onion, sliced

500g skinless chicken thigh fillets, cut into bite-size pieces

2 cups (500ml) dashi stock

4 tbsps tamari

3 tbsps mirin

3 tbsps brown sugar

4 eggs

2 tbsps chopped spring onion, to garnish

STEPS

1. Cook the rice according to packet directions. Set aside.

2. Heat oil in a pan over medium heat. Add onion and cook for 3-5 minutes, stirring regularly, until soft and translucent.

3. Add chicken and cook for 5 minutes, until brown. Pour in the stock ensuring it covers the chicken, then add tamari, mirin and sugar. Bring to the boil and simmer for 4 minutes, until the liquid is slightly reduced.

4. Whisk the eggs in a bowl. Pour the eggs over the chicken and onion. Turn the heat to low and cover with a lid. Once egg is cooked turn off heat.

5. Spoon the chicken and egg over the cooked rice and top with chopped spring onion to serve.

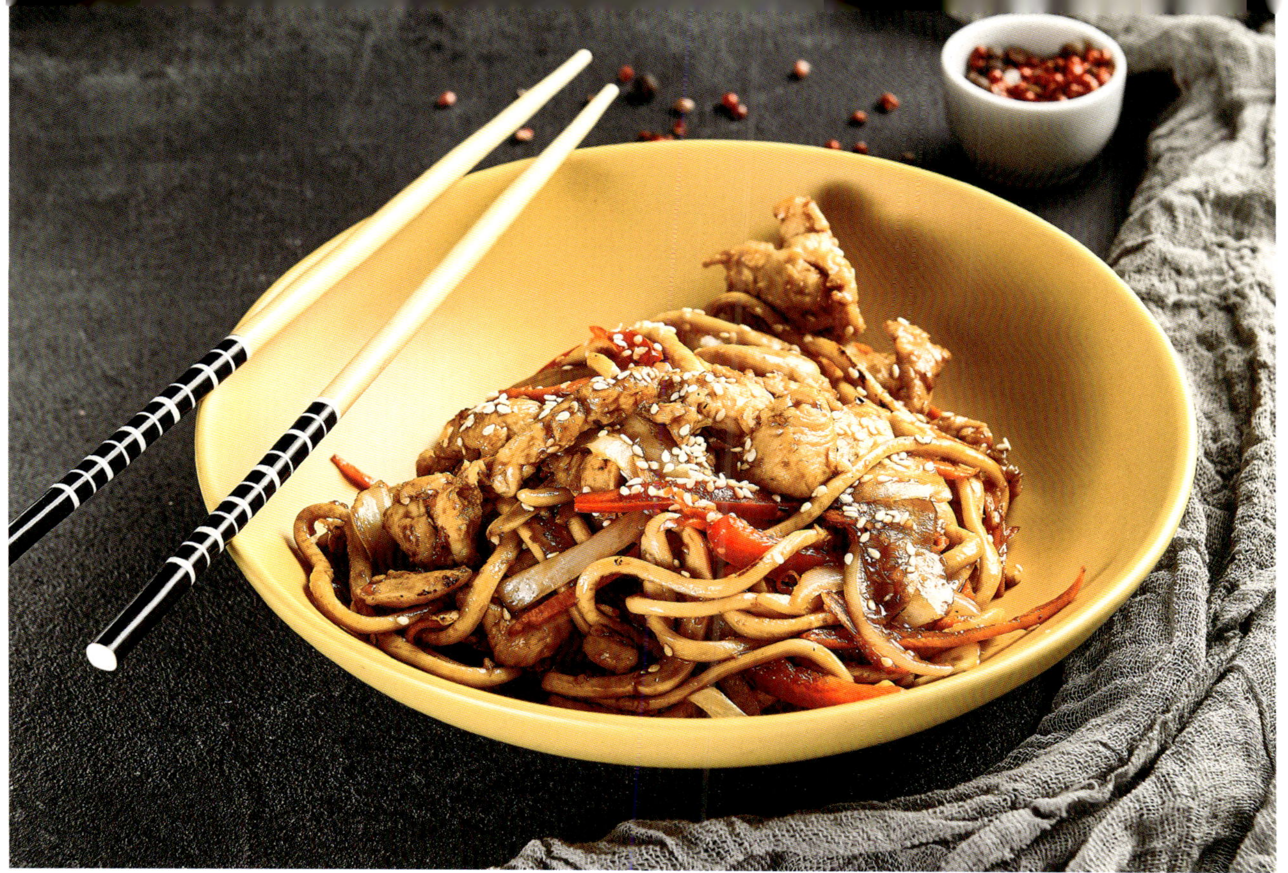

SERVES 4 | PREP + COOK TIME: 30 MINS | DAIRY FREE |

STICKY CHICKEN NOODLE STIR-FRY

2 tbsps vegetable oil

1 onion, thinly sliced

2 red capsicums, sliced

2 large chicken breasts, cut into thin strips

450g Hokkien noodles, cooked according to packet instructions

1 tsp sesame seeds

SAUCE

½ cup (125ml) soy sauce

⅓ cup (80ml) chicken stock

¼ cup (60ml) pineapple juice

¼ cup (55g) packed light brown sugar

2 cloves garlic, minced

Small piece fresh ginger, minced

2½ tsps cornflour

STEPS

1. Whisk together sauce ingredients in a medium bowl. Set aside.

2. Heat 1 tablespoon oil in a wok or large frying pan over medium-high heat. Add onion and capsicum and cook, stirring constantly, for 3 minutes until vegetables are tender-crisp. Transfer to a bowl and set aside.

3. Add the remaining oil to the pan. Add chicken and stir-fry for 3 minutes until it is no longer pink. Push chicken to the edges of the pan then add the prepared sauce to the centre of the pan. Bring to a boil and cook for 3 minutes until thick and syrupy.

4. Return vegetables to the pan along with the noodles, tossing to combine. Scatter with sesame seeds to serve.

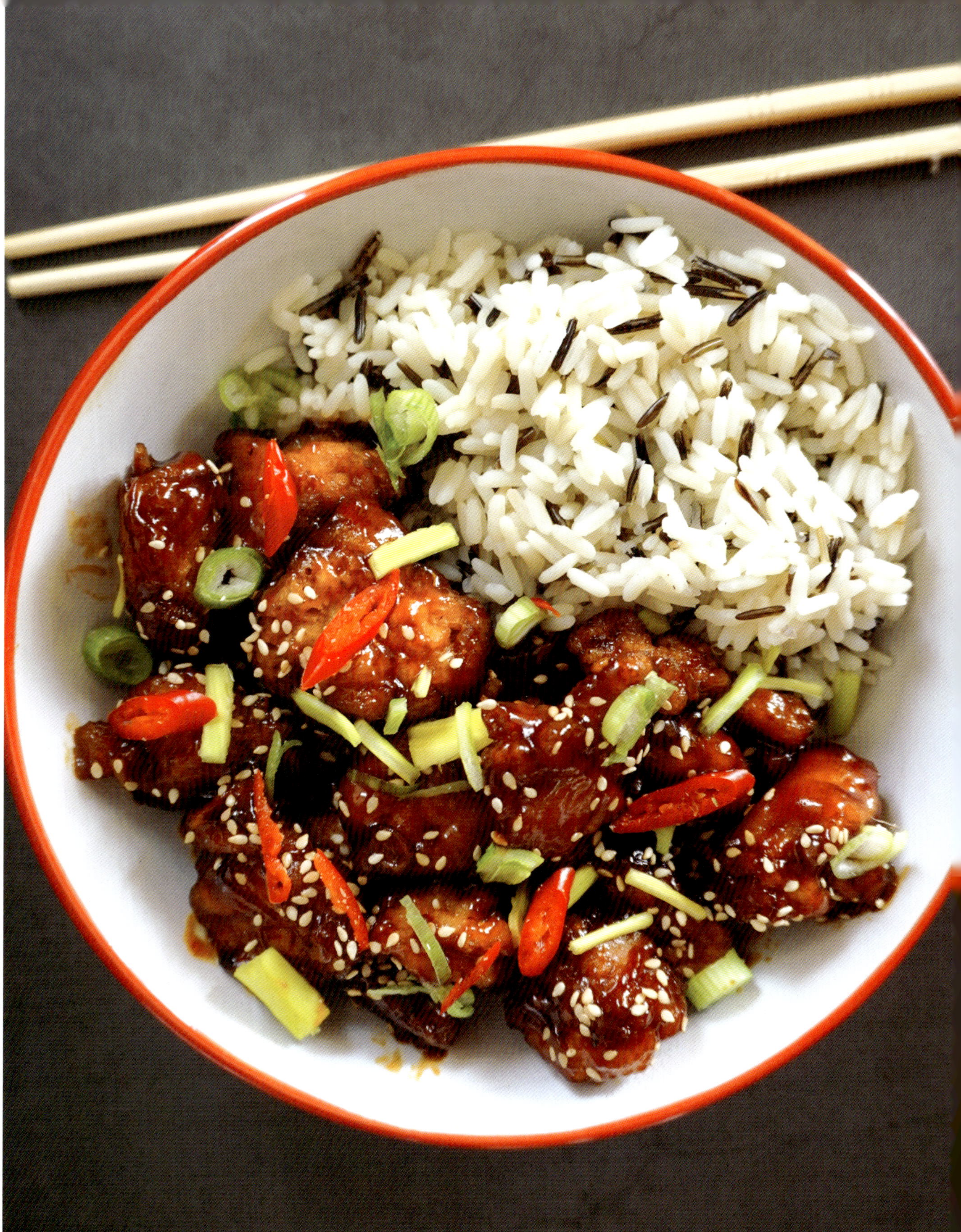

SWEET & SOUR CAULIFLOWER

SERVES 4 | PREP + COOK TIME: 30 MINS | VEG | DAIRY FREE |

1 head cauliflower, cut into bite-size pieces
Salt and pepper to taste
⅓ cup (80ml) + 3 tbsps oil
½ cup (75g) cornflour
2 tbsps sesame seeds
2 spring onions, chopped
1 red chilli, thinly sliced
Steamed rice to serve (optional)

SAUCE

½ cup (125ml) apple cider vinegar
¼ cup (60ml) tomato sauce
2 tbsps soy sauce
⅓ cup (80ml) maple syrup
1 clove garlic, minced
1 tsp salt
1 tbsp cornflour
2 tbsps water

STEPS

Preheat oven to 220°C.

1. Place the cauliflower in a large bowl. Add the salt, pepper and 3 tablespoons oil. Toss to combine. Add the cornflour. Toss again until well coated.
2. Heat remaining oil in a frying pan over a medium-high heat. Fry the cauliflower for about 5 minutes, flipping to cook on all sides. Place on a lined baking tray.
3. In a small bowl whisk together the sauce ingredients. Pour over the cauliflower and toss to coat.
4. Bake for 15 minutes until crispy. Sprinkle with sesame seeds, spring onions and chilli slices. Serve with steamed rice if desired.

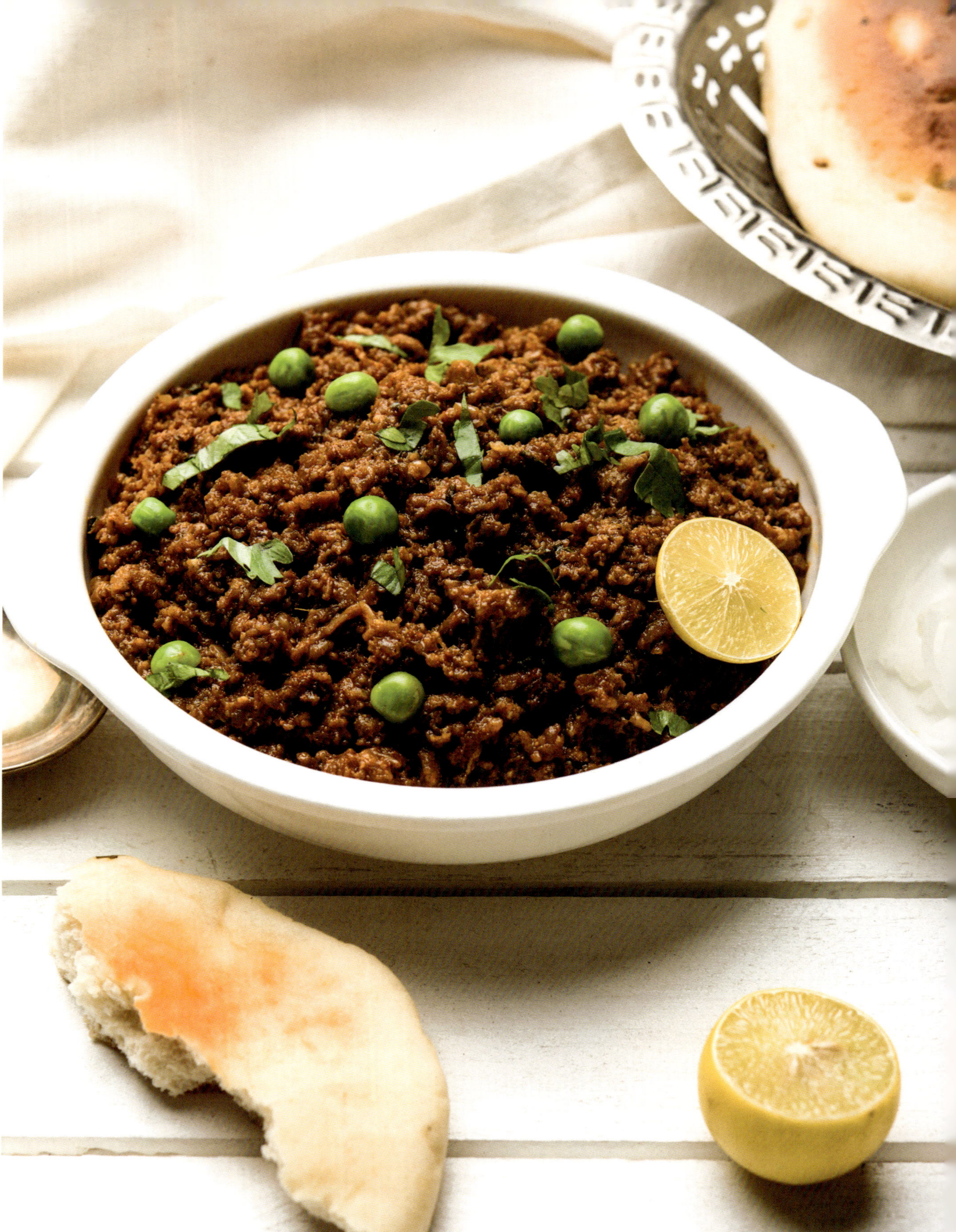

SPICED MINCED LAMB (KHEEMA PAAV)

SERVES 4 | PREP + COOK TIME: 50 MINS | GLUTEN FREE | DAIRY FREE |

Small piece ginger, minced
4 cloves garlic, minced
700g lamb mince
2 tbsps vegetable oil
5-7 curry leaves
2 onions, finely chopped
2 medium tomatoes, finely chopped
1-3 green chillies (to taste), deseeded and finely chopped
1 tbsp finely chopped coriander + more for garnish
1 tsp chilli powder
½ tsp ground turmeric
⅔ cup (150ml) water
¾ cup (180ml) coconut milk
1 cup (170g) peas
2 tbsps ground coriander
1 tsp garam masala
1 tsp brown sugar
2 tbsps vinegar
Salt to taste
1 tbsp lime juice

STEPS

1. Mix the ginger and garlic with the lamb mince and set aside.
2. Heat the oil in a large, heavy-bottomed pan over medium-high heat. Add the curry leaves and cook for 30 seconds until fragrant.
3. Add onions and fry for 5-7 minutes until soft and golden brown. Add the tomatoes and cook for a further 5 minutes. Add the green chillies, chopped coriander, chilli powder and turmeric. Stir well and cook for 1 minute.
4. Add the lamb. Cook, stirring, for 5 minutes then add the water. Bring to a boil then reduce heat and simmer, partially covered, for 20 minutes until all the liquid is absorbed.
5. Add coconut milk, peas, ground coriander and garam masala. Simmer for a further 5-7 minutes. Add sugar and vinegar and salt to taste. Squeeze over lime juice and garnish with extra fresh coriander to serve.

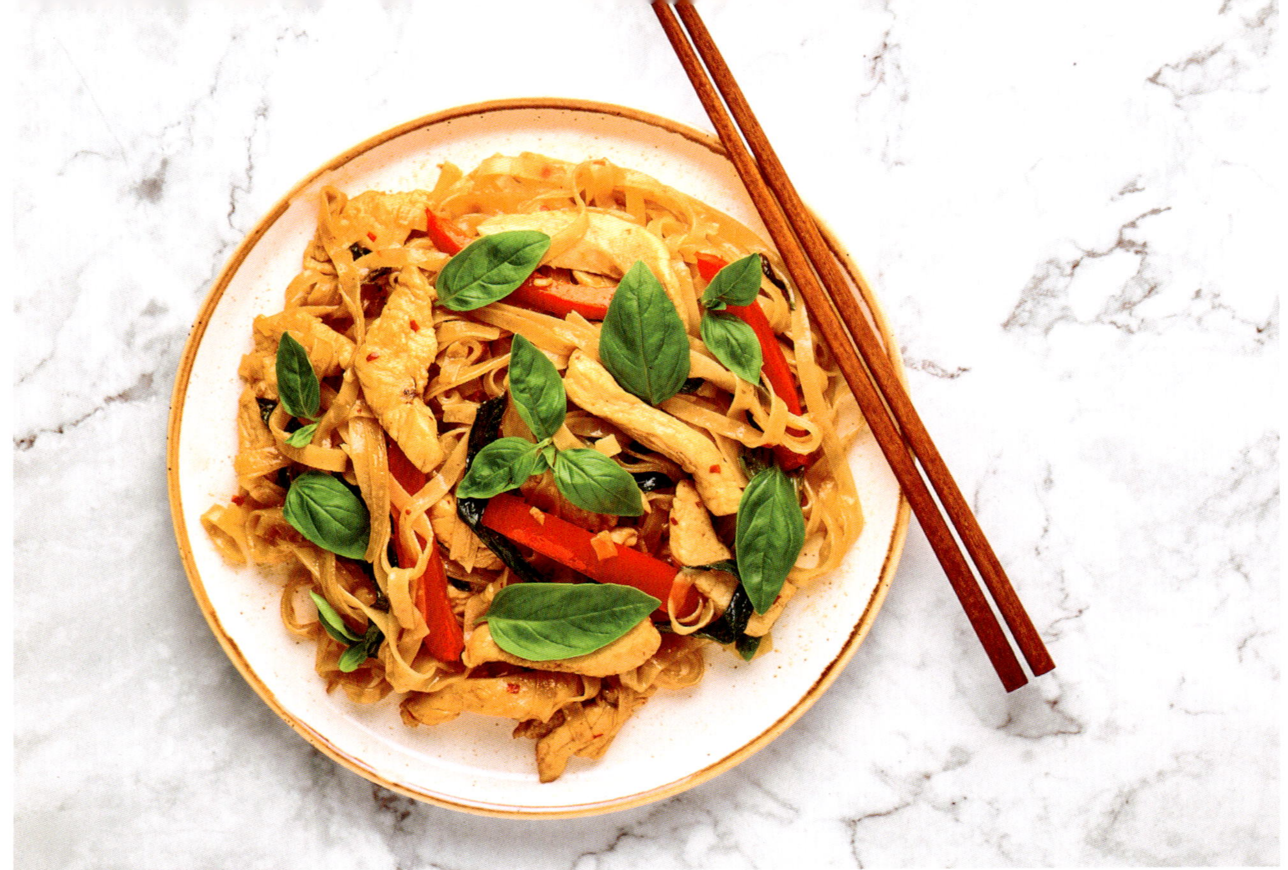

PAD KEE MAO DRUNKEN NOODLE

- 4 tbsps fish sauce
- 2 tbsps dark sweet soy sauce
- 1 tsp rice wine vinegar
- 3 tbsps vegetable oil
- 6 cloves garlic, minced
- 3 Thai chillies, chopped
- 1 onion, sliced
- 500g chicken thighs, sliced
- 450g flat rice noodles, soaked according to the packet instructions
- 2 red capsicums, sliced
- Handful of basil leaves

STEPS

1. Stir together the fish sauce, soy sauce and vinegar, and set aside.
2. Heat a wok or large frying pan over medium-high heat. When hot, add the oil, garlic, chillies and onion. Cook, stirring constantly, for about 30 seconds until fragrant.
3. Add the chicken and a splash of the sauce. Stir-fry for about 5 minutes, until cooked through.
4. Add the soaked noodles to the pan along with the capsicum. Increase the heat to high, and add the sauce. Cook for 5 minutes, or until all ingredients are coated with the sauce and vegetables are just tender.
5. Stir through half of the basil leaves, then scatter with the remaining basil to serve.

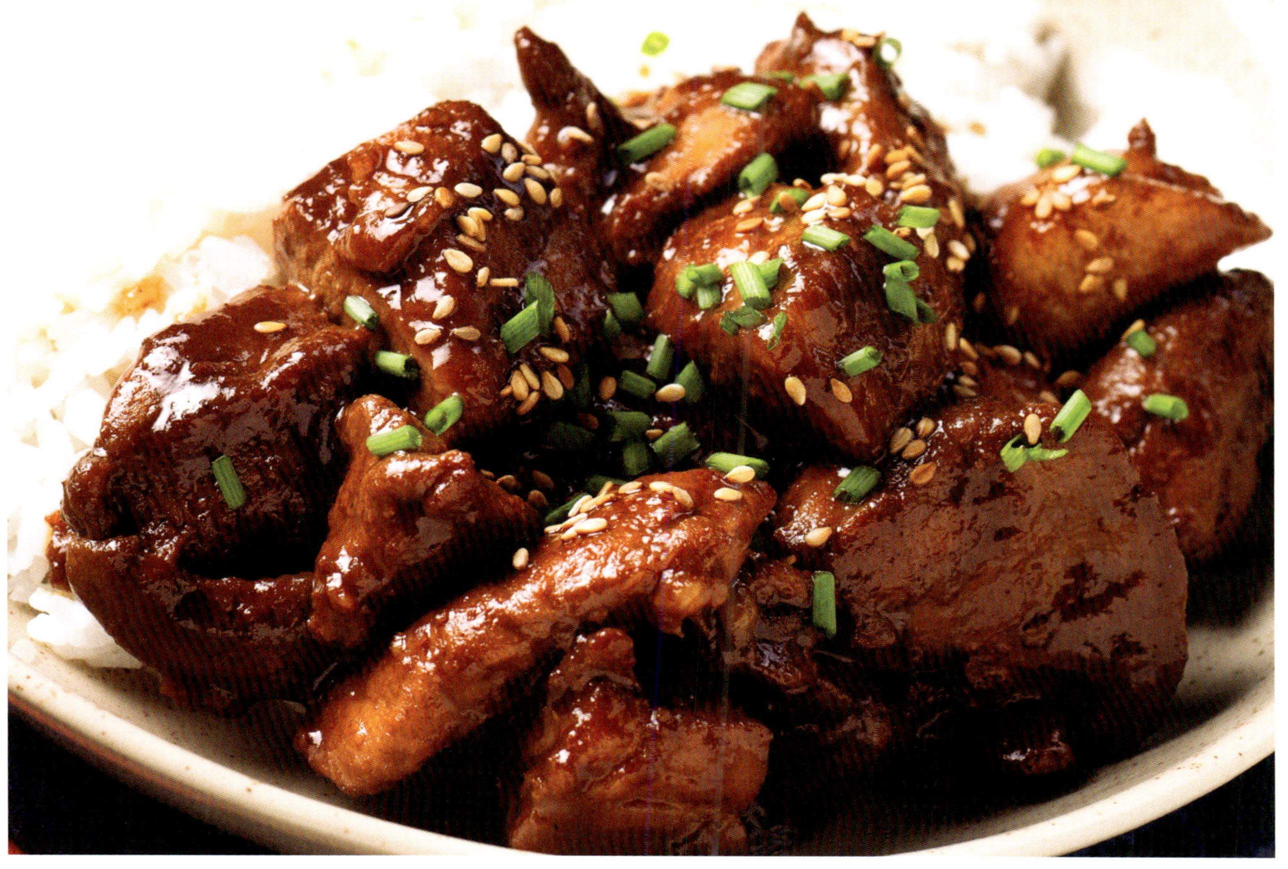

SERVES 4 | PREP + COOK TIME: 25 MINS | GLUTEN FREE | DAIRY FREE |

STICKY GARLIC & GINGER PORK

½ cup (180g) honey

2-4 tbsps Sriracha to taste

1 tbsp rice wine vinegar

1 tbsp peanut oil + extra if needed

750g boneless pork loin chops, cut into bite-size pieces

½ tsp salt

½ tsp pepper

5 cloves garlic, minced

Large piece ginger, grated

Cooked rice to serve

1 tbsp toasted sesame seeds

1 tbsp chopped chives

STEPS

1. In a small bowl, whisk together the honey, Sriracha and rice wine vinegar. Set aside.
2. Heat the oil in a heavy-bottomed pan over medium-high heat.
3. Season the pork with salt and pepper. Carefully add the pork to the pan, working in batches to avoid overcrowding. When pork is browned on all sides, transfer it to a plate.
4. Add the garlic and ginger to the pan. Stir for 30 seconds until fragrant. Increase the heat to high and pour in the sauce. Bring to a boil, stirring frequently.
5. Return the pork to the pan and continue to cook for a few minutes, stirring constantly, until the sauce is thick and sticky. Serve with rice, garnished with sesame seeds and chives.

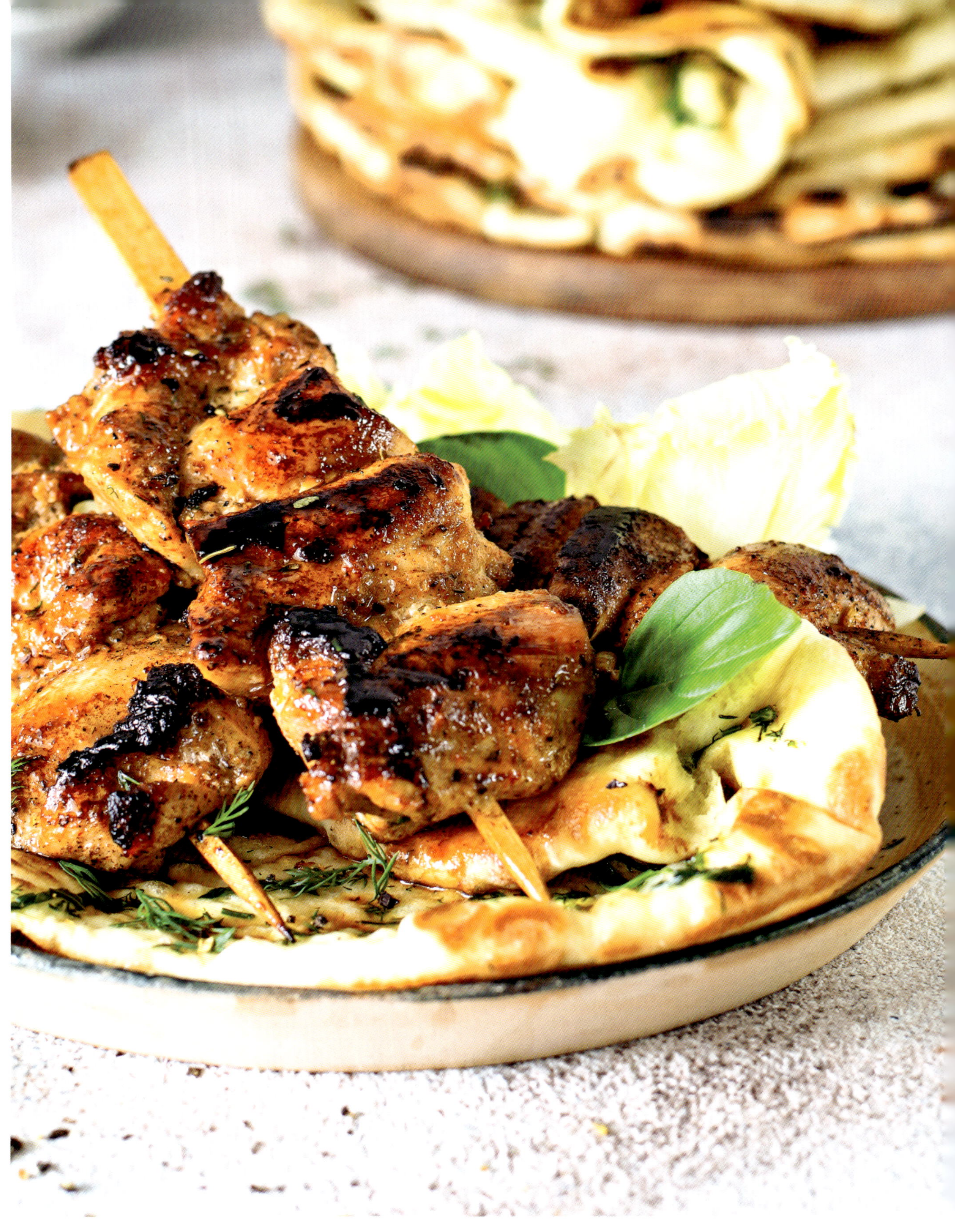

TANDOORI CHICKEN SKEWERS

1 cup (250ml) plain yoghurt

2 cloves garlic, minced

Medium piece ginger, minced

1 tsp smoked paprika

1 tsp ground coriander

1 tsp ground cumin

1 tsp ground turmeric

½ tsp ground cloves

½ tsp cayenne pepper

Salt and pepper to taste

1kg boneless, skinless chicken thighs, cut into 5cm pieces

4 large naan breads, warmed

YOGHURT SAUCE

⅓ cup (15g) roughly chopped mint leaves

⅓ cup (15g) roughly chopped coriander leaves and stalks

Pinch of caster sugar

1 tbsp white wine vinegar

1 cup (250ml) plain yoghurt

STEPS

1. In a large bowl, whisk together yoghurt, garlic, ginger and spices. Season with salt and pepper to taste. Place chicken cubes in marinade and stir to coat. Cover and transfer to the fridge to marinate for at least 1 hour (or overnight if convenient).
2. Remove chicken from marinade and thread onto wooden skewers (see note).
3. Cook chicken on a barbecue or grill pan over medium-high heat for 4-5 minutes on each side, turning occasionally until chicken is cooked through.
4. Combine the yoghurt sauce ingredients in a blender and pulse until smooth.
5. Serve chicken skewers on warm naan bread with yoghurt sauce.

NOTE: For best results, soak skewers in water for 30 minutes first to prevent them from burning or breaking while cooking.

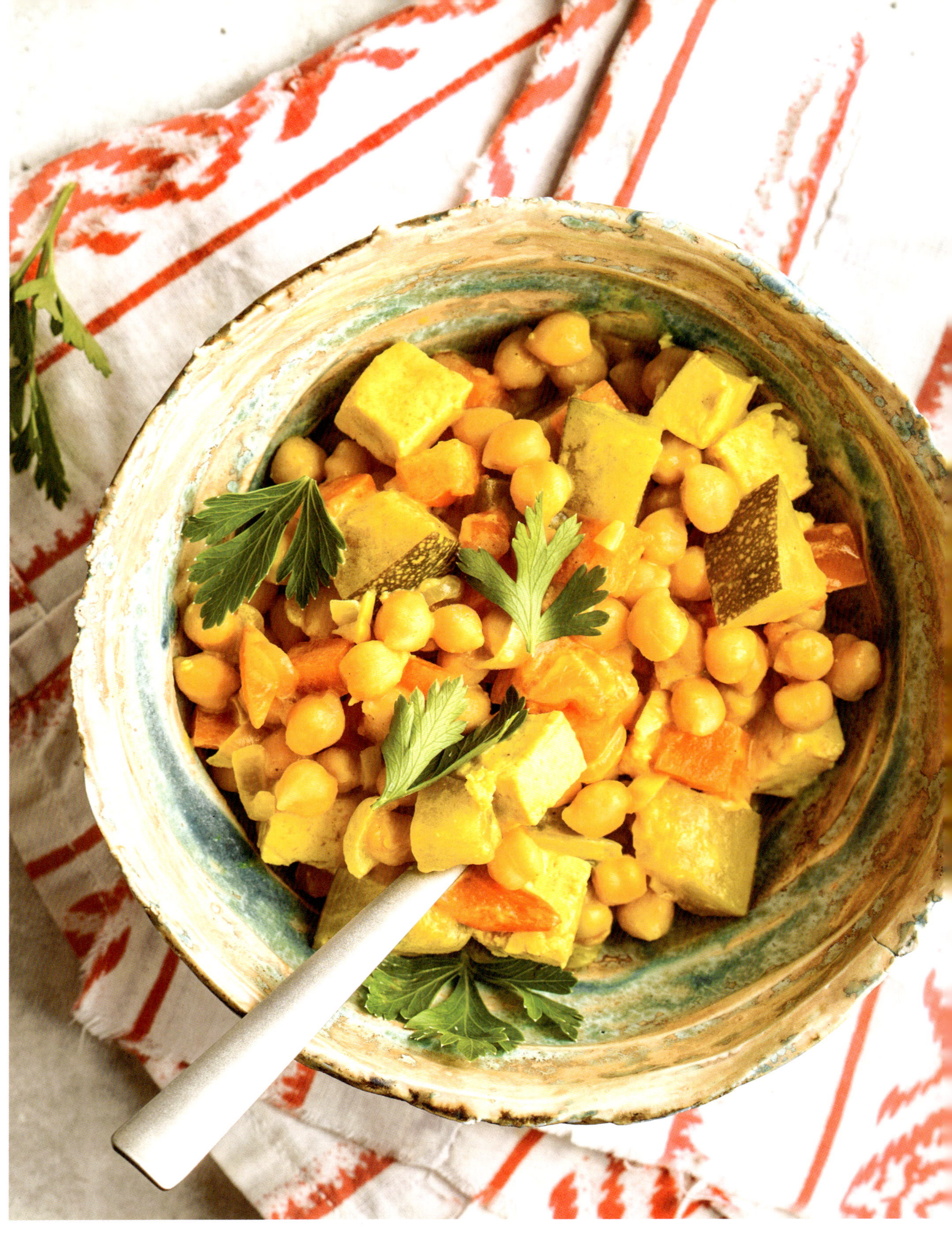

CURRIED TOFU & VEGETABLES

2 tbsps olive oil

300g firm tofu, cut into 3cm pieces

1 onion, finely chopped

1 zucchini, cut into the 1cm-thick slices, then cut into quarter moons

1 red capsicum, diced

1 x 400g can chickpeas, drained and rinsed

⅓ cup (100g) korma curry paste

1 x 270ml can coconut milk

½ cup (125ml) warm water

STEPS

1. Heat half the oil in a wok or large frying pan over medium-high heat. Stir-fry the tofu for 3 minutes or until golden. Transfer to a plate.

2. Heat the remaining oil in the pan and place over medium heat. Cook the onion, stirring, for 5-7 minutes until soft. Add the zucchini and capsicum and continue to cook for a further 5 minutes until vegetables are soft. Add the chickpeas and cook for 2 minutes or until lightly browned.

3. Add the curry paste and cook, stirring, for 2 minutes until fragrant. Add the coconut milk and warm water. Stir to combine. Bring to the boil.

4. Reduce heat to low. Return the tofu to the pan. Cook, partially covered, for 8 minutes or until the sauce thickens. Serve immediately.

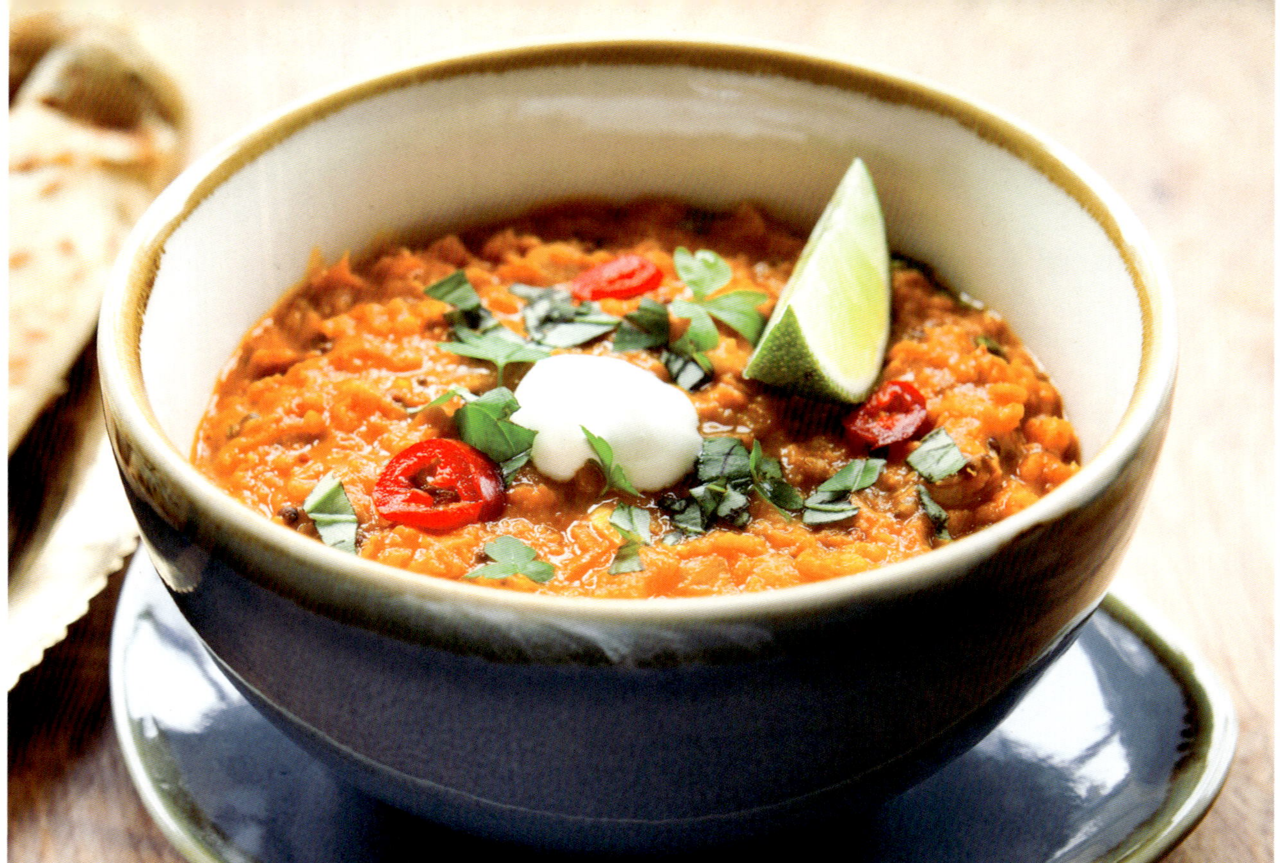

CLASSIC DHAL

2 tbsps ghee or peanut oil
½ tsp mustard seeds
1 onion, finely chopped
2 cloves garlic, finely chopped
Large piece ginger, finely chopped
4 cups (1L) water or vegetable stock
1 cup (185g) dried red lentils
1 tsp ground cumin
1 tsp ground coriander
1 tsp ground turmeric
½ tsp ground cardamon
¼ tsp ground cinnamon
⅛ tsp cayenne pepper
1 tsps salt or to taste
1 tbsp tomato paste
¼ cup (60ml) yoghurt to serve
1 red chilli, sliced, to serve
¼ cup (10g) chopped coriander to serve
Lime wedges to serve

STEPS

1. Heat ghee or oil in a large pan over medium heat. Add mustard seeds and allow them to sizzle for 30 seconds. Add onion, garlic and ginger. Cook, stirring often, for 5-7 minutes until onion is soft and translucent.

2. Stirring constantly, add water or stock, lentils, spices and salt. Bring to a low boil, then reduce heat to low. Cover and simmer for 20 minutes or until lentils are very tender.

3. Stir in tomato paste and cook for 4-5 minutes more, adding more water if needed.

4. Top with a dollop of yoghurt and scatter with sliced chilli and coriander leaves. Serve with lime wedges.

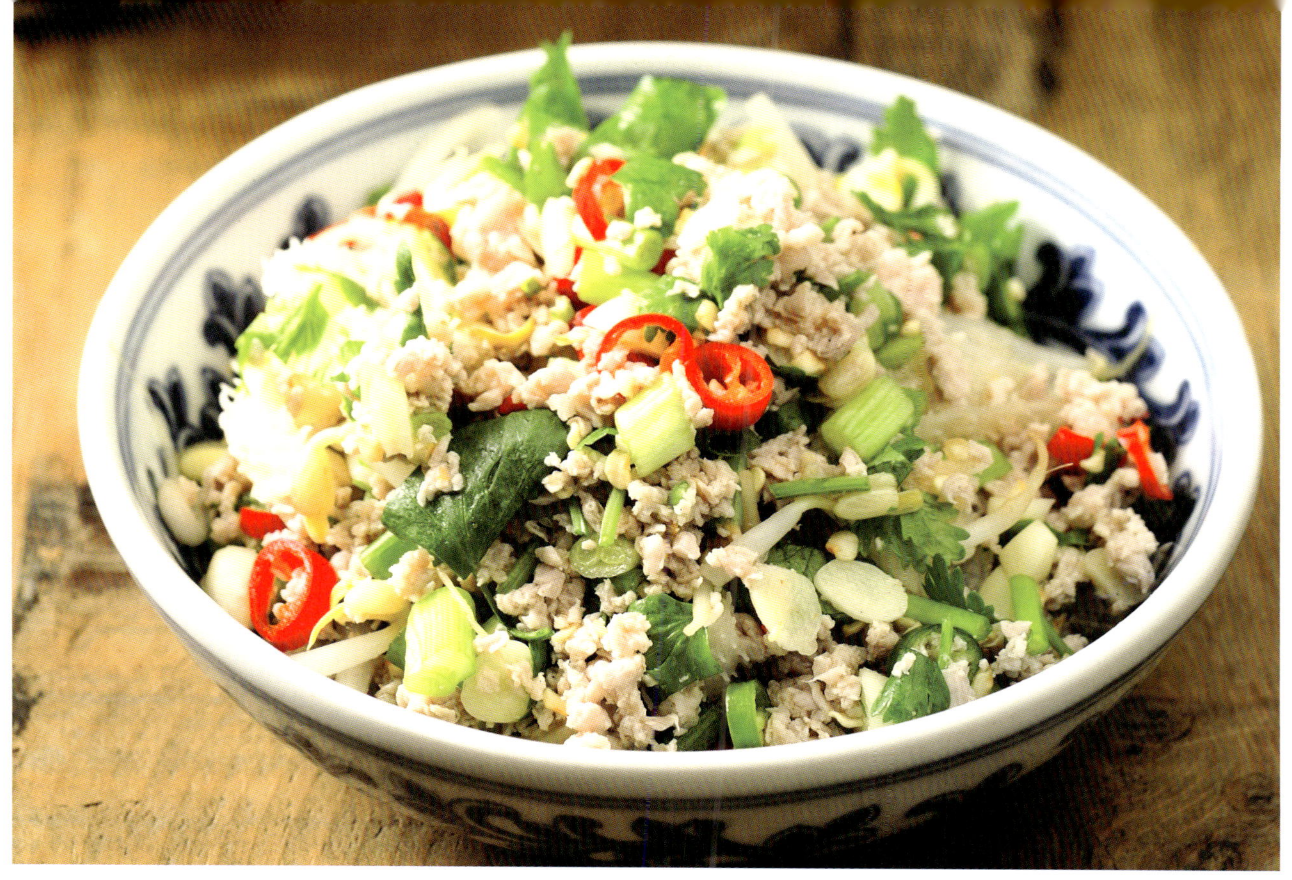

SERVES 4 | PREP + COOK TIME: 20 MINS | GLUTEN FREE | DAIRY FREE |

CHICKEN LARB

400g chicken mince

¼ cup (60ml) fresh lime juice

2 tsps rice wine

1 tsp brown sugar

2 tbsps fish sauce

⅔ cup (150ml) chicken stock

2 cloves garlic, thinly sliced

2 spring onions, sliced

2 tbsps fresh ginger, grated

½ cup (20g) fresh coriander, chopped

1 cup (100g) bean sprouts, rinsed

1 tbsp toasted rice powder (optional)

1 red chilli, sliced

STEPS

1. Heat a large wok or frying pan to medium-high heat.
2. Cook the chicken for 6 minutes, stirring to break up any lumps. Add the lime juice, rice wine, brown sugar, fish sauce, stock, garlic, spring onion and ginger and stir through for 2 minutes.
3. Remove from the heat and strain the chicken, reserving the liquid.
4. In a large bowl, toss together the chicken mixture, coriander, bean sprouts and toasted rice powder, if using. Toss through the reserved liquid, as much as desired. Garnish with fresh chilli and serve warm.

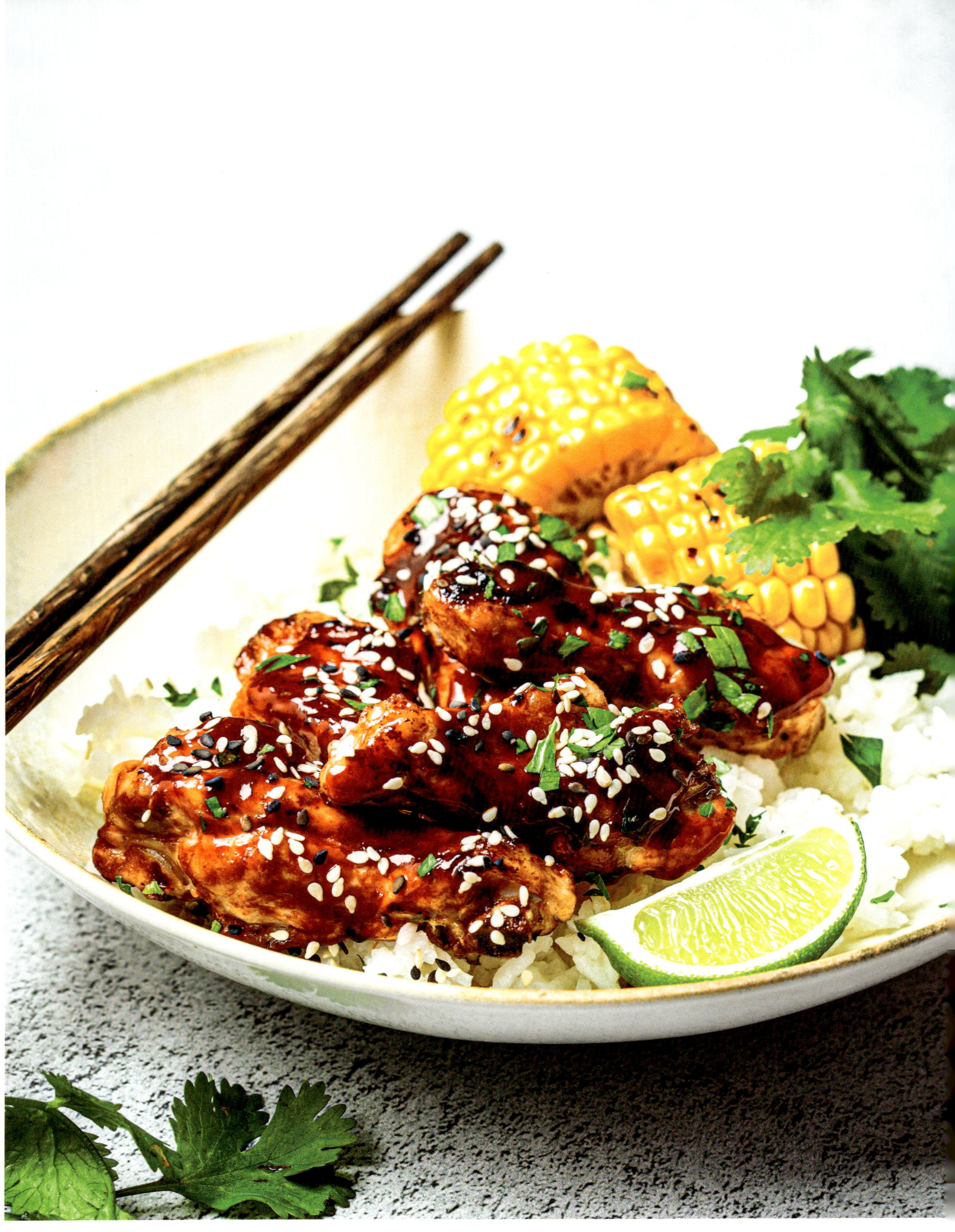

STICKY SESAME CHICKEN

2 corn cobs

1 tbsp olive oil

2 eggs, lightly beaten

3 tbsps cornflour

10 tbsps plain flour

½ tsp salt

½ tsp pepper

½ tsp garlic salt

2 tsps paprika

1kg chicken drumettes

5 tbsps peanut oil or vegetable oil

1 tbsp sesame oil

2 cloves garlic, minced

1 tbsp rice wine vinegar

2 tbsps honey

2 tbsps sweet chilli sauce

3 tbsps tomato ketchup

2 tbsps brown sugar

4 tbsps soy sauce (use tamari for gluten-free)

Boiled rice to serve

Handful fresh coriander leaves + 2 tbsps chopped coriander

Lime wedges to serve

2 tbsps black and white sesame seeds

STEPS

1. Brush the corn cobs with olive oil. Place cobs in a large frying pan over medium-high heat and cook, turning frequently, for 10 minutes or until corn is nicely charred. Remove from heat and set aside.

2. Place the egg in one shallow bowl, the cornflour in another and combine the flour, salt, pepper, garlic salt and paprika in a third shallow bowl. Dredge the chicken pieces in the cornflour, then dip in the egg, and finally dredge in the seasoned flour.

3. Heat the oil in a wok or large frying pan until very hot. Add chicken to the wok and stir-fry on a high heat for 6-7 minutes, until well browned. You may need to cook in two batches. Remove from the pan and place on a paper towel-lined plate.

4. Add the sesame oil, garlic, vinegar, honey, chilli sauce, ketchup, sugar and soy sauce to the hot wok. Stir and bubble on a high heat for 2-3 minutes until the sauce reduces by about a third. Add the chicken back in and toss in the sauce to coat. Cook for 1-2 minutes.

5. Cut corn into small sections. Serve chicken with corn, boiled rice, coriander leaves and lime wedges. Top with sesame seeds and chopped coriander.

SERVES 4 | PREP + COOK TIME: 30 MINS | DAIRY FREE |

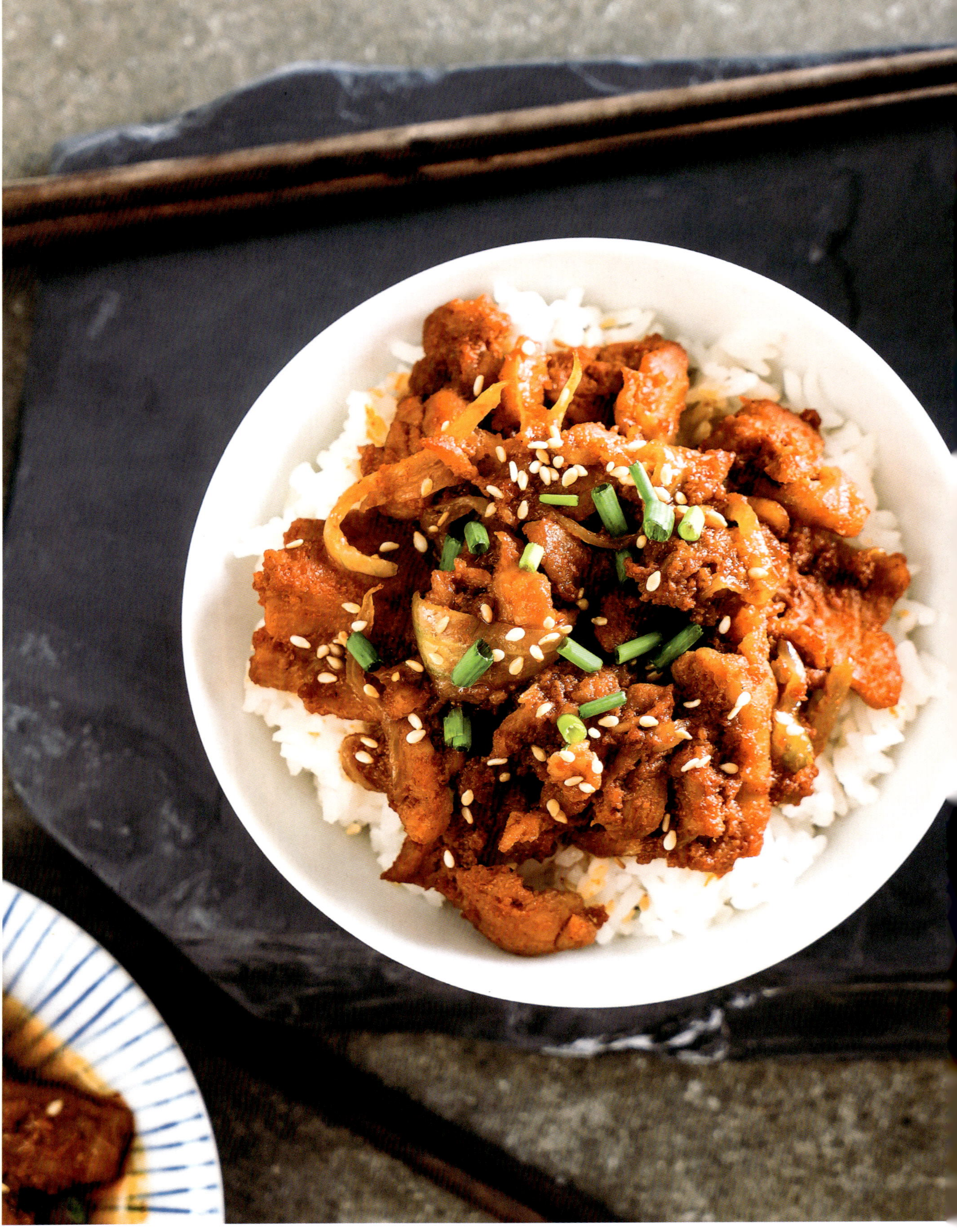

SPICY KOREAN PORK

1kg pork shoulder or butt, thinly sliced

1 medium onion, sliced

2 spring onion tops, chopped, reserving some for garnish

2 tbsps oil

Steamed rice to serve

2 tsps sesame seeds

MARINADE

6 tbsps gochujang (Korean chilli paste)

1-2 tbsps gochugaru (Korean chilli flakes)

3 tbsps soy sauce

3 tbsps rice wine or mirin

2 tbsps sugar

1 tbsp honey

2 tbsps sesame oil

2 tbsps minced garlic

Medium piece ginger, grated

½ small apple, grated

STEPS

1. Combine the marinade ingredients in a large bowl and mix well.

2. Add the pork and stir to coat. Add the onions and spring onions and stir once more. Set aside to marinate for 30 minutes.

3. Heat half of the oil in large frying pan over medium-high heat. Add half of the meat and onions and cook, stirring occasionally, for 5-7 minutes until slightly caramelised. Repeat with the remaining oil and meat.

4. Serve over steamed rice and scatter with sesame seeds and chopped spring onions.

SERVES 4 | PREP + COOK TIME: 45 MINS + MARINATING | DAIRY FREE |

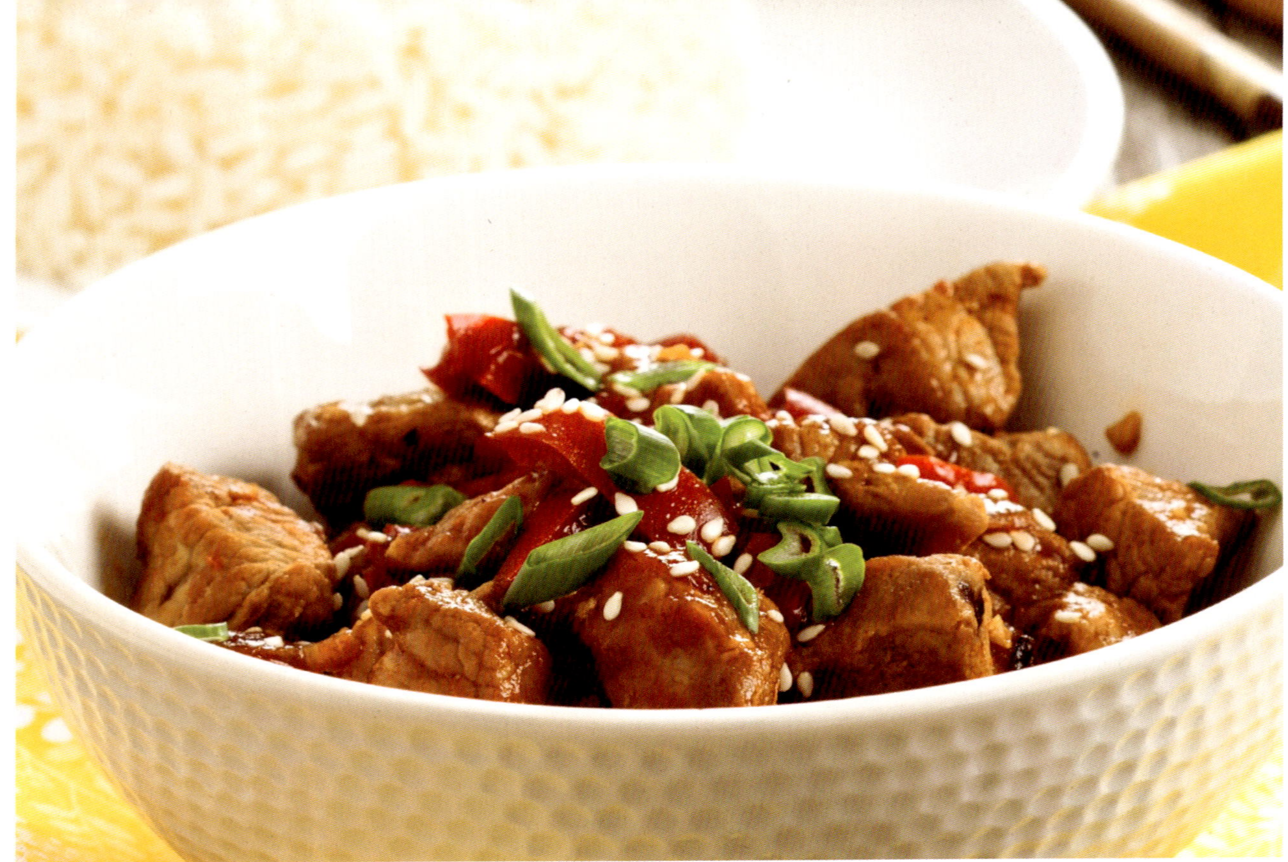

HONEY-SESAME PORK

- 6 tbsps dark soy sauce
- 3 tbsps honey
- 2 tbsps Shaoxing wine
- 1 tbsp sesame oil
- 1 tbsp cornflour
- 1 tbsp vegetable oil
- 500g lean pork, cut into thin strips
- 1 clove garlic, crushed
- 1 small piece ginger, finely chopped
- ½ red chilli, finely chopped + 1 red chilli, sliced, to garnish
- 1 tbsp sesame seeds, to garnish
- 2 spring onions, sliced, to garnish
- 1 tsp toasted sesame oil
- Boiled rice to serve

STEPS

1. In a small bowl, mix the soy sauce, honey and Shaoxing wine with the sesame oil. Add the cornflour to the mixture and stir well to combine.
2. Heat a wok or large frying pan over a high heat. Add the vegetable oil and then add the pork. Stir-fry for 5 minutes, until brown and almost cooked through.
3. Add the garlic, ginger and chilli and stir-fry for 1 minute until fragrant.
4. Add the honey-sesame sauce and cook for 2-3 minutes.
5. Garnish with sesame seeds, sliced chilli and spring onion and drizzle with toasted sesame oil. Serve with boiled rice.

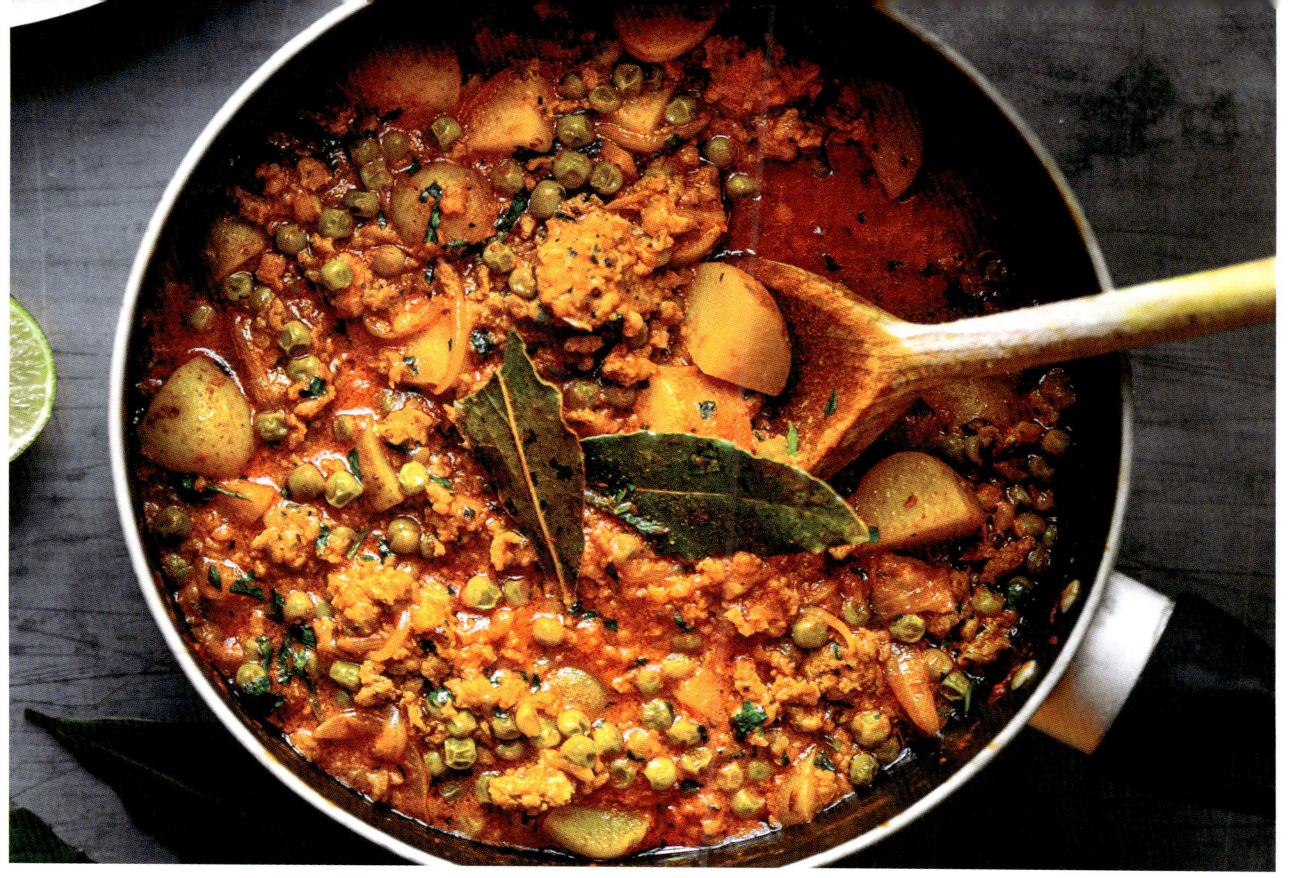

ALOO KHEEMA

1 tbsp vegetable oil
500g beef mince
Salt and pepper to taste
1 large onion, chopped
2 cloves garlic, chopped
Small piece ginger, finely chopped
2 tbsps hot curry powder
3 potatoes, cut into 3cm chunks
2 tbsps tomato paste
2 medium tomatoes, grated
2 bay leaves
2 cups (500ml) vegetable stock
1 cup peas
2 tbsps chopped coriander leaves

STEPS

1. Heat 1 teaspoon of the oil in a large saucepan over a high heat. Add the mince and season with salt and pepper. Cook for 3-5 minutes until browned, breaking up with a spoon. Remove from the pan and set aside. Drain and discard any fat.

2. Heat the remaining oil in the same pan over medium heat. Cook the onion, garlic and ginger for 7-8 minutes until soft. Add the curry powder and potatoes; cook for 3-4 minutes more.

3. Stir in the tomato paste, grated tomatoes, bay leaves and vegetable stock. Return the beef to the pan. Simmer for 15 minutes.

4. Add peas and cook for a further 5 minutes until the peas are cooked and potatoes are tender.

5. Stir in chopped coriander to serve.

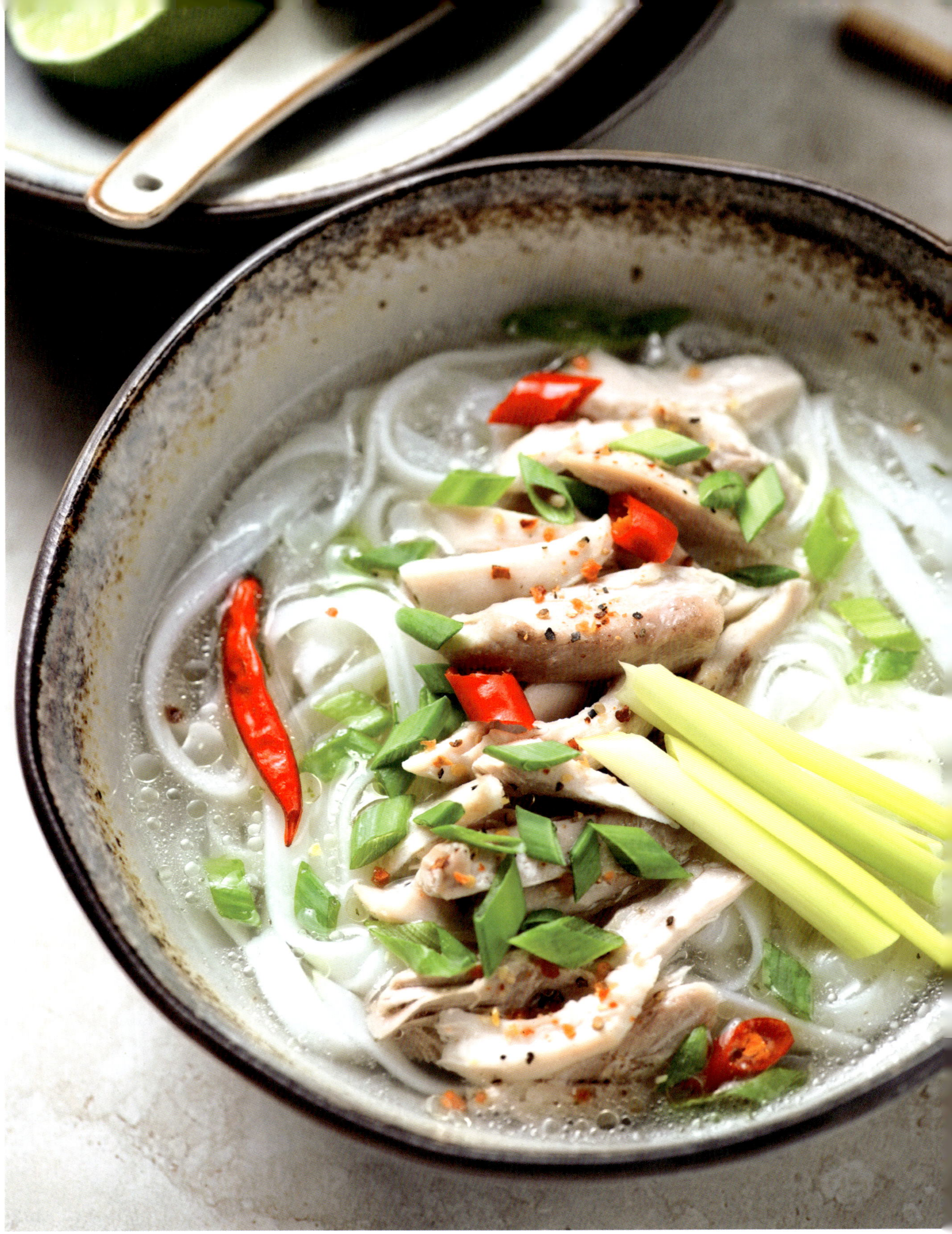

SLOW-COOKED CHICKEN PHO

8 cups (2L) water
1 chicken (about 1.8kg), fat trimmed
1 onion, coarsely chopped
¼ cup (60ml) dark soy sauce
Small piece ginger, thinly sliced
4 cloves garlic, halved
2 long red chillies, coarsely chopped
1 tbsp fish sauce
1 star anise
1 tsp white peppercorns
200g dried flat rice noodles
2 spring onions, chopped
1 tsp dried chilli flakes
1 red chilli, thickly sliced (optional)
1 stalk lemongrass, chopped into 5cm pieces, to garnish (optional)

STEPS

1. Place water, chicken, onion, soy sauce, ginger, garlic, chilli, fish sauce, star anise and peppercorns in a slow cooker. Cover and cook on high for 4½ hours or until chicken is cooked through and very tender. Remove chicken with tongs and a large spatula and set aside to cool slightly in a large bowl.
2. Meanwhile, strain stock through a fine sieve into a large saucepan. Add any liquid that has collected around the cooling chicken.
3. When chicken is cool enough to handle, remove meat from carcass (discard bones). Thinly slice breast meat and set aside for garnish. Add dark meat to stock and reheat over medium heat until just simmering.
4. Meanwhile, cook noodles in boiling salted water according to packet directions until just tender. Drain and divide between serving bowls. Ladle soup and dark meat over noodles, then top with reserved breast meat.
5. Scatter with spring onions, dried chilli flakes, red chilli and lemongrass, if desired.

SERVES 4 | PREP + COOK TIME: 5 HOURS | DAIRY FREE |

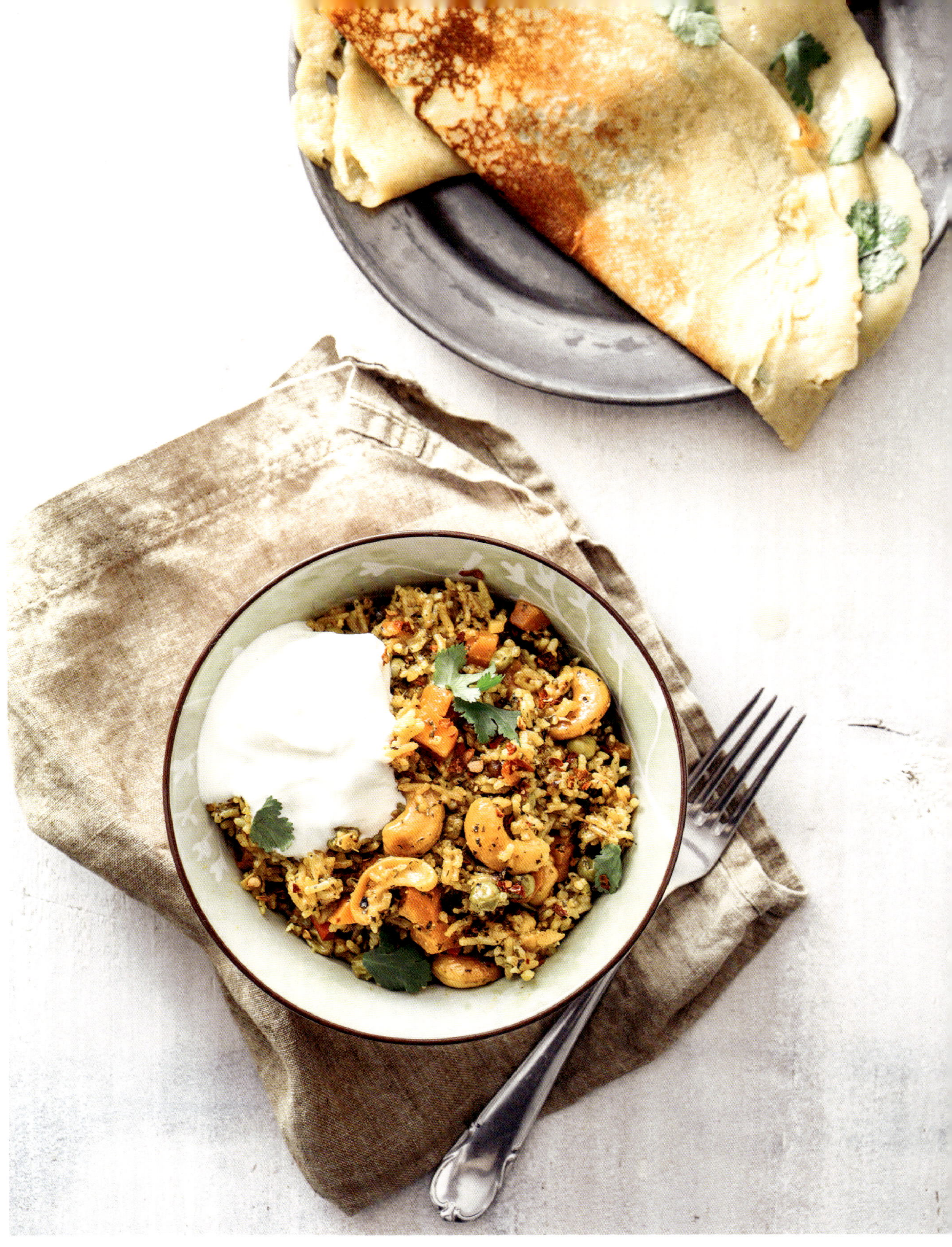

BIRYANI WITH PUMPKIN & CASHEW NUTS

2 tbsps sunflower oil

1 large onion, halved and thinly sliced

Medium piece ginger, shredded

3 tbsps korma curry paste

1 cinnamon stick

4 green cardamon pods

2 star anise

125g potatoes, diced

1 small butternut pumpkin, diced

¾ cup (200ml) water

½ cup (125ml) Greek yoghurt + more for serving

¾ cup (125g) peas

Salt to taste

Pinch of saffron

¼ tsp rosewater

3 tbsps boiling water

1⅔ cups (250g) basmati rice, rinsed and soaked for 30 minutes

Butter for greasing

1 cup (125g) roasted, salted cashews nuts

STEPS

1. Heat oil in a large saucepan over medium-high heat. Add onion and cook for 3-5 minutes, stirring regularly, until soft. Add the ginger and cook for 2 more minutes. Stir in the curry paste, followed by the whole spices. Cook for 1 minute then add in the potatoes and pumpkin. Pour in the water, cover and boil for about 5-7 minutes until the vegetables are just tender. Stir in the yoghurt and peas with a pinch of salt.
2. In a small bowl mix the saffron and rosewater with 3 tablespoons boiling water. Stir well to combine.
3. Drain the soaked rice and add to a pan of boiling, salted water. Simmer for 5-10 minutes until almost tender. Drain.
4. Butter the base of a lidded ovenproof dish. Add the curried vegetables into the dish, scatter over the roasted cashew nuts, then top with the rice. Drizzle over the rosewater mixture, cover with foil and the lid.
5. Cook for 45 minutes to 1 hour at 180°C until thoroughly heated through. Scatter with coriander leaves and serve with yoghurt.

SERVES 4 | PREP + COOK TIME: 1 HOUR 30 MINS | VEG | GLUTEN FREE |

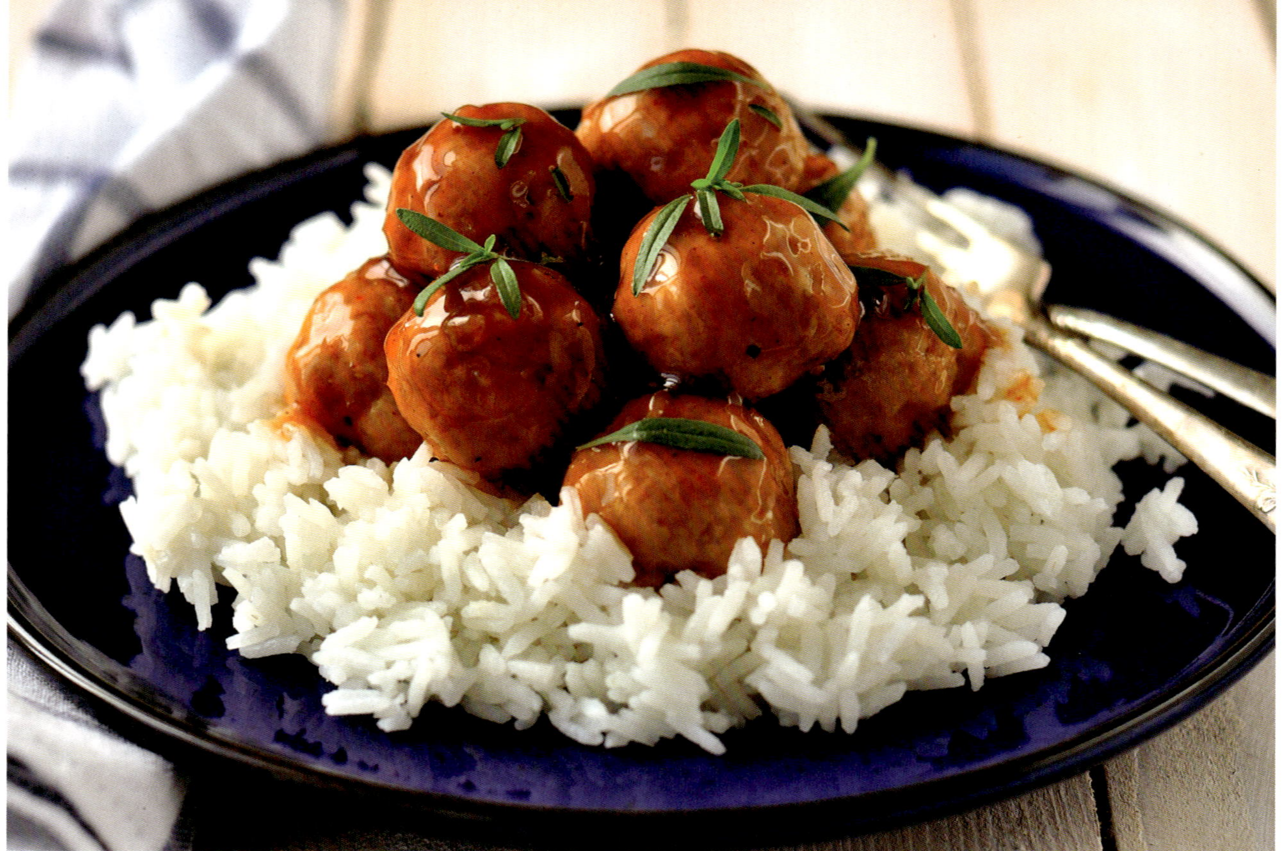

SWEET & SPICY GLAZED MEATBALLS

MEATBALLS

500g beef mince

4 spring onions, chopped

⅓ cup (40g) breadcrumbs

3 cloves garlic, minced

1 egg

1½ tbsps Sriracha

Small piece ginger, grated

Salt and pepper to taste

GLAZE

½ cup (160g) apricot jam

Zest of 1 orange

Juice of 1 lime

1 tbsp soy sauce

2 tbsps Sriracha

½ red chilli, chopped

TO SERVE

Steamed rice

STEPS

Preheat oven to 200°C.

1. In a large bowl, add all the meatball ingredients and mix with your hands to combine. Form into walnut-sized meatballs.
2. Arrange the meatballs on a lined baking tray and bake for 20-25 minutes or until cooked through.
3. Meanwhile, in a small pan whisk together all the glaze ingredients. Heat gently over low heat until just bubbling.
4. Pour glaze over meatballs and serve immediately with steamed rice.

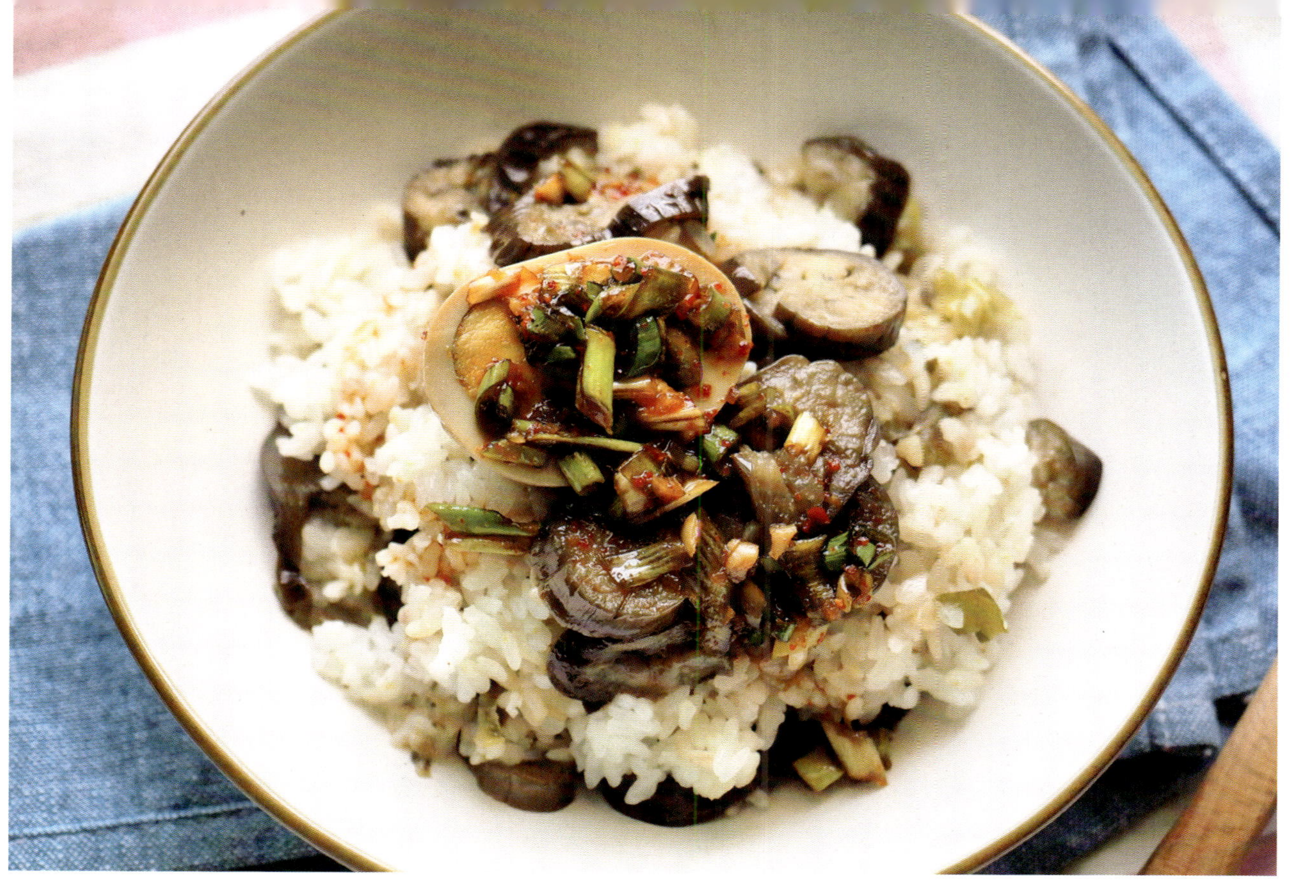

SERVES 4 | PREP + COOK TIME: 50 MINS + SOAKING | VEG | GLUTEN FREE | DAIRY FREE |

EGGPLANT WITH STICKY RICE

2 cups (310g) glutinous rice, soaked overnight

4 long Japanese eggplants, sliced into 1cm-thick discs

3 cloves garlic, minced

1 small red chilli, minced

Medium piece of ginger, grated

2 tbsps tamari

2 tsps toasted sesame oil

¼ tsp sugar

½ tsp gochugaru (Korean chilli flakes)

1 spring onion, chopped

2 hard boiled eggs, halved

STEPS

1. Drain rice and place in a steamer basket lined with greaseproof paper. Steam over a pan of simmering water for 35-45 minutes or until sticky and tender.
2. Place eggplants in a steamer over a pan of boiling water on high heat. Cook, covered, for 3 minutes until soft. Transfer to a bowl to cool.
3. Place the garlic, chilli, ginger, tamari, sesame oil, sugar and gochugaru in a small bowl. Whisk or stir to combine. Add spring onion and stir through.
4. Pour the mixture over the eggplant. Add egg halves and gently stir to coat.
5. Divide the rice between bowls. Top with eggplant mixture.

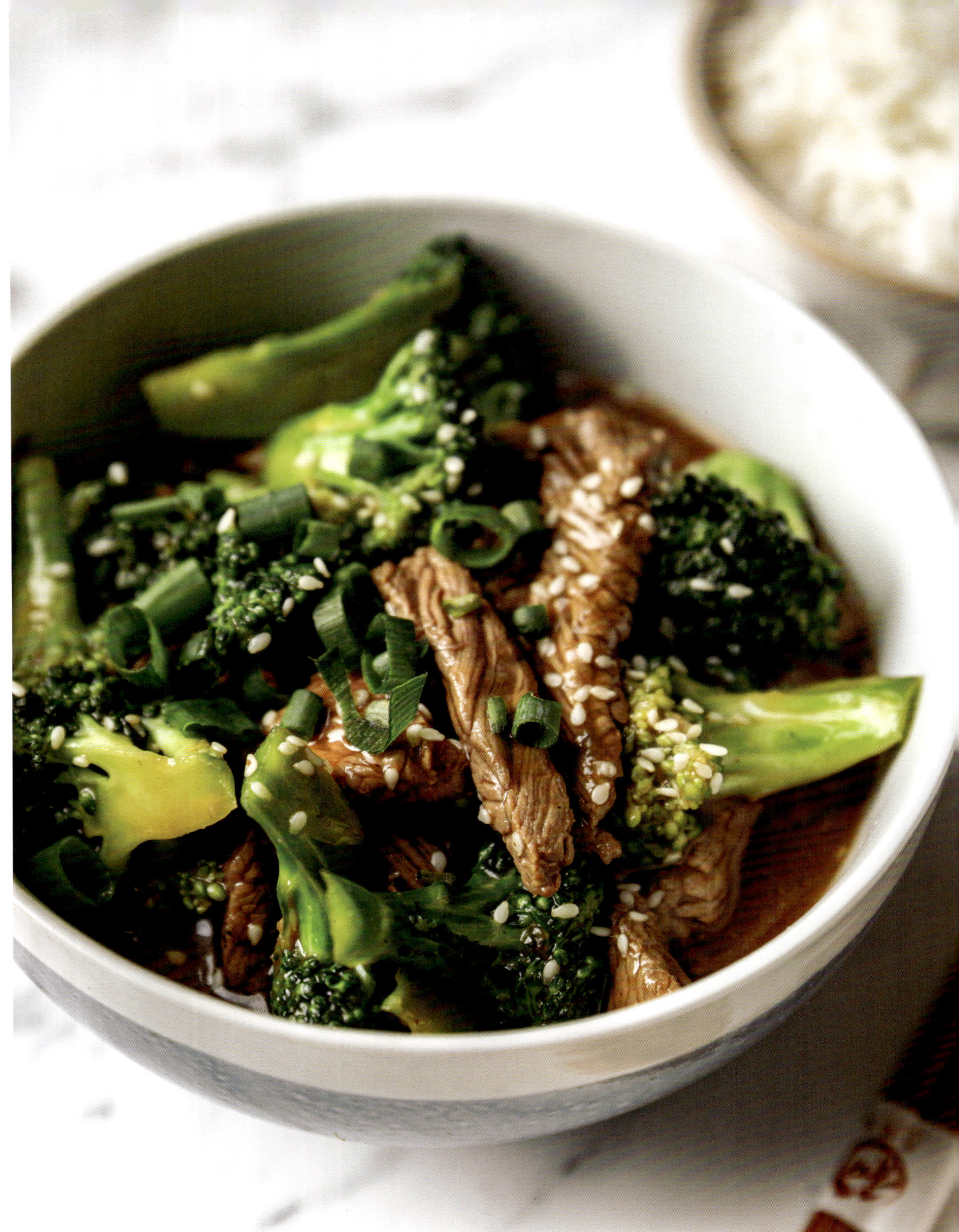

SERVES 4 | PREP + COOK TIME: 30 MINS | DAIRY FREE |

CHINESE BEEF & BROCCOLI

1 head broccoli, broken into florets

2 tbsps cornflour

1¼ cups (310ml) water

1 tsp sugar

2 tbsps soy sauce

1 tbsp Shaoxing wine

⅛ tsp Chinese five-spice powder

360g beef flank or rump, cut into bite-size pieces

2 tbsps peanut oil

1 clove garlic, finely chopped

Small piece ginger, finely chopped

2 spring onion tops, sliced

1 tsp sesame seeds

STEPS

1. Place the broccoli into a pan of boiling water. Cook for 1 minute from when water returns to a boil, until tender. Drain and set aside.
2. Place cornflour and ¼ cup of the water in a bowl and mix into a slurry. Add sugar, soy sauce, Shaoxing wine and five-spice powder. Stir to combine.
3. Place the beef and 2 tablespoons of the sauce into a bowl and set aside.
4. Heat oil in a frying pan over high heat. Add beef and cook for 1 minute until browned. Add garlic and ginger. Stir for another 30 seconds until fragrant. Pour sauce and remaining water into the pan and quickly mix. When the sauce starts bubbling, add broccoli and stir to coat. Simmer for 1 minute or until sauce is thickened.
5. Scatter with spring onions and sesame seeds to serve.

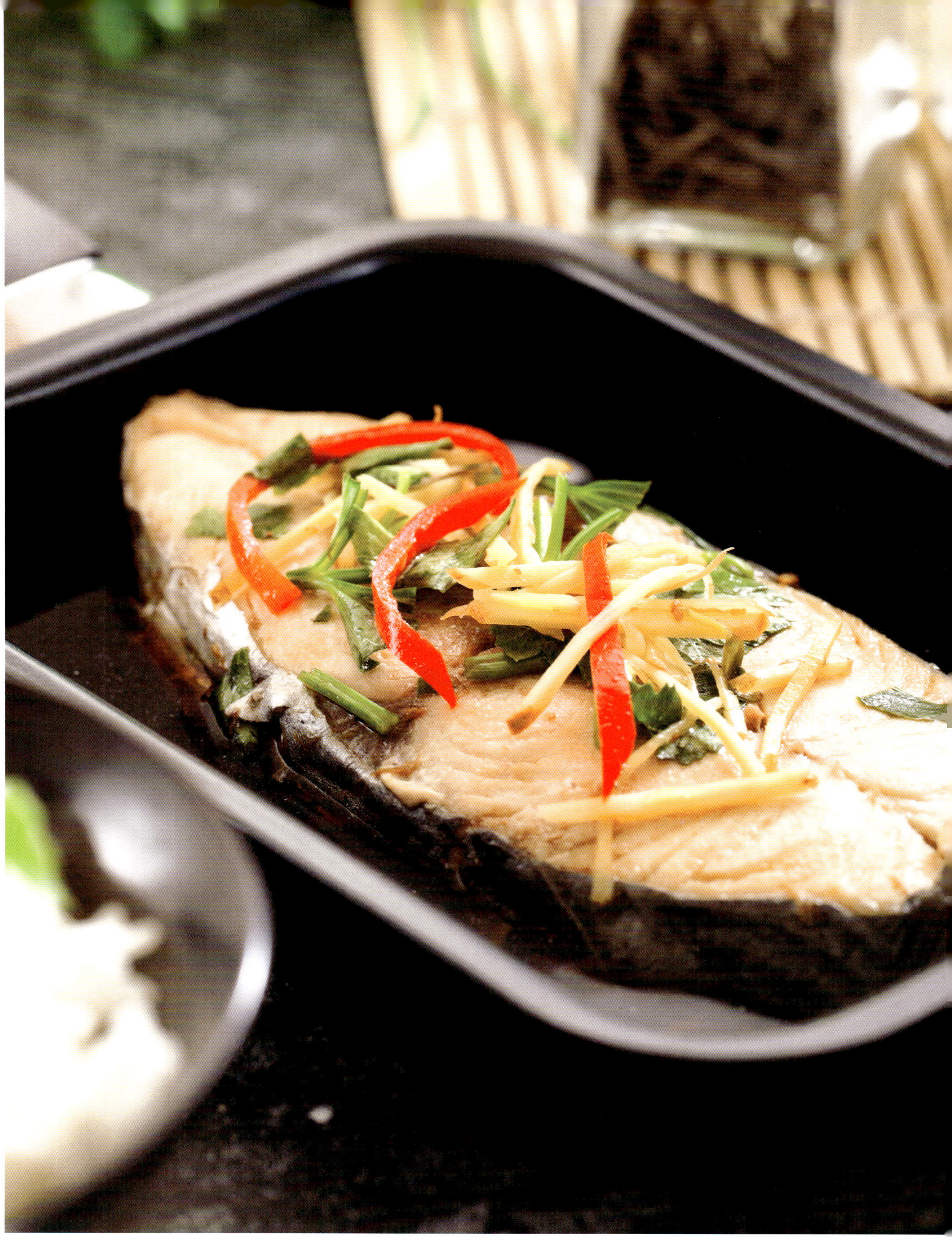

GINGER SOY MACKEREL

2 x 180g mackerel steaks
Medium piece ginger, julienned
¼ long red chilli, julienned
1 tbsp Shaoxing wine
1 tbsp soy sauce
1 tsp peanut oil
2 tsps sesame oil
Handful of coriander leaves, chopped

STEPS

1. Place mackerel steaks on a heatproof plate that fits into a large steamer. Scatter over ginger and chilli. Drizzle with Shaoxing wine and soy sauce. Cover and steam over a pan or wok of boiling water for 10 minutes until fish is cooked through.

2. Heat peanut oil and sesame oil in a small saucepan for 1-2 minutes until smoking.

3. Transfer fish to serving plates, drizzle over juices, then pour over hot oil. Scatter with coriander leaves to serve.

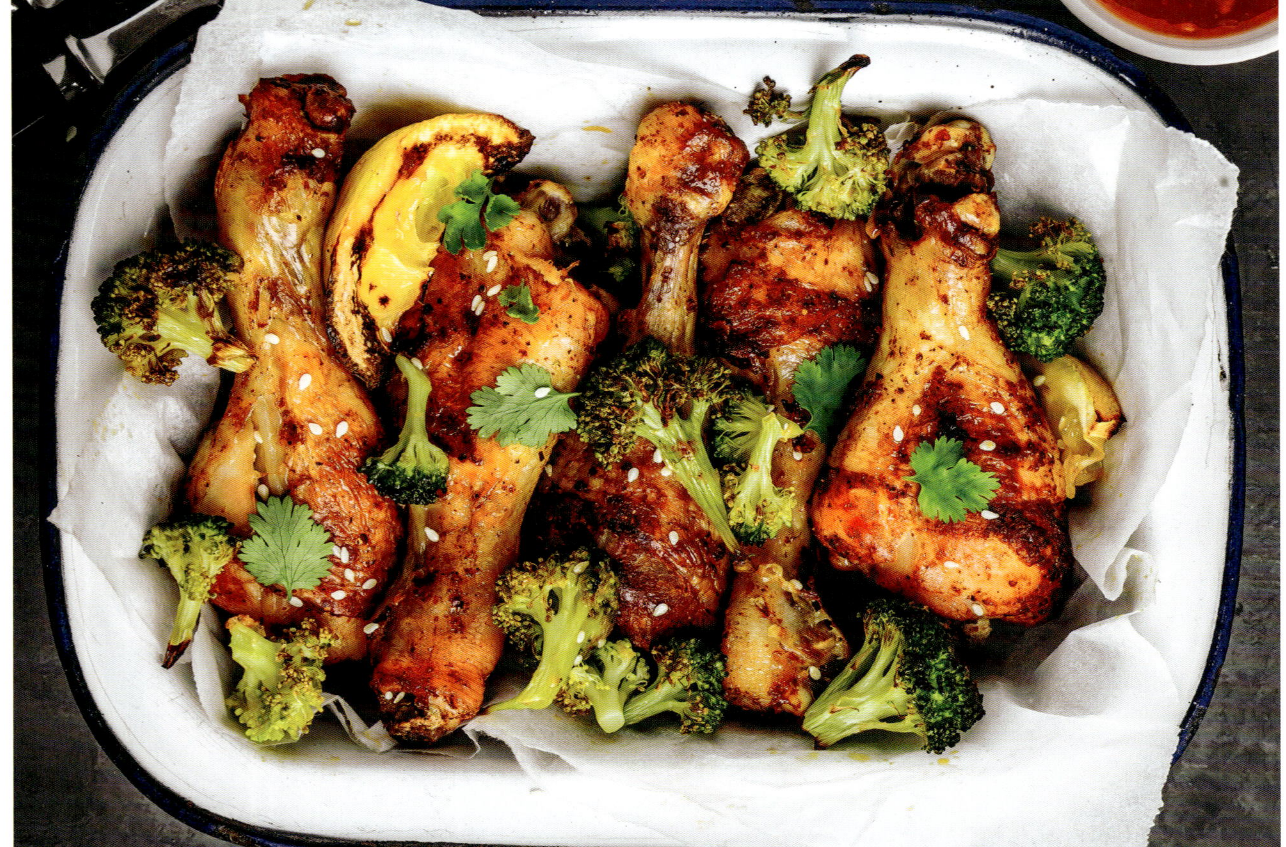

CHILLI ROAST BROCCOLI & CHICKEN

- 1 long red chilli, deseeded and finely chopped
- 1 tsp dried chilli flakes
- 2 tsps lemon zest
- 2 cloves garlic, crushed
- ½ tsp salt
- 2 tsps + 2 tbsps olive oil
- 8 chicken drumsticks
- 2-4 lemon wedges
- 1 head broccoli, cut into florets
- 1 tsp sesame seeds
- 2 tbsps coriander leaves

STEPS

Preheat oven to 200°C.

1. Combine chilli, chilli flakes, lemon zest, crushed garlic, salt and 2 teaspoons of oil in a small bowl and mix well. Place chicken in an ovenproof dish. Rub evenly with the chilli mixture. Cover and place in the fridge for 1 hour to marinate.
2. Drizzle chicken with the remaining oil and toss to coat. Nestle the lemon wedges into the dish around the chicken.
3. Roast for 15 minutes, then add broccoli to the dish. Turn the chicken and toss to coat the broccoli. Cook for a further 15 minutes until chicken is cooked though and broccoli is tender.
4. Scatter with sesame seeds and coriander leaves to serve.

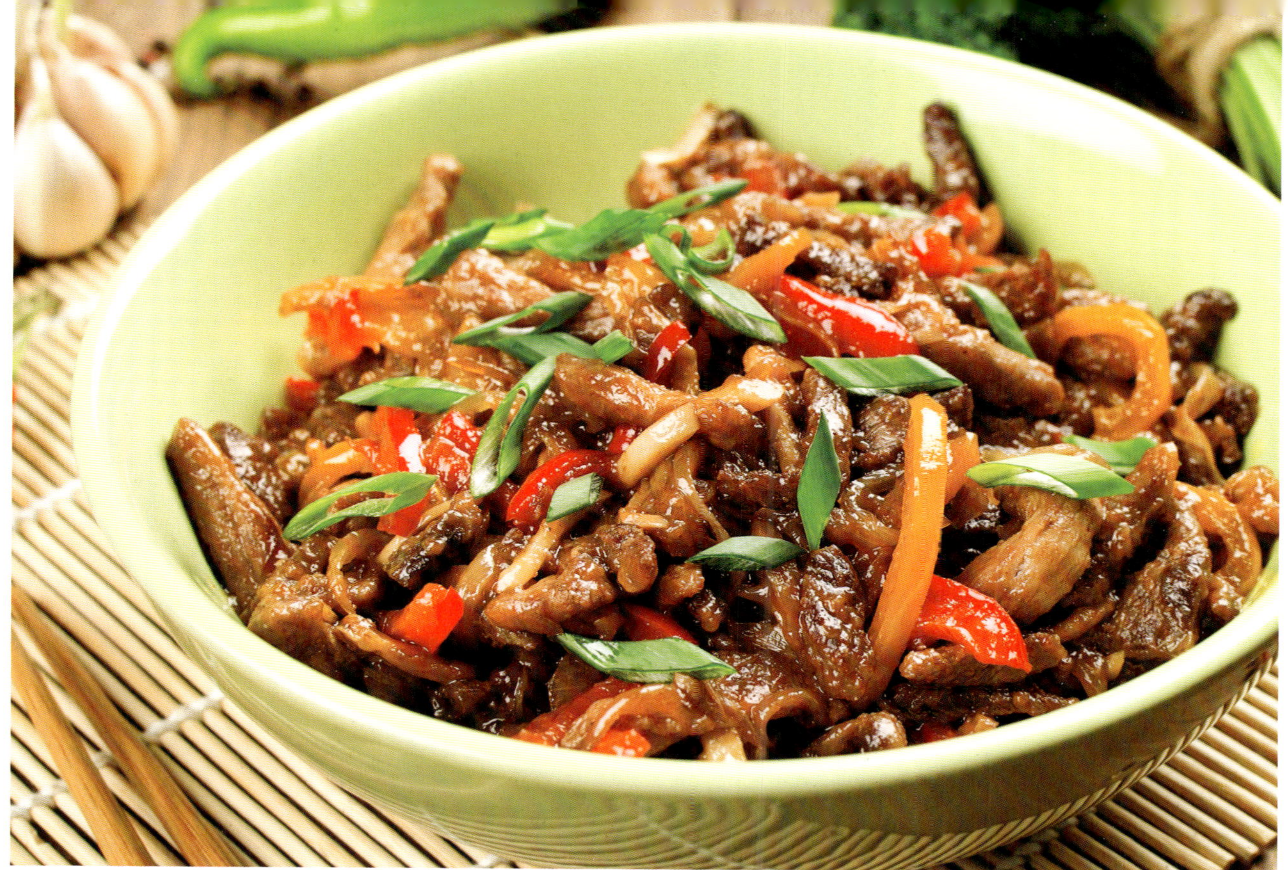

JAPANESE PORK STIR-FRY

500g pork loin or pork tenderloin, thinly sliced

2 tbsps tamari

2 tbsps mirin

1 tbsp sake or dry white wine

1 tbsp vegetable oil

1 red capsicum, thinly sliced

1 yellow capsicum, thinly sliced

1 onion, thinly sliced

2 cloves garlic, minced

Medium piece ginger, grated

2 tbsps oyster sauce

1 tbsp cornflour dissolved in 2 tbsps water

Spring onions, chopped, for garnish

STEPS

1. In a bowl, combine the sliced pork, tamari, mirin, and sake. Mix well and let it marinate for about 10-15 minutes.

2. Heat oil in a large frying pan or wok over medium-high heat. Add pork and stir-fry for 2-3 minutes, or until the pork is cooked through. Remove the pork from the pan and set aside.

3. In the same pan, add the sliced capsicums, onion, minced garlic and grated ginger. Stir-fry for about 3-4 minutes until the vegetables are tender-crisp.

4. Return the cooked pork to the pan and add oyster sauce. Stir-fry for another 2-3 minutes to coat the pork and vegetables with the sauce. Pour in the cornflour mixture and cook for an additional minute, stirring continuously, until the sauce thickens. Serve garnished with spring onions.

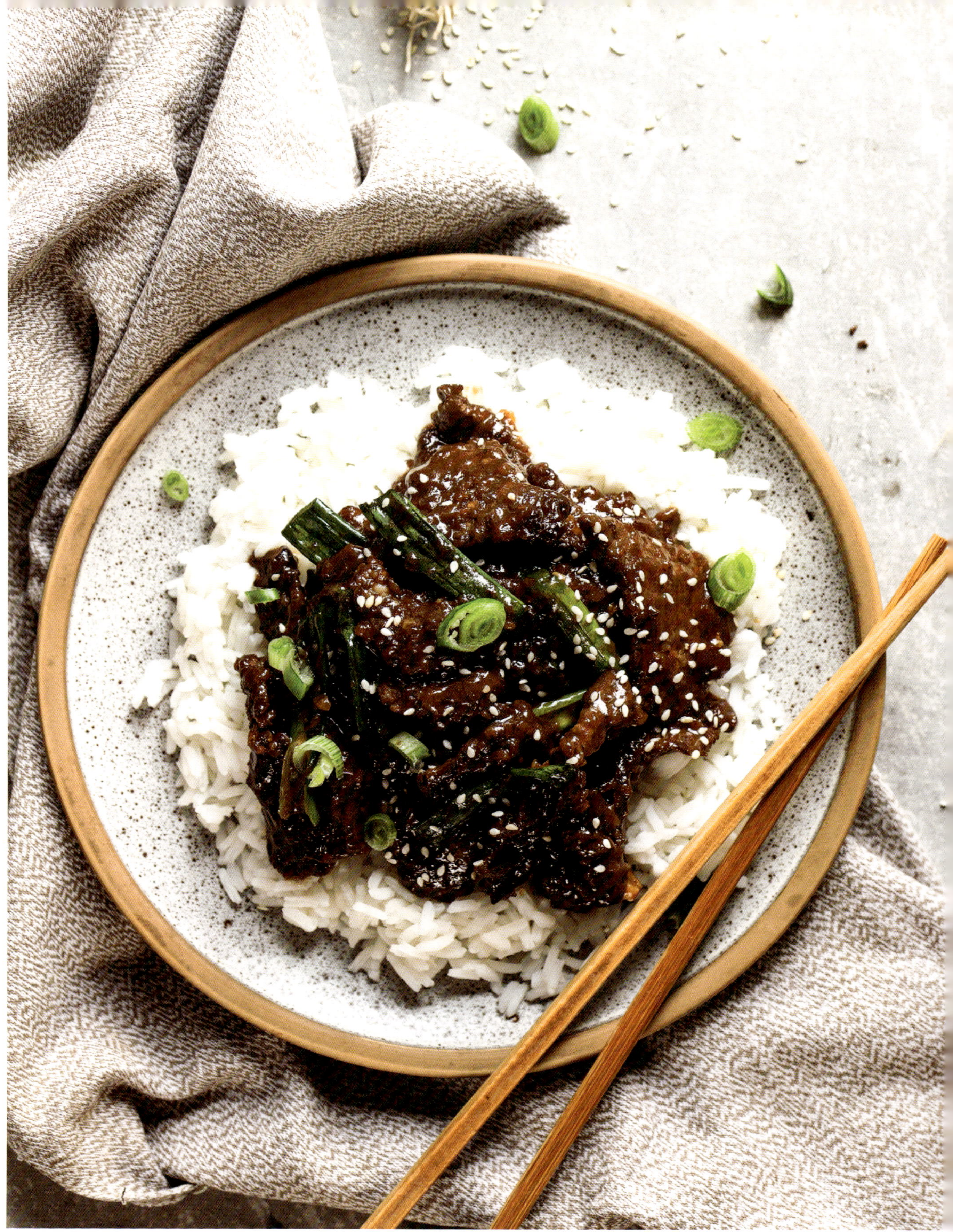

MONGOLIAN BEEF BOWL

1 tsp sesame oil

½ cup (125ml) soy sauce

⅓ cup (40g) cornflour

Pinch of salt and pepper

600g beef sirloin fillet, sliced

⅓ cup (80ml) peanut or other neutral-flavoured oil

½ tsp ginger, finely grated

3 cloves garlic, crushed

½ tsp chilli flakes

6 spring onions; 5 sliced into 4cm sections, 1 thinly sliced to garnish

½ cup (125ml) chicken stock

1 tbsp brown sugar

Steamed rice to serve

STEPS

1. In a large bowl, whisk the sesame oil, 1 teaspoon of the soy sauce and 1 tablespoon of the cornflour. Set aside.
2. Season remaining cornflour with salt and pepper and toss the beef in the flour mix to coat.
3. Heat the peanut oil in a wok over medium-high heat. Add the ginger, garlic and chilli and fry for 30 seconds until fragrant. Add the beef and spring onion and stir-fry for 3 minutes.
4. Add the rest of the soy sauce and the stock and once it's simmering, add the brown sugar and stir until dissolved.
5. Serve with steamed rice and scatter with sesame seeds and chopped spring onions.

SERVES 4 | PREP + COOK TIME: 20 MINS | DAIRY FREE |

MALAI KOFTA

KOFTAS

200g paneer (Indian cottage cheese), grated

2 medium potatoes, boiled and mashed

2 tbsps plain flour

1 tbsp cornflour

1 tsp ginger-garlic paste

1 tsp chilli powder

½ tsp garam masala

Salt to taste

Oil for frying

SAUCE

2 tbsps ghee or vegetable oil

1 large onion, finely chopped

1 clove garlic, minced

Small piece ginger, minced

2 tomatoes, grated

½ tsp ground turmeric

1 tsp chilli powder

1 tsp ground coriander

½ tsp ground cumin

¼ cup (30g) cashew nuts, soaked in water for 30 minutes and ground to a paste

½ cup (125ml) + 2 tbsps cream

Salt to taste

STEPS

1. In a mixing bowl, combine grated paneer, mashed potatoes, flour, cornflour, garlic-ginger paste, chilli powder, garam masala and salt. Mix well then shape into 12-15 round koftas.

2. Heat 5-10cm oil in a deep pan over medium heat. When the oil is hot, gently drop the koftas into the oil and fry until they turn golden brown. Remove with a slotted spoon and place on a plate lined with paper towel.

3. In a separate pan, heat ghee or vegetable oil over medium heat. Add onion and saute for 5-7 minutes until golden. Add garlic and ginger and saute for 1 minute until fragrant. Add the tomatoes and cook until the oil starts to separate from the masala. Reduce the heat to low and add turmeric, chilli powder, coriander and cumin. Mix well and cook for 2-3 minutes.

4. Stir in the cashew nut paste and cook for another 2 minutes. Add ½ cup cream and mix well. Season with salt. Simmer for 5-7 minutes.

5. Add the koftas to the sauce and simmer for a few minutes until heated through. Drizzle with cream to serve.

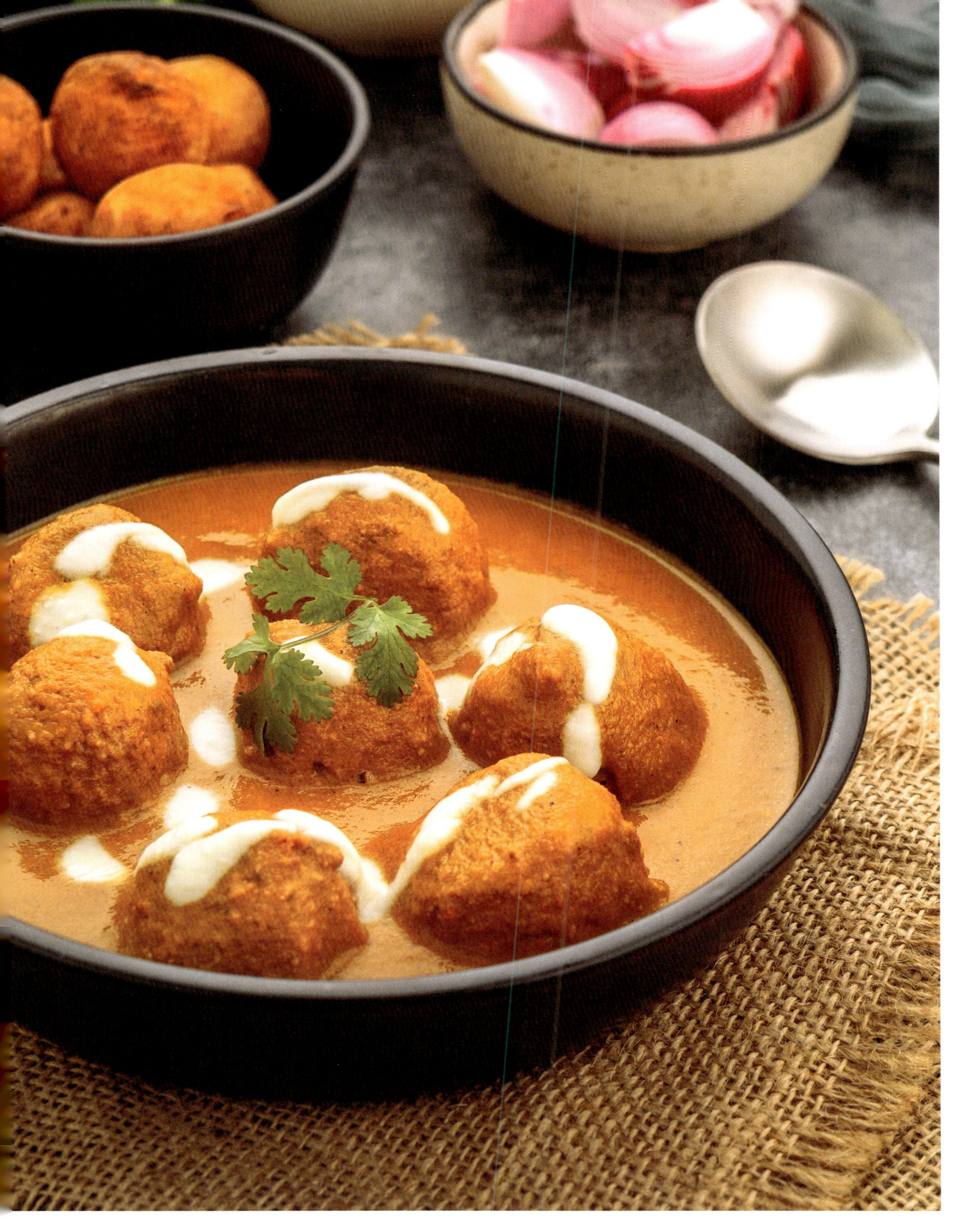

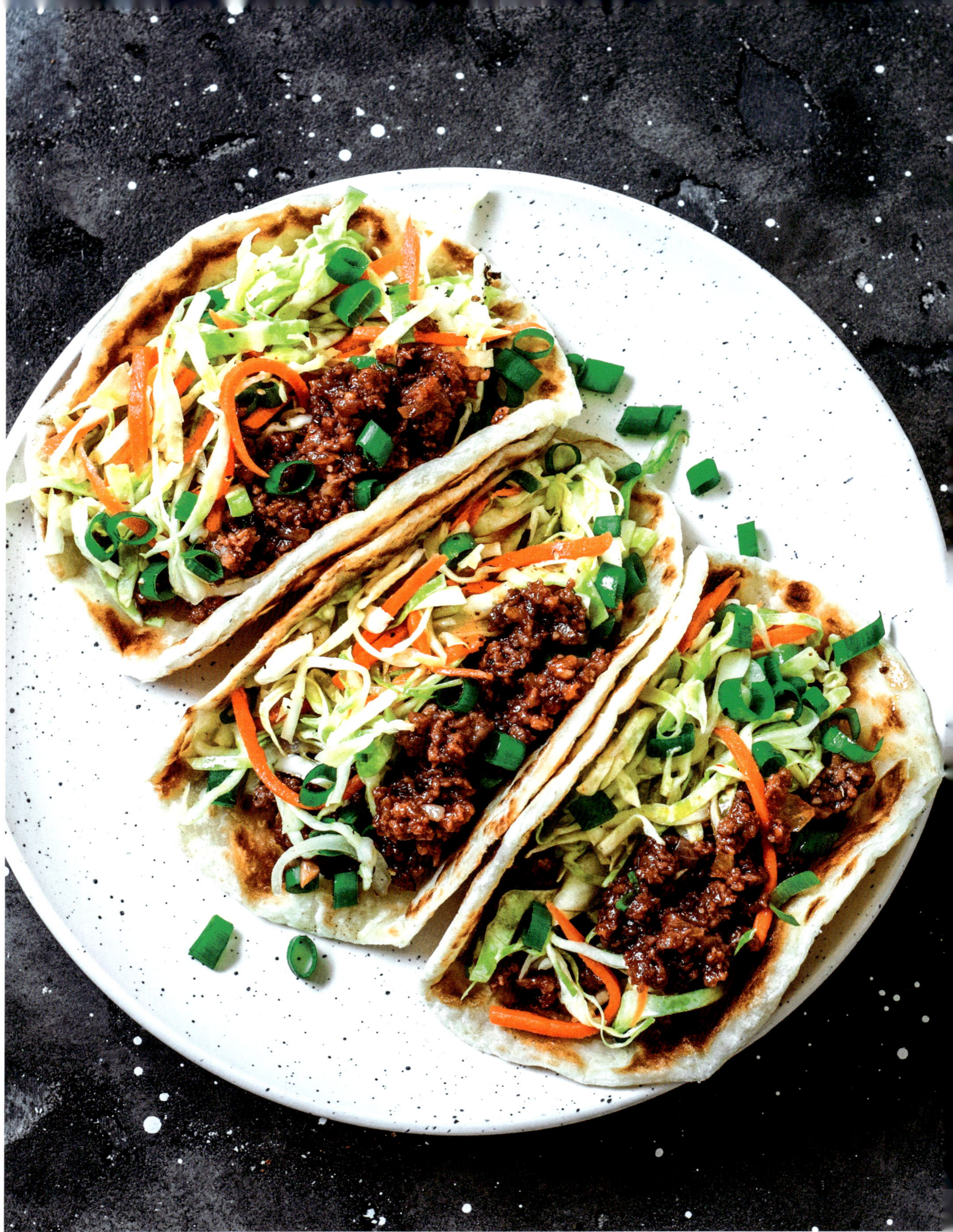

KOREAN BEEF TACOS

4 large or 8 small flatbreads or flour tortillas

500g green cabbage, thinly sliced

1 large carrot, julienned

2 tbsps rice wine vinegar

¼ tsp dried chilli flakes

1 tsp maple syrup

1 tsp + 1 tbsp sesame oil

Medium piece ginger, grated

4 cloves garlic, minced

500g beef mince

¾ cup (110g) brown sugar

¼ cup (60ml) soy sauce

1 tsp Sriracha

2 spring onions, chopped, to garnish

STEPS

Preheat the oven to 180°C.

1. Wrap the flatbreads in foil and place in the preheated oven to warm through.
2. Place the cabbage and carrot in a large bowl. Pour over vinegar, chilli, syrup, 1 teaspoon sesame oil, half the ginger and a quarter of the garlic. Toss to combine. Stand for 10 minutes.
3. Heat a large pan over medium-high heat. Stir-fry the meat with 1 tablespoon sesame oil, remaining garlic and ginger, for 5 minutes, until browned. Add brown sugar, soy sauce and Sriracha. Cook until the liquid has reabsorbed and the meat is shiny.
4. Spoon into warm flatbreads along with the cabbage salad. Top with spring onions and serve.

SERVES 4 | PREP + COOK TIME: 30 MINS | DAIRY FREE |

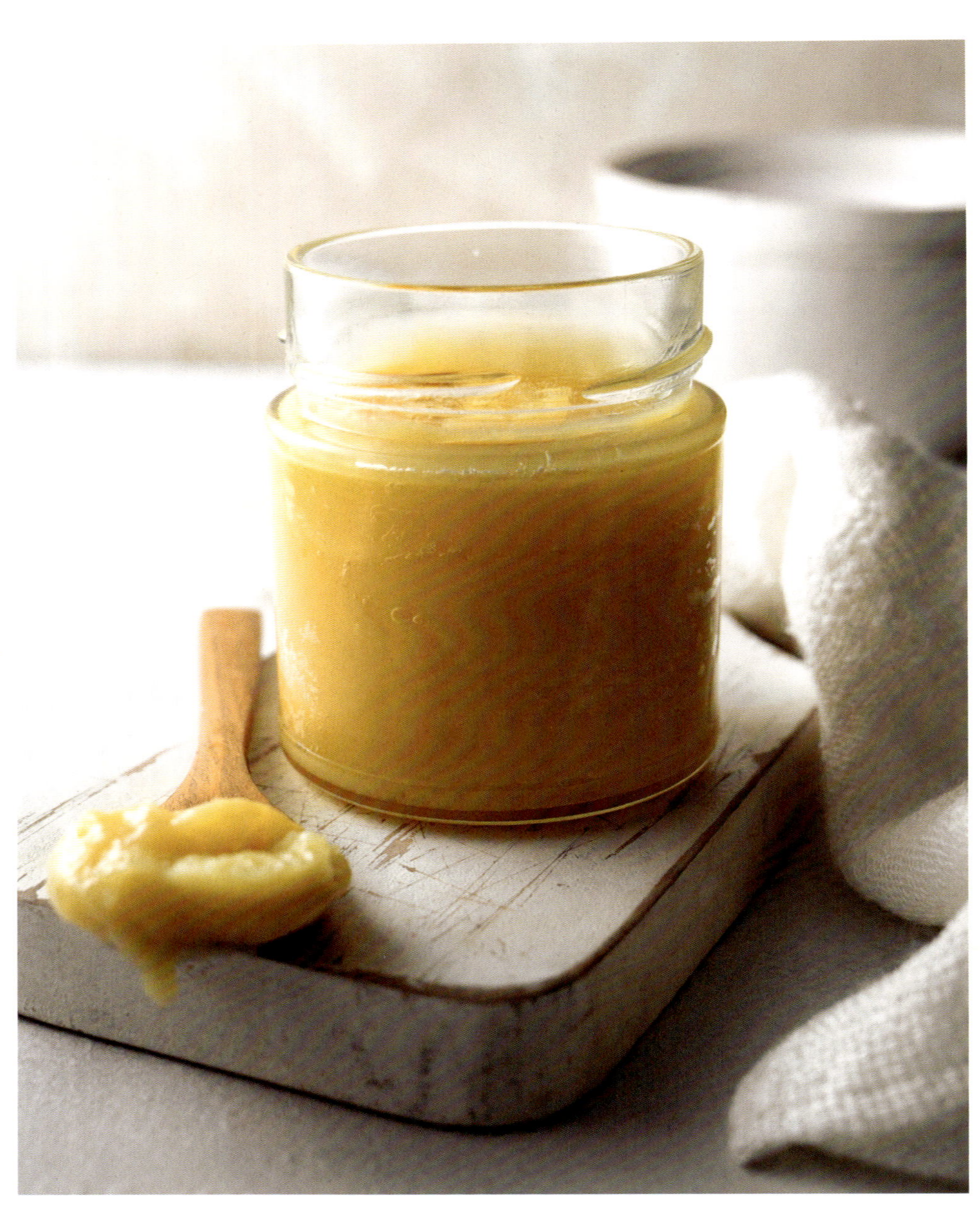

GRILLED, FRIED & BAKED

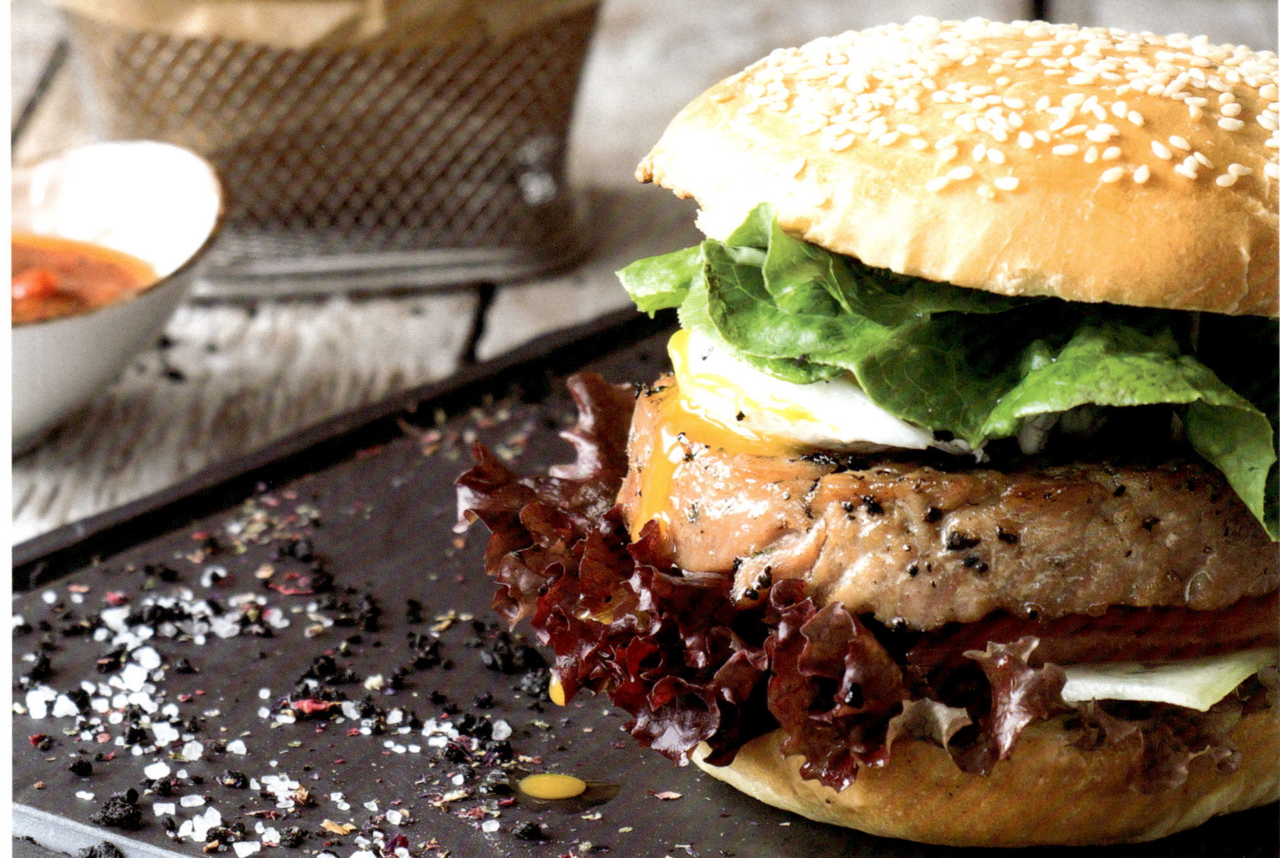

SEARED TUNA STEAK BURGERS

WASABI MAYONNAISE

4 tbsps mayonnaise

2 tsps wasabi paste

BURGERS

4 thick tuna steaks

3 tbsps olive oil

Salt and pepper to taste

4 eggs

4 burger buns

4 butter lettuce leaves

4 lollo rosso leaves or other bitter lettuce

1 Lebanese cucumber, sliced

2 Roma tomatoes, sliced

STEPS

1. Combine the mayonnaise and wasabi in a small bowl. Mix well, then cover and refrigerate until ready to use.
2. Brush the tuna steaks lightly with a little of the olive oil and season with salt and pepper. Heat a grill pan or nonstick frying pan over medium-high heat. When hot cook the tuna steaks for 1-2 minutes on each side depending on thickness.
3. Heat remaining oil in a large frying pan. Break the eggs into the pan and cook for 3-4 minutes until the whites are cooked and the yolk is runny.
4. Serve tuna steaks and fried eggs in burger buns with butter lettuce, lollo rosso, cucumber, tomato, a big dollop of wasabi mayonnaise and a sprinkling of salt and pepper.

SERVES 4 | PREP + COOK TIME: 35 MINS | DAIRY FREE |

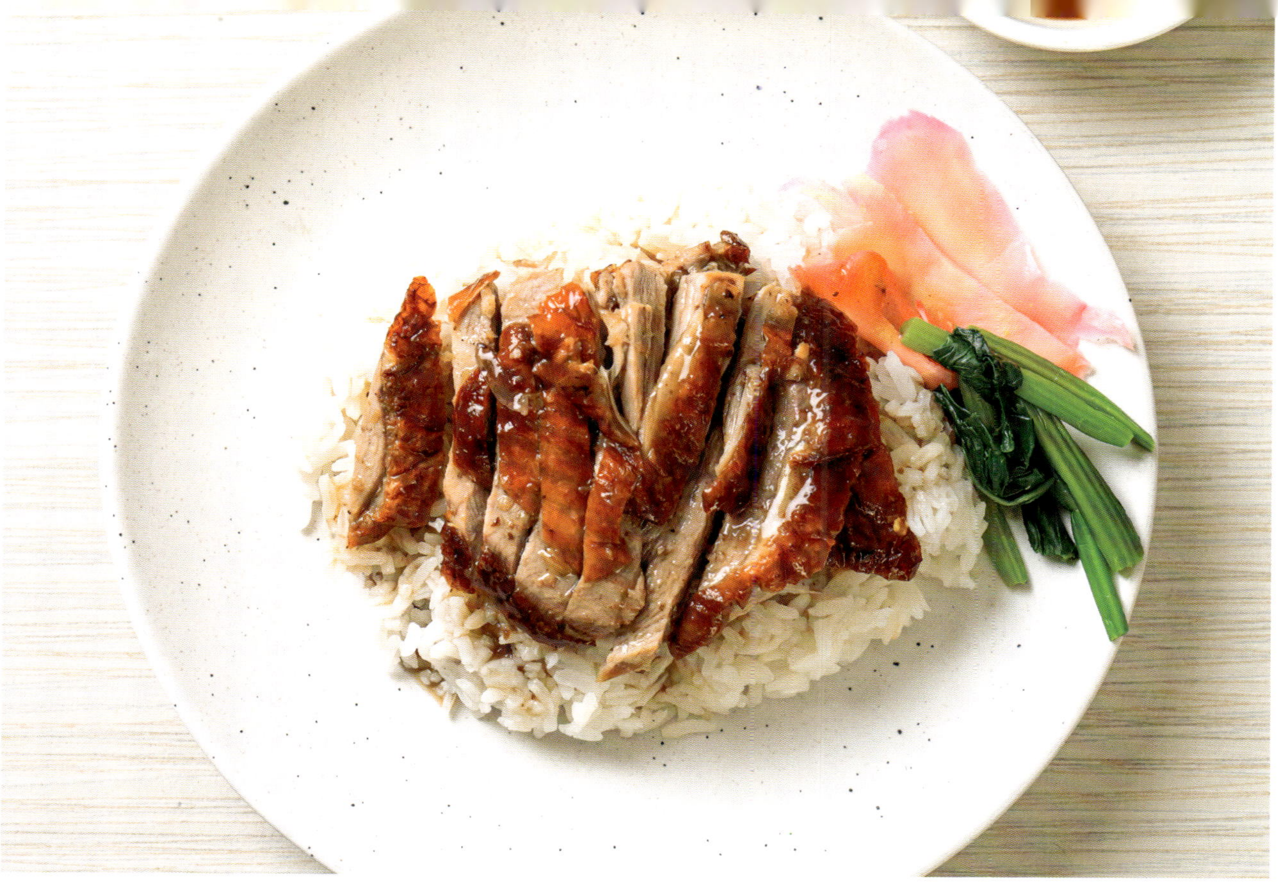

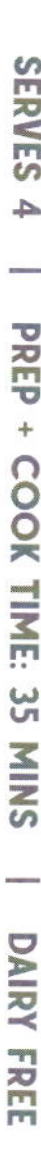

HOISIN ROASTED DUCK

4 duck breasts (boneless, skin-on)

2 tsps salt

1 tsp pepper

SAUCE

2 tsps sesame oil

4 cloves garlic, grated

Medium piece ginger, grated

4 tbsps hoisin sauce

2 tbsps honey

2 tbsps soy sauce

TO SERVE

Cooked rice, steamed greens and pickled ginger

STEPS

Preheat oven to 200°C.

1. Pat duck dry with paper towel. Score duck skin lightly and season with salt and pepper.
2. Place duck skin-side down in a frying pan. Place over medium-low heat and let the fat render out. Cook for 6-8 minutes, until the skin becomes crispy. Turn over and seal the meat for 1 minute.
3. Place the duck breast skin-side down on a lined baking tray. Bake for 8-10 minutes, flipping halfway through. Set aside to rest for 6-3 minutes.
4. Meanwhile heat sesame oil in a small saucepan over low heat. Add garlic and ginger and stir for few seconds. Add hoisin sauce, honey and soy sauce. Simmer and reduce until the sauce thickens.
5. Slice duck and serve with sauce, rice, steamed greens and pickled ginger.

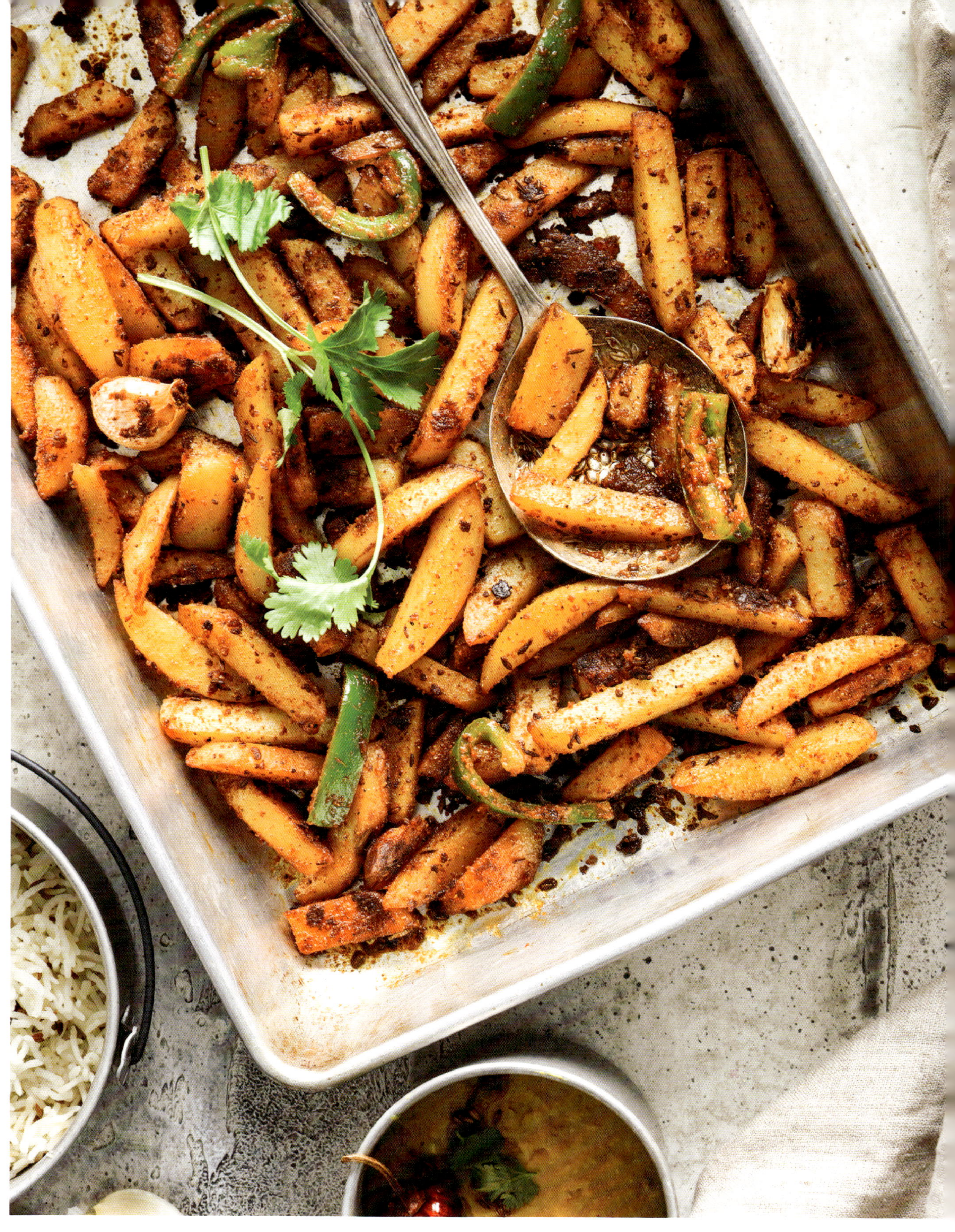

MASALA FRIES

½ tsp garam masala

½ tsp chilli powder

½ tsp dried mango powder (amchur powder)

½ tsp salt

3 tbsps olive oil

750g potatoes

1 green capsicum, sliced

4 cloves garlic, whole

1 tsp lemon juice

Handful fresh coriander leaves to serve

STEPS

Preheat oven to 200°C.

1. Place the garam masala, chilli powder, dried mango powder and salt in a large bowl along with the olive oil. Mix well and set aside.
2. Peel the potatoes. Wash and cut into fries. Soak in water for about 5-10 minutes to remove excess starch. Drain and pat dry.
3. Add potatoes, capsicum and garlic cloves to the bowl with the sauce mix. Toss to coat.
4. Transfer to a roasting tin. Bake for 40-45 minutes, until tender, turning once.
5. Drizzle with lemon juice and scatter with coriander leaves to serve.

SERVES 4 | PREP + COOK TIME: 1 HOUR | VEG | GLUTEN FREE | DAIRY FREE |

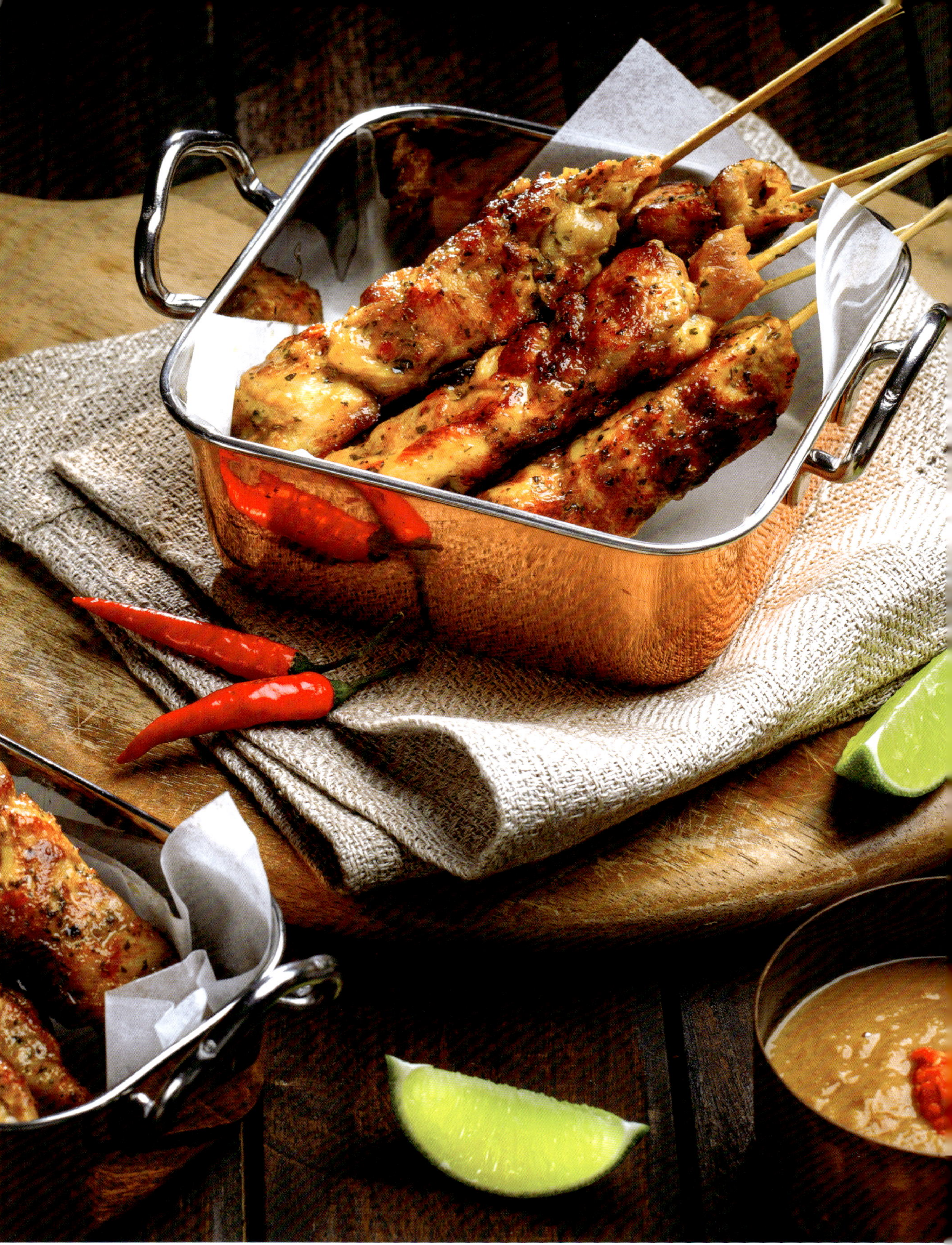

BARBECUE CHILLI PORK SKEWERS

500g pork fillets, cut into 2cm pieces
Medium piece ginger, grated
¼ tsp dried chilli flakes
2 tsps chilli paste
¼ cup (60ml) peanut oil
1 tsp sesame oil
3 cloves garlic, minced
4 tbsps tamari

PEANUT DIPPING SAUCE

¾ cup (190g) peanut butter
¼ cup (60ml) rice wine vinegar
⅓ cup (80ml) tamari
3 tbsps honey
Small piece ginger, grated
1 clove garlic, minced
2 tsps Sriracha, or to taste
2-4 tbsps coconut milk

STEPS

1. Place pork into a shallow dish. Combine ginger, chilli flakes, chilli paste, peanut oil, sesame oil, garlic and tamari. Whisk to combine. Pour over pork. Toss to coat. Cover and refrigerate for at least 1 hour or overnight.
2. Drain pork, reserving marinade. Thread pork onto skewers (see note). Preheat a barbecue plate on medium-high.
3. Barbecue skewers for 8 minutes or until cooked through, turning and basting with marinade often.
4. Whisk together the dipping sauce ingredients, adding enough coconut milk to reach your desired consistency. Serve with the cooked skewers.

NOTE: For best results, soak skewers in water for 30 minutes first to prevent them from burning or breaking while cooking.

SERVES 4 | PREP + COOK TIME: 25 MINS + MARINATING | GLUTEN FREE | DAIRY FREE |

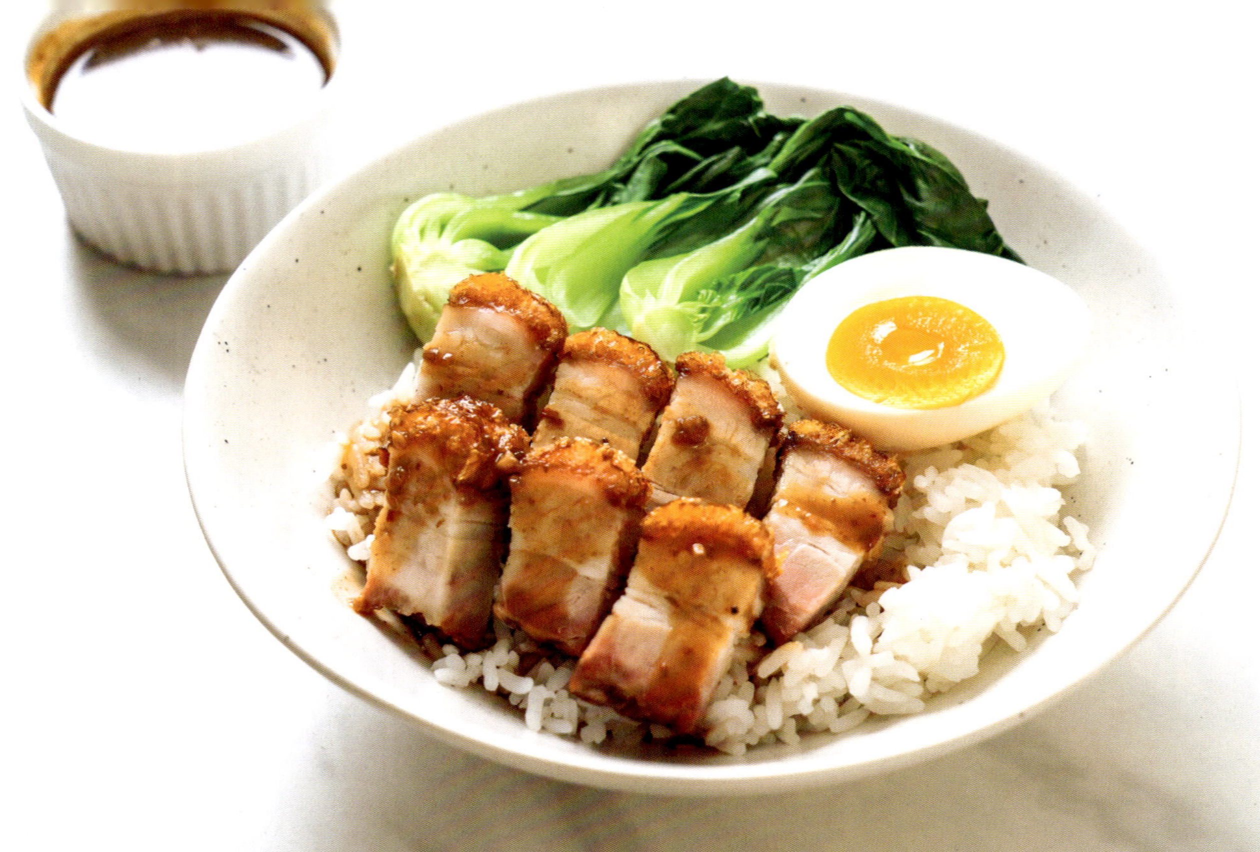

CRISPY PORK BELLY

1 tbsp Chinese five-spice powder

1 tbsp oil

1kg pork belly, dried and scored all over

2 tsps salt

Cooked rice, steamed bok choy and hard-boiled egg halves to serve

CARAMELISED CHILLI SAUCE

1 tbsp oil

3 cloves garlic, chopped

1 large shallot, finely chopped

4 red chillies, finely chopped

Large piece ginger, finely chopped

1 cup (250ml) white wine

¼ cup (60ml) hoisin sauce

1½ tbsps soy sauce

½ cup (125ml) water or chicken stock

¼ cup (50g) brown sugar

STEPS

Preheat oven to 220°C.

1. Mix five-spice and oil together to form a paste. Rub paste into meat side of pork belly. Rub salt into skin side.
2. Place pork skin-side down on a rack in a tray. Roast for 15 minutes, then turn pork over and roast for 25-30 minutes, or until the skin crackles.
3. To make the sauce, heat oil in a frying pan and add garlic, shallot, chilli and ginger. Saute for 3-4 minutes, then add wine and allow to bubble before adding the remaining ingredients. Simmer sauce for 5 minutes until sticky.
4. Cut pork belly into small pieces. Pour over sauce. Serve with rice, bok choy and hard-boiled egg halves.

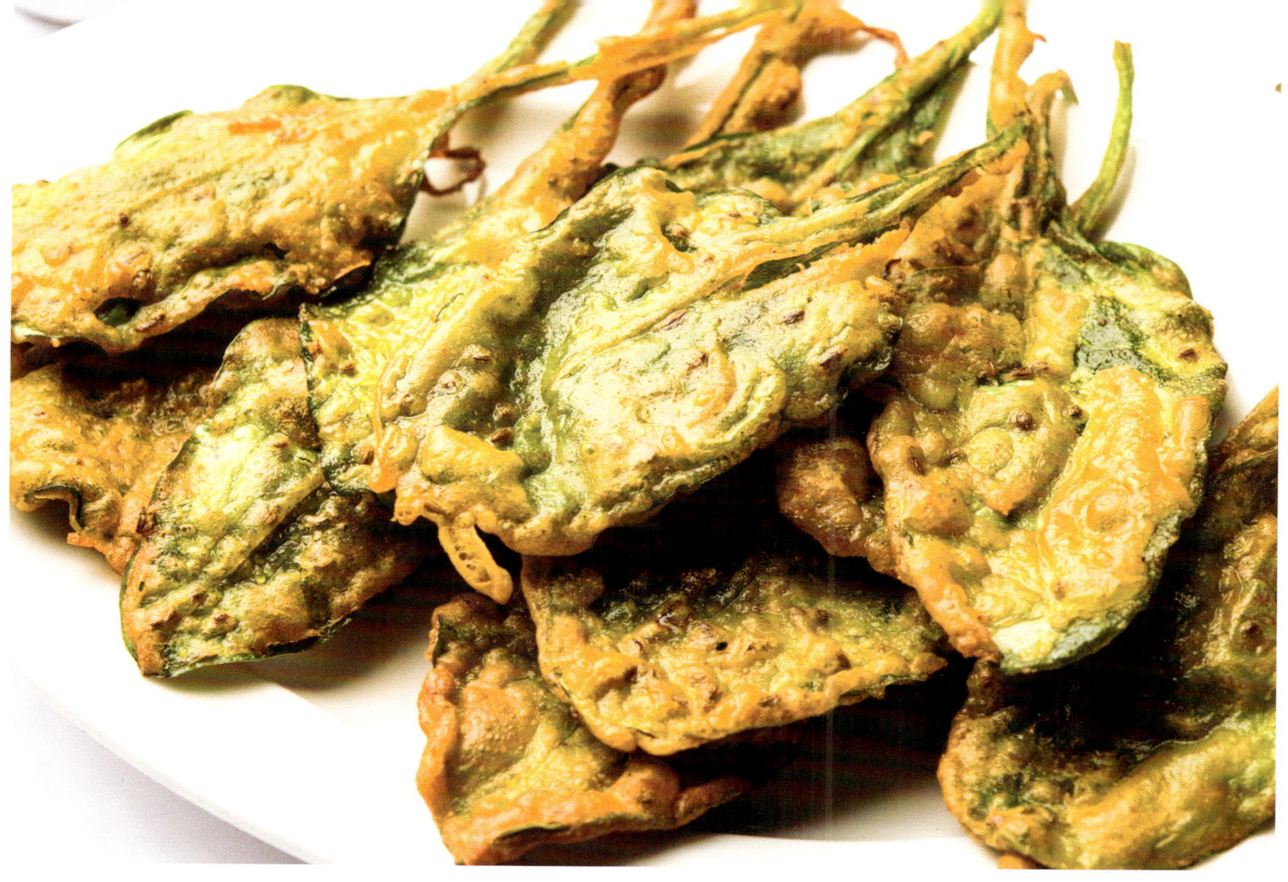

SERVES 4 | PREP + COOK TIME: 20 MINS | VEG | GLUTEN FREE | DAIRY FREE |

CRISPY PALAK

½ cup (45g) besan (chickpea flour)
1 tsp ground turmeric
½ tsp asafoetida
½ tsp chilli powder
½ tsp ground fennel seeds
¼ tsp ajwain seeds
½ tsp salt
1 tbsp rice flour
⅓ cup (100ml) water
1¼ cups (300ml) vegetable oil
100g spinach leaves, washed and dried

STEPS

1. Place the besan, turmeric, asafoetida, chilli powder, ground fennel seeds, ajwain seeds, salt and rice flour in a bowl and mix well. Add water and mix to a smooth batter.
2. Heat the oil in a wok or wide, deep frying pan. When hot, dip each spinach leaf into the batter, shake off the excess and drop into the oil. Work in batches making sure you don't overcrowd the pan. Cook for 2-3 minutes until golden and crisp.
3. Transfer to a plate lined with paper towel using a slotted spoon to drain before serving.

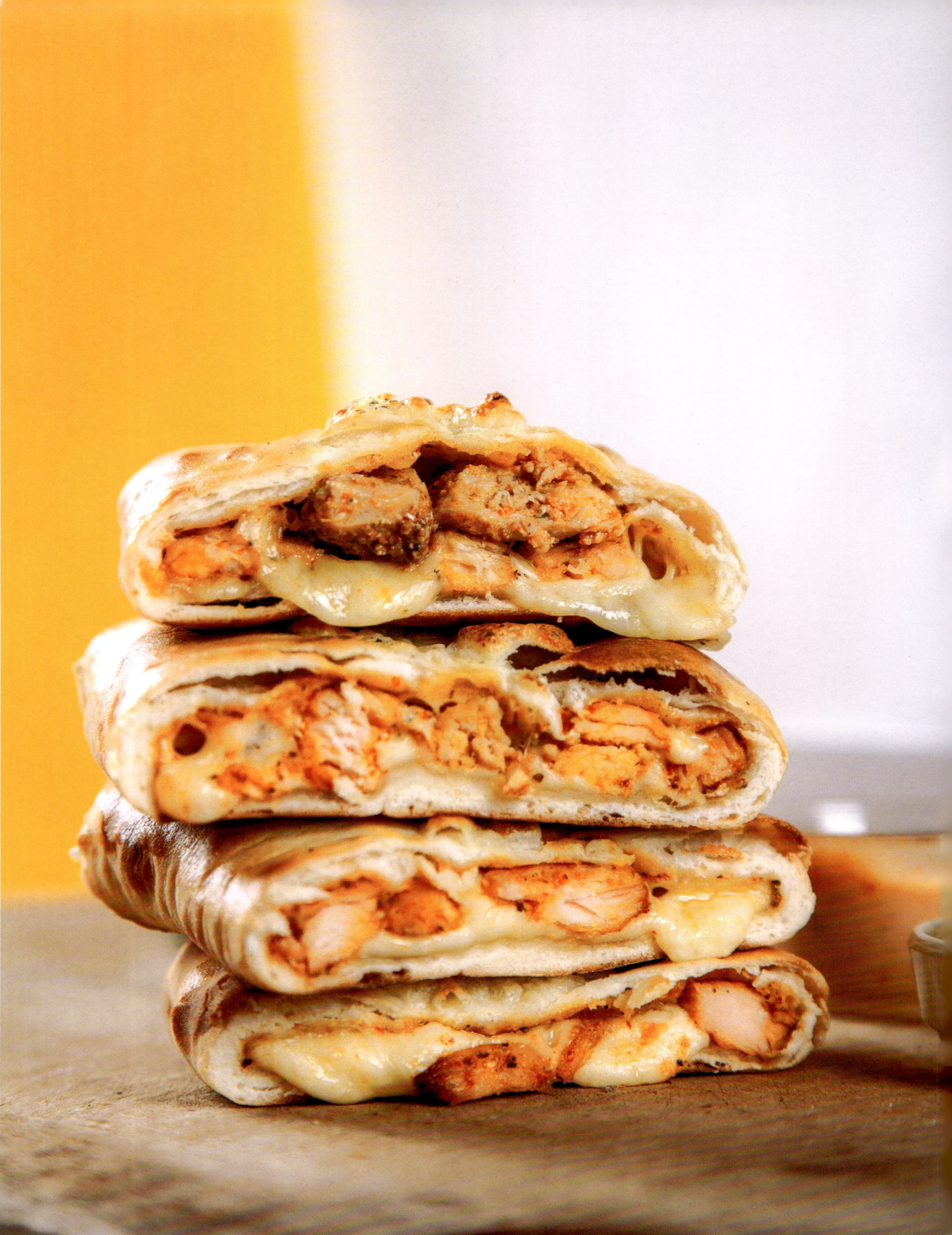

TANDOORI CHICKEN NAAN WRAPS

500g chicken breast or boneless, skinless chicken thighs, cubed

3 tbsps olive oil + 1 tbsp for frying

¼ cup (60ml) plain yoghurt

Medium piece fresh ginger, minced

4 cloves garlic, minced

2 tsps garam masala

2 tsps cumin

2 tsps mild chilli powder

½ tbsp ground turmeric

1 tsp ground coriander

1 tsp paprika

¼ tsp cayenne pepper

1 tsp salt

Juice of 1 lime

4 large naan breads

1 cup (125g) mozzarella cheese, shredded

STEPS

1. Add the chicken to a large bowl along with the olive oil, yoghurt, ginger, garlic, spices and lime juice. Mix well. Leave to marinate for at least 30 minutes or overnight in the fridge.
2. Preheat oven to 175°C.
3. Heat oil in a large cast-iron frying pan over medium-high heat. Add the chicken and cook for 4-5 minutes on each side until a nice brown crust develops. Reduce the heat to low and cook for a minute or two more until cooked through.
4. Spoon the chicken into the centre of each naan. Sprinkle with cheese. Fold the naan around the chicken and cheese. Wrap each naan tightly in foil.
5. Place the wrapped naan in the oven and heat for 10-15 minutes until the bread is warm and the cheese is melted. Serve immediately.

SERVES 4 | PREP + COOK TIME: 30 MINS + MARINATING |

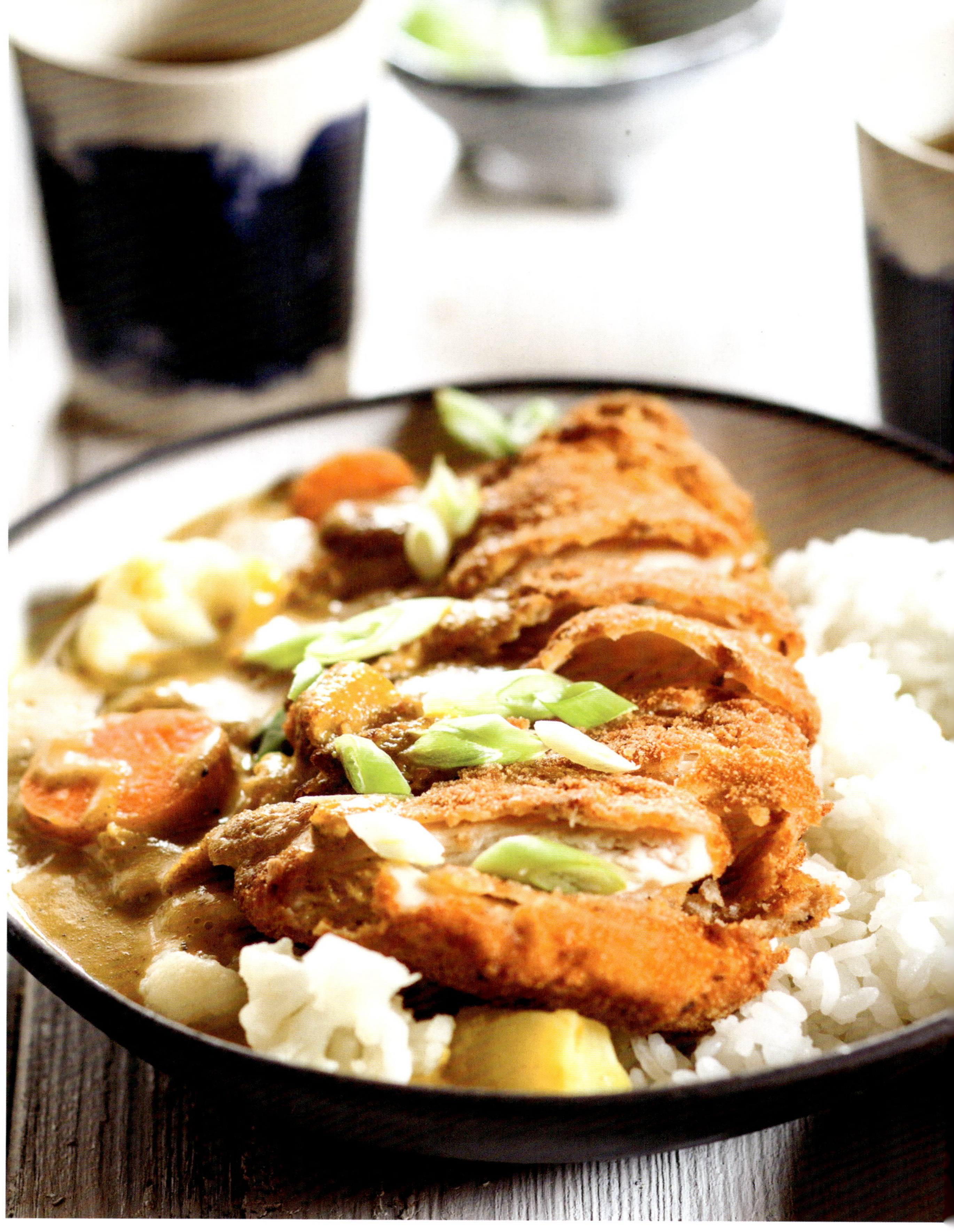

CHICKEN KATSU CURRY

4 chicken breast fillets, halved lengthways

Salt to taste

1 cup (125g) plain flour

2 eggs, lightly whisked

2 cups (250g) panko breadcrumbs

Vegetable oil for shallow frying

CURRY SAUCE (SEE NOTE)

2 tbsps vegetable oil

1 onion, finely diced

2 cloves garlic, finely chopped

1 tbsp plain flour

1 tbsp curry powder

1 tsp garam masala

2 tsps rice wine vinegar

2 tsps honey

2 cups (500ml) chicken stock

¾ cup (185ml) apple juice

1 tbsp finely grated ginger

1 carrot, thinly sliced

1 cup (100g) cauliflower florets

2 tbsps cornflour mixed with 2 tbsps water

Salt to taste

TO SERVE

Steamed rice

Chopped spring onion

STEPS

1. To make the curry sauce, heat the vegetable oil in a saucepan over medium-high heat. Add the onion and cook, stirring, for 8-10 minutes until golden. Add the garlic and cook for another minute. Add flour and cook, stirring, for another minute. Stir through the curry powder and garam masala. Add vinegar, honey, chicken stock, apple juice and ginger. Stir until well combined. Add the carrot and cauliflower and simmer for 20 minutes until vegetables are tender. Then stir through the cornflour mixture. Simmer for a further minute to thicken. Season with salt to taste. Keep warm.

2. Meanwhile season each piece of chicken with salt. Place the flour, eggs and breadcrumbs in separate shallow dishes. Coat each piece of chicken first in flour, then egg and then in the breadcrumbs.

3. Heat about 2cm of oil in the bottom of a large frying pan over medium-high heat. When the oil is hot, add the chicken in batches and cook for about 4 minutes each side or until golden and the chicken is cooked through. Transfer to a plate lined with paper towel to drain. Season with salt.

4. Cut the chicken into slices. Serve the curry sauce with rice and top with chicken slices and scatter with chopped spring onion.

NOTE: You can buy pre-made katsu curry sauces at most supermarkets. Choose this option to save time and effort.

SERVES 4 | PREP + COOK TIME: 55 MINS | DAIRY FREE |

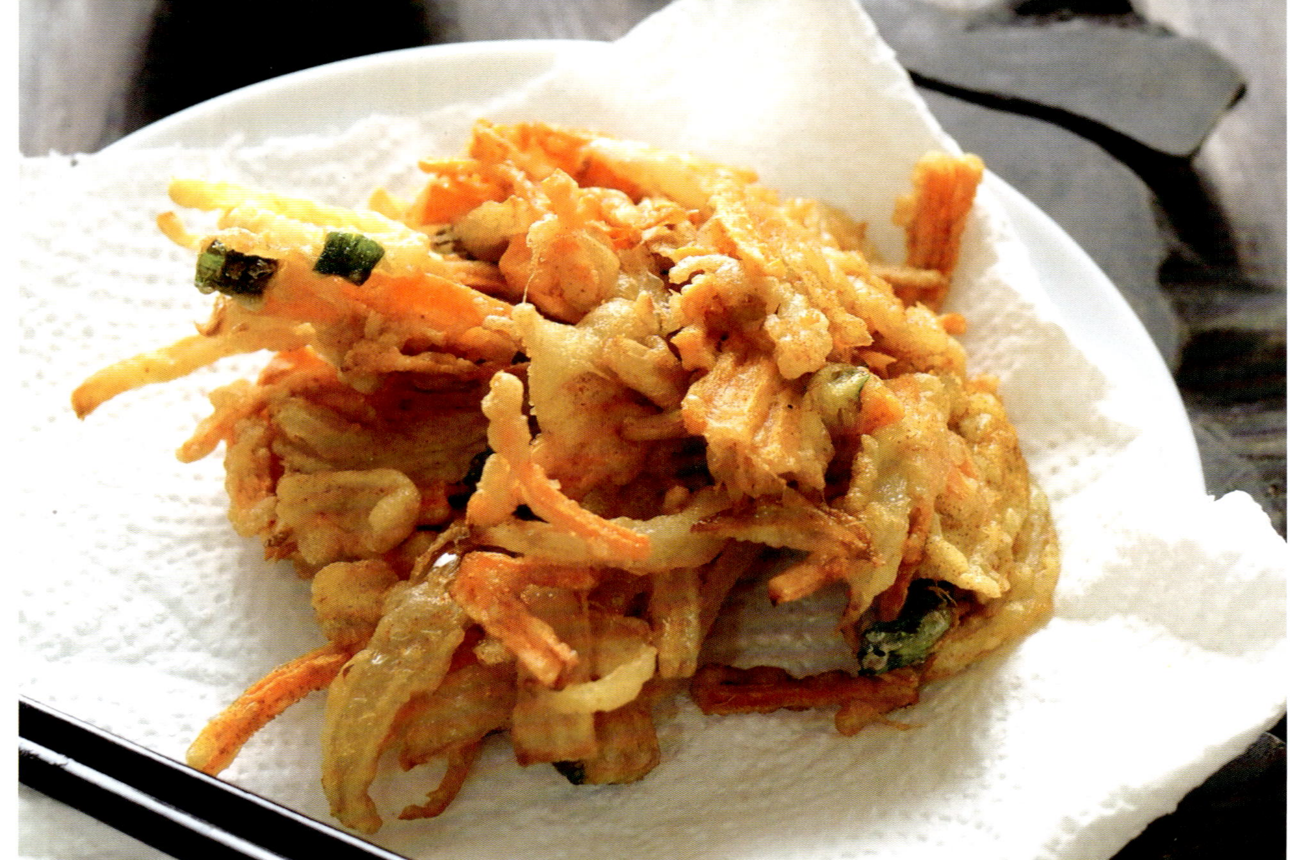

KAKIAGE TEMPURA

1 onion, thinly sliced

1 carrot, julienned

¼ sweet potato, julienned

3 shiso leaves, thinly sliced (optional)

7 tbsps plain flour

Salt to taste

⅓ cup (100ml) water

¼ cup (50ml) oil

STEPS

1. Place the sliced vegetables in a bowl with 2 tablespoons flour. Toss to coat.
2. Place the remaining flour and ½ teaspoon salt in a separate bowl and pour in the water, mix together until just combined. Add the sliced vegetables and stir to coat.
3. Heat oil in a deep frying pan to 170°C. Scoop small amounts of the mixture with a ladle. Use a pair of chopsticks to gently slide the mixture into the oil. Deep fry the batter till golden brown on both sides.
4. Remove with a slotted spoon and drain on a plate lined with paper towel. Season with salt to serve.

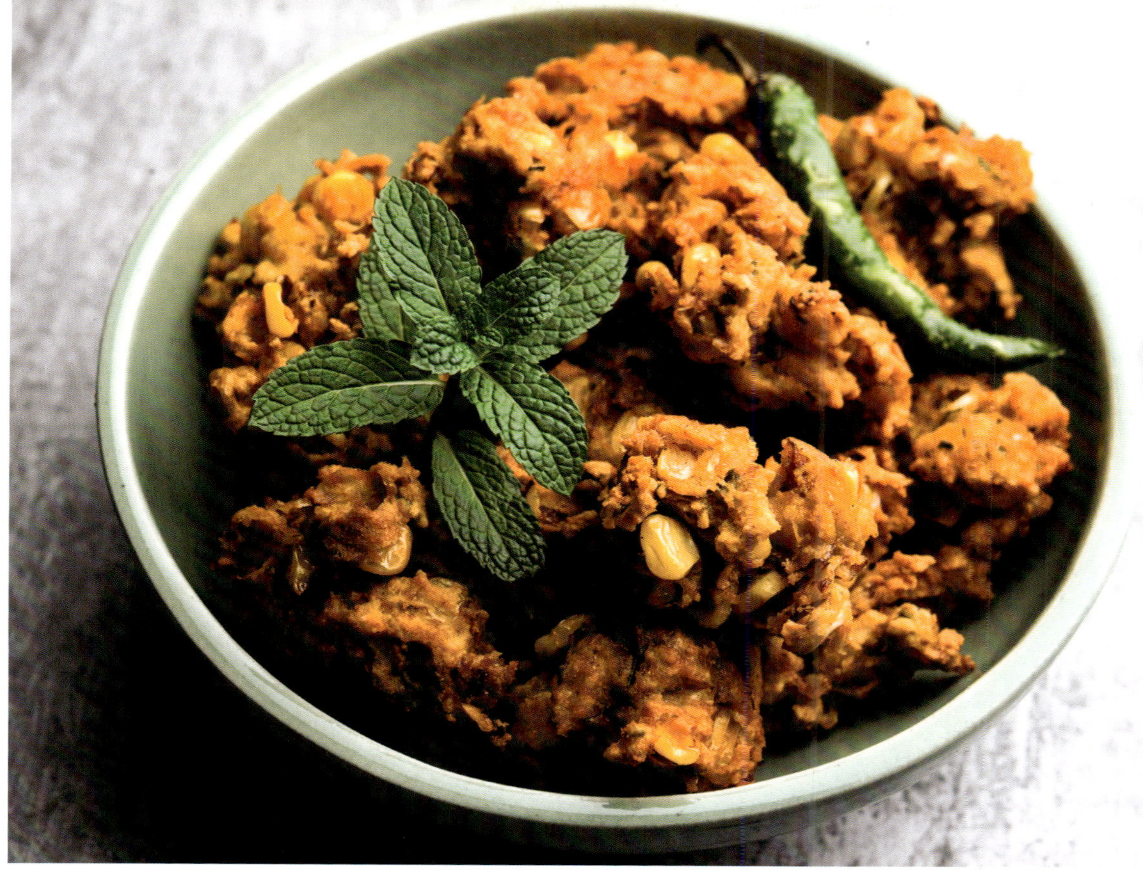

SERVES 4 | PREP + COOK TIME: 30 MINS | VEG | GLUTEN FREE | DAIRY FREE |

CORN PAKORAS

1½ cups (260g) corn kernels

2 gloves garlic, minced

Small piece ginger, grated

½ tsp cumin seeds

3 tbsps besan (chickpea flour)

2 tbsps rice flour

1-2 tsps garam masala

1 small red onion, sliced

2 green chillies, chopped

1 tbsp chopped coriander leaves

½ tsp salt

⅛ tsp ground turmeric

½ tsp chilli powder

Oil for frying

STEPS

1. Steam the corn over a pan of simmering water for 7-8 minutes until tender. Set aside to cool for 5 minutes.
2. Add corn to a large bowl along with all the remaining ingredients except oil. Mix and squash with your hands.
3. Heat at least 5cm oil in a heavy-bottomed saucepan over medium heat. When the oil is hot drop small amounts of the mixture into the oil and cook undisturbed for 3-4 minutes until crisp and golden brown.
4. Remove with a slotted spoon and drain on a plate lined with paper towel before serving.

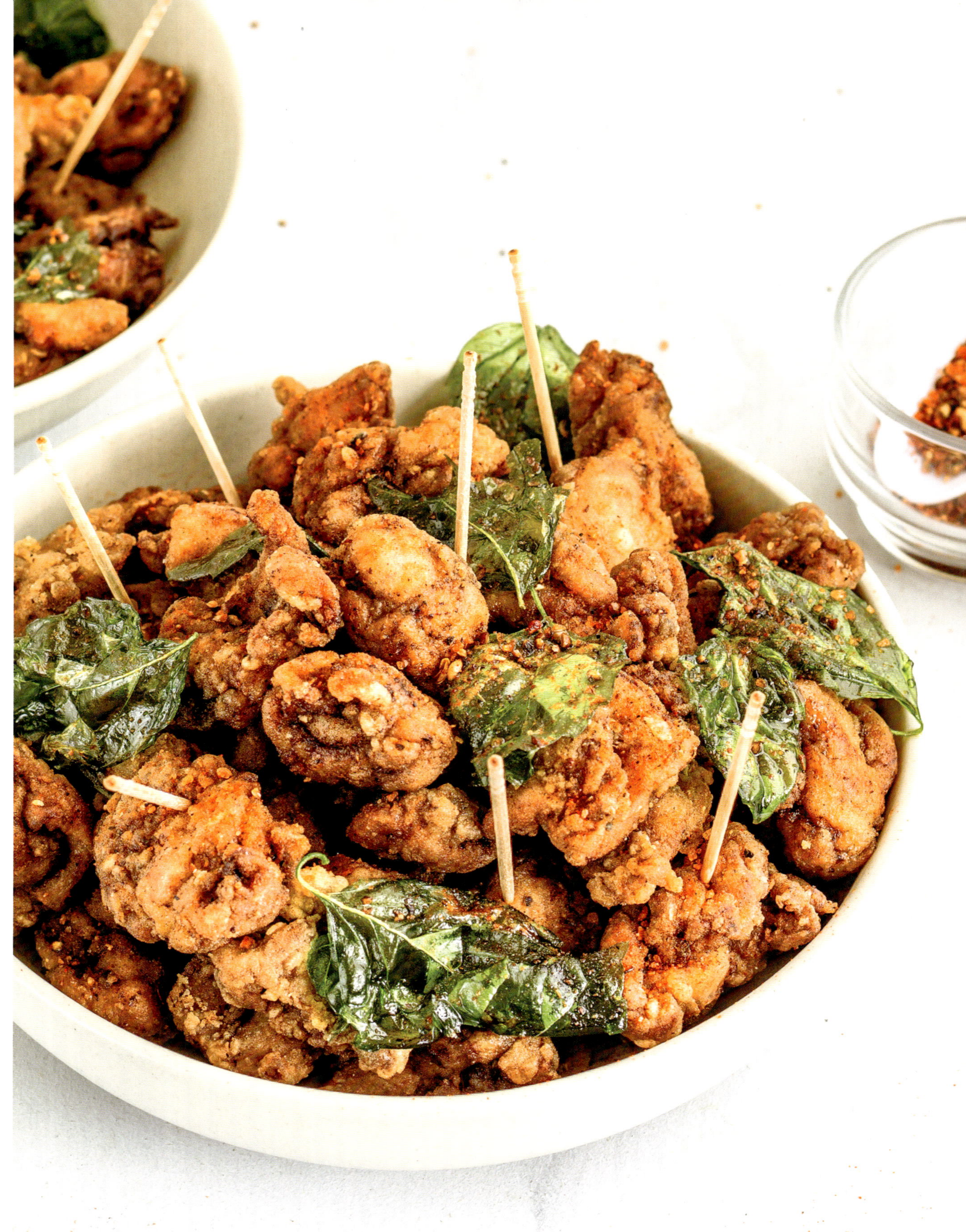

TAIWANESE FRIED CHICKEN

750g boneless, skinless chicken thighs, cut into 3cm pieces

2 tbsps soy sauce

1 tbsp Shaoxing wine

1 tsp sugar

1½ tsps Chinese five-spice powder

1 tsp white pepper

2 tsps salt

1 tbsp whole Sichuan or black peppercorns

1 cup (115g) tapioca flour

1 tbsp water

6 cups (1.5L) vegetable oil

1 cup (15g) fresh basil leaves

STEPS

1. Place the chicken in a large bowl along with soy sauce, Shaoxing wine, sugar, five-spice powder, white pepper and 1 teaspoon salt. Set aside to marinate about 1 hour.

2. Coarsely grind the peppercorns in a spice grinder or mortar and pestle and mix with the remaining salt. Set aside.

3. Place tapioca flour and water in a shallow dish. Dredge chicken in the flour mixture.

4. Heat vegetable oil in a large, heavy-bottomed pan to 180°C. Working in batches, add the battered chicken to the hot oil and fry for 5-7 minutes until golden brown and crisp. Using a slotted spoon transfer to a plate lined with paper towel to drain. Scatter with salt and ground peppercorns.

5. Fry basil leaves for 1 minute until crisp. Serve with fried chicken.

SERVES 4 | PREP + COOK TIME: 30 MINS + MARINATING | DAIRY FREE |

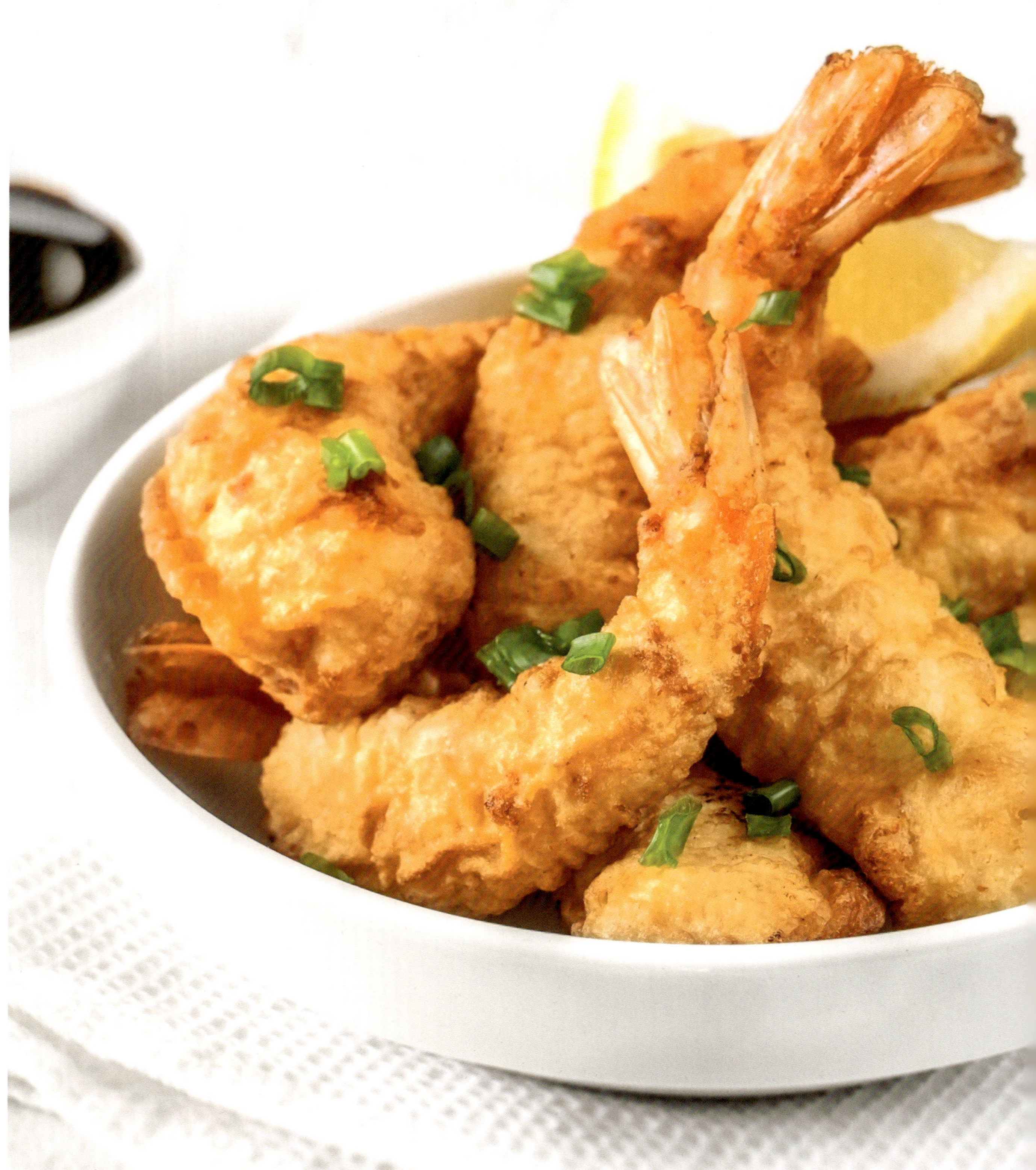

TEMPURA PRAWNS

3 cups (750ml) neutral-flavoured oil

1 cup (125g) plain flour

1 large egg

¾ cup (185ml) iced water

12 large tiger prawns, peeled and deveined, tails intact

Cornflour for dusting

TEMPURA DIPPING SAUCE

1 tsp dashi powder

3 tbsps soy sauce

2 tbsps mirin

2 tsps sugar

STEPS

1. To make the sauce, combine the dashi, soy sauce, mirin, and sugar in a small saucepan. Bring it to a simmer and let the sugar dissolve completely. Remove from the heat and set aside.
2. Heat oil in a wok or saucepan to 180°C. Test this by dipping in a wooden spoon and if bubbles appear the oil is hot enough.
3. While the oil is heating, sift the flour into a large bowl. Add the egg and iced water to a jug and whisk to combine. Pour egg mixture into the flour and stir until just incorporated.
4. Dust the prawns in cornflour, then dip into the batter.
5. Fry the prawns in the hot oil for 2 minutes until golden brown. Serve with tempura dipping sauce.

SERVES 4 | PREP + COOK TIME: 30 MINS | DAIRY FREE |

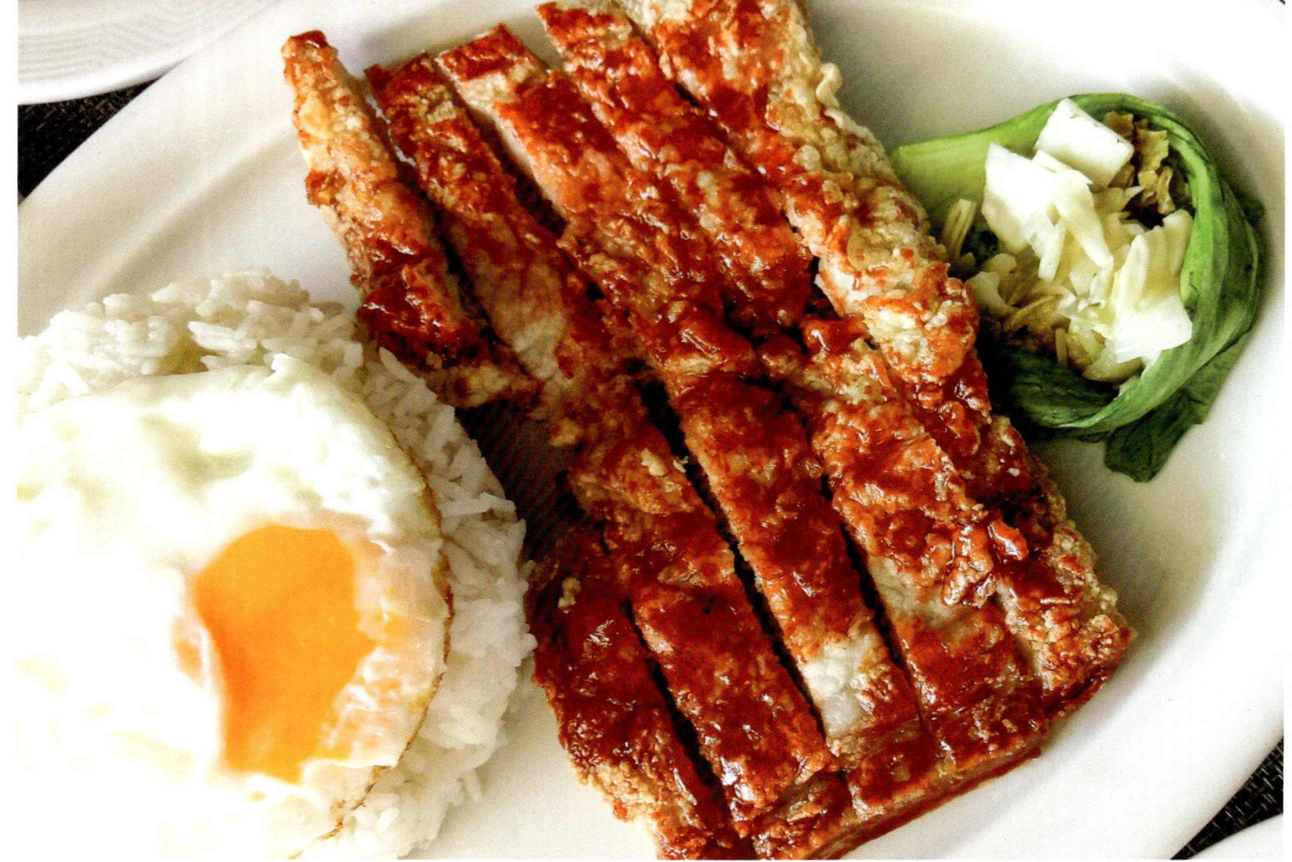

PORK CHOPS IN PEKING SAUCE

2 tbsps cornflour
1 cup (125g) panko breadcrumbs
4 pork loin chops, cut into strips
½ cup (125ml) vegetable oil

PEKING SAUCE

1 clove garlic, minced
Pinch of ground ginger (optional)
½ tsp Chinese five-spice powder
3 tbsps brown sugar
2 tbsps Worcestershire sauce
4 tbsps hoisin sauce
1 tbsp white vinegar
8 tbsps tomato ketchup
1 tbsp cornflour
1 cup (250ml) water

TO SERVE

Steamed rice
Fried eggs

STEPS

1. Place the cornflour and breadcrumbs on two separate plates.
2. Dredge the pork strips first through the cornflour, and then through the breadcrumbs. Shake to remove any excess.
3. Heat the oil in a large frying pan or wok until sizzling (to test, dip a wooden spoon in the oil and look for bubbles). Carefully add in the pork. Fry for 4 minutes each side until lightly golden. Set aside to drain on paper towels.
4. In a small bowl, whisk together the sauce ingredients until well combined.
5. Using the same pan set over medium heat, pour in the sauce. Bring to a gentle simmer. Add the crispy pork to the pan and gently stir to coat in the sauce. Remove from the pan. Serve with rice and fried eggs.

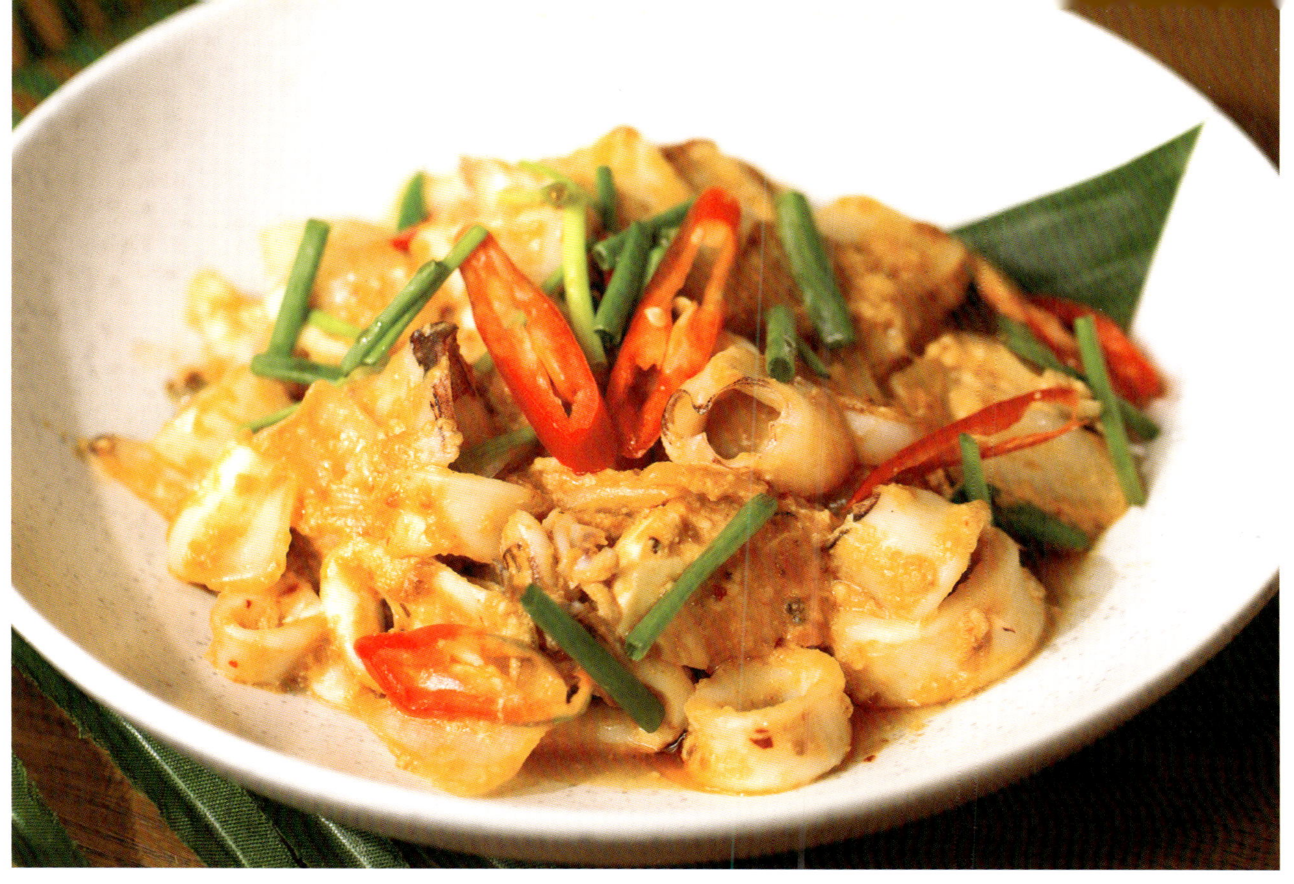

FRIED SQUID WITH SALTED EGGS

2 tbsps peanut oil

1 onion, sliced into thin wedges

2 cloves garlic, chopped

300g squid, cleaned and cut into bite-size pieces

2 salted egg yolks (available in Asian grocery stores), crushed

2 tsps fish sauce

1 tbsp chilli paste

¼ tsp pepper

2 spring onions, cut into 5cm lengths

1 red chilli, sliced

STEPS

1. Heat oil on a pan on medium heat. Add onion and cook, stirring regularly, for 3-5 minutes until soft and translucent. Add garlic and cook, stirring, for 1 minute until fragrant.

2. Add squid. Stir-fry for about 30 seconds, taking care not to let it overcook.

3. Add salted egg yolks, lightly pressing on the yolks to dissolve them. Add fish sauce, chilli paste and pepper. Stir to mix well. Transfer to a plate.

4. Sprinkle with spring onions and chillies to serve.

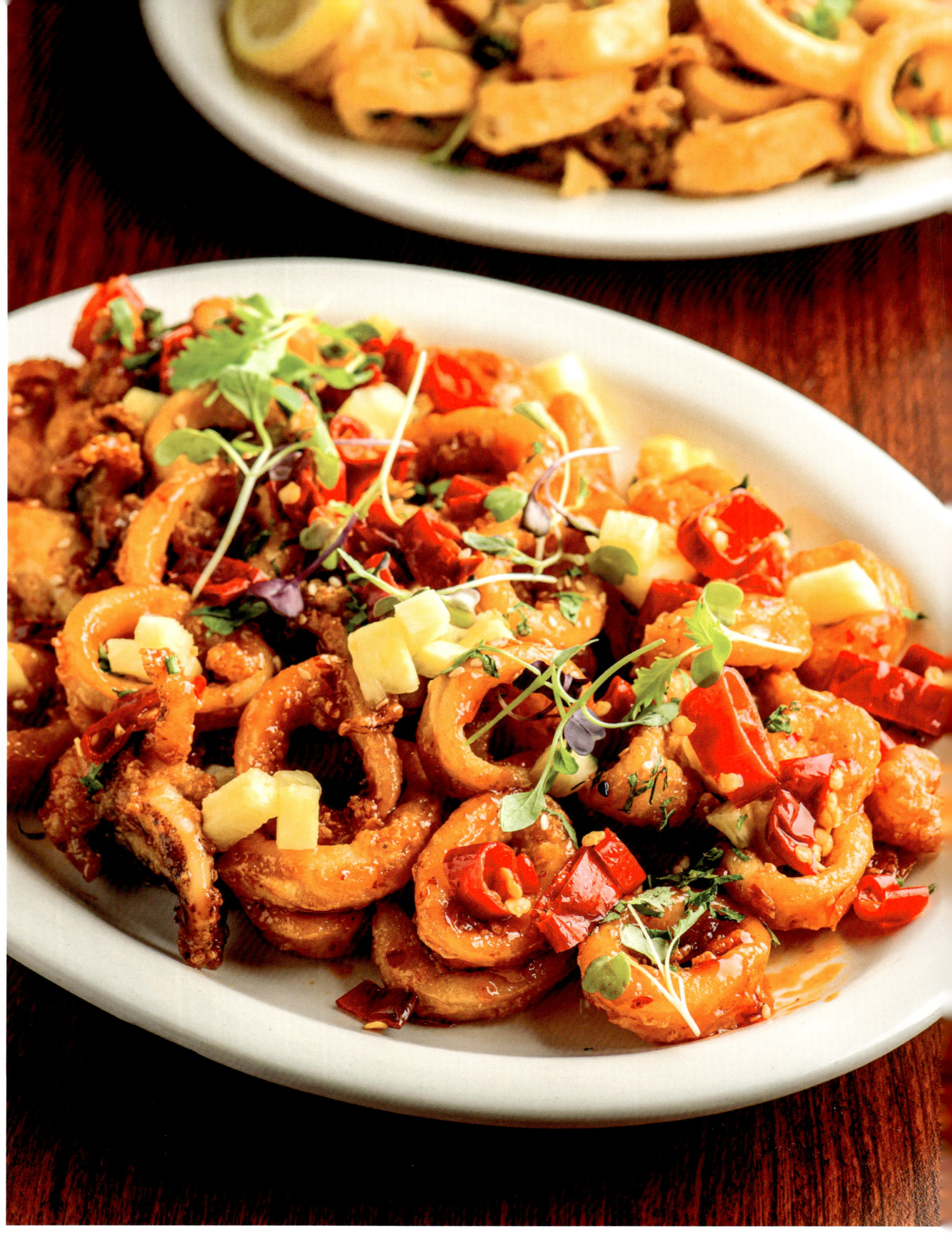

SWEET CHILLI CALAMARI

1 cup (125g) plain flour

1 tsp paprika

½ tsp salt

¼ tsp pepper

500g calamari rings

Vegetable oil for frying

STICKY CHILLI SAUCE

½ cup (125ml) sweet chilli sauce

2 tbsps soy sauce

2 tbsps lime juice

2 tbsps honey

2 cloves garlic, minced

Small piece ginger, grated

TO SERVE

1 cup (200g) pineapple chunks

1 red chilli, sliced

Micro herbs to garnish

STEPS

1. In a mixing bowl, combine the flour, paprika, salt and pepper. Mix well. Coat the calamari rings in the flour mixture, shaking off any excess.

2. Heat 3cm vegetable oil in a deep pan or deep fryer to about 180°C.

3. Carefully add the calamari rings to the hot oil and fry in batches for 2-3 minutes, or until they turn golden brown and crispy. Remove from the oil with a slotted spoon and drain on a plate lined with paper towel.

4. In a small saucepan, combine sweet chilli sauce, soy sauce, lime juice, honey, minced garlic and grated ginger. Heat the sauce over medium heat, stirring continuously, until it thickens slightly and all the flavours are well combined. Remove from heat.

5. In a serving dish, combine the fried calamari, pineapple chunks and sliced chilli. Drizzle with sweet chilli sauce and gently toss to coat. Garnish with micro herbs.

SERVES 4 | PREP + COOK TIME: 45 MINS | DAIRY FREE |

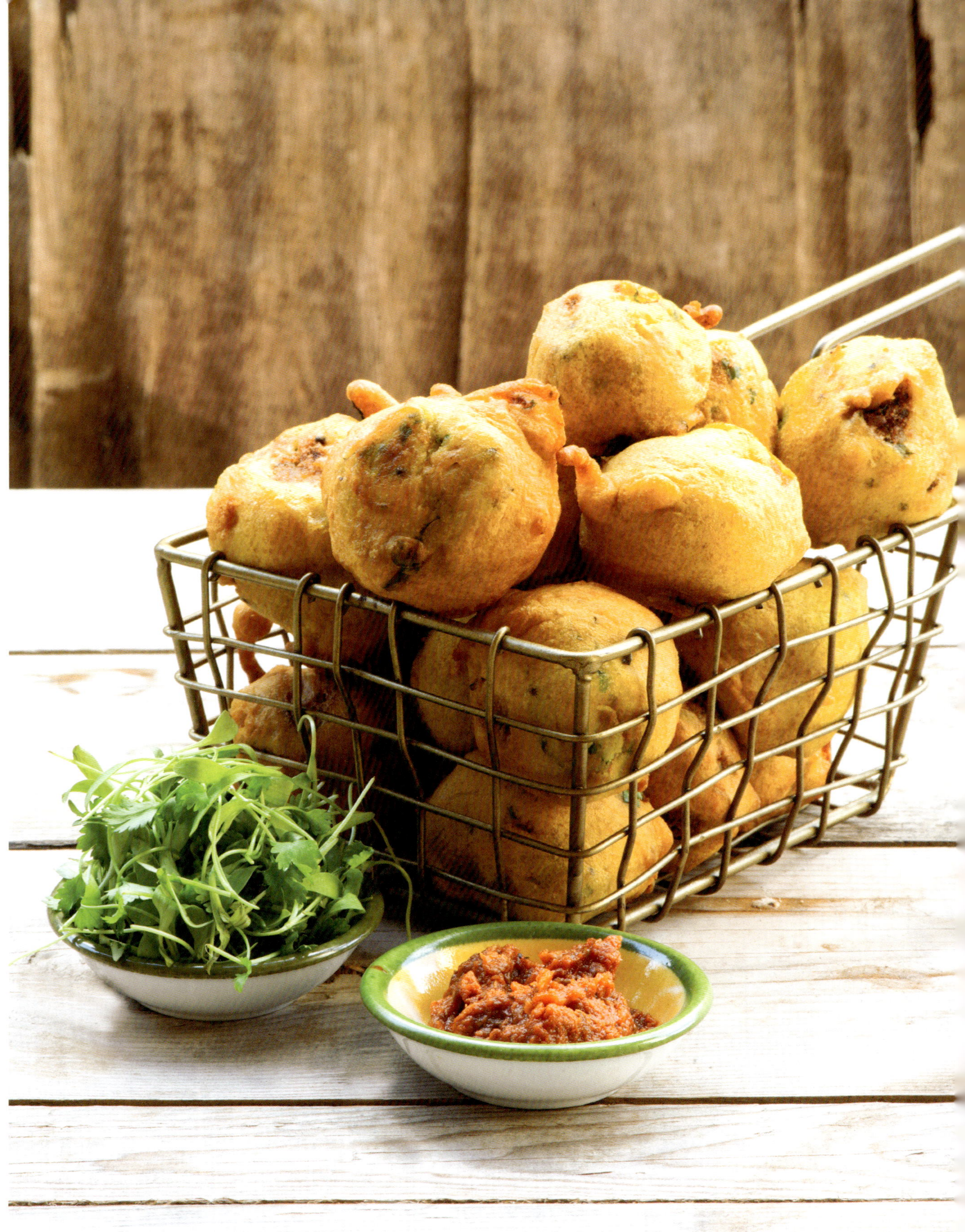

BATATA VADA (SPICED POTATO BALLS)

1 tbsp oil
Small piece ginger, grated
1 small green chilli, minced
¼ tsp ground turmeric
1 tbsp chopped coriander leaves
2 cups (520g) mashed potatoes
2 tsps lemon juice
2 tsps sugar
Salt to taste
2 cups (500ml) oil for deep frying

BATTER

1 cup (95g) besan (chickpea flour)
¼ tsp chilli powder
1 tbsp oil
Pinch of asafoetida
Pinch of bicarbonate of soda
Salt to taste
¾ cup (185ml) water

STEPS

1. Heat the oil in a frying pan over medium heat. Add the ginger and chilli and cook for 30 seconds until fragrant. Add the turmeric followed by the coriander, mashed potatoes, lemon juice, sugar and salt to taste. Saute for 3-4 minutes. Remove from the heat and set aside to cool.
2. When cool enough to handle, divide the mixture into 10 equal portions. Roll each portion into a ball.
3. Place the besan, chilli powder, oil, asafoetida, bicarb and salt in a large bowl. Add a little water at a time and whisk until smooth.
4. Heat oil for deep-frying in a wide pan over medium heat to 180°C. Dip each potato ball first into the batter and then carefully add to the hot oil. Cook in batches to avoid overcrowding the pan. Cook for a few minutes, turning occasionally with a slotted spoon, until golden brown all over.
5. Remove from the pan with a slotted spoon and drain on a plate lined with paper towel before serving.

MAKES 10 | PREP + COOK TIME: 35 MINS | VEG | GLUTEN FREE | DAIRY FREE |

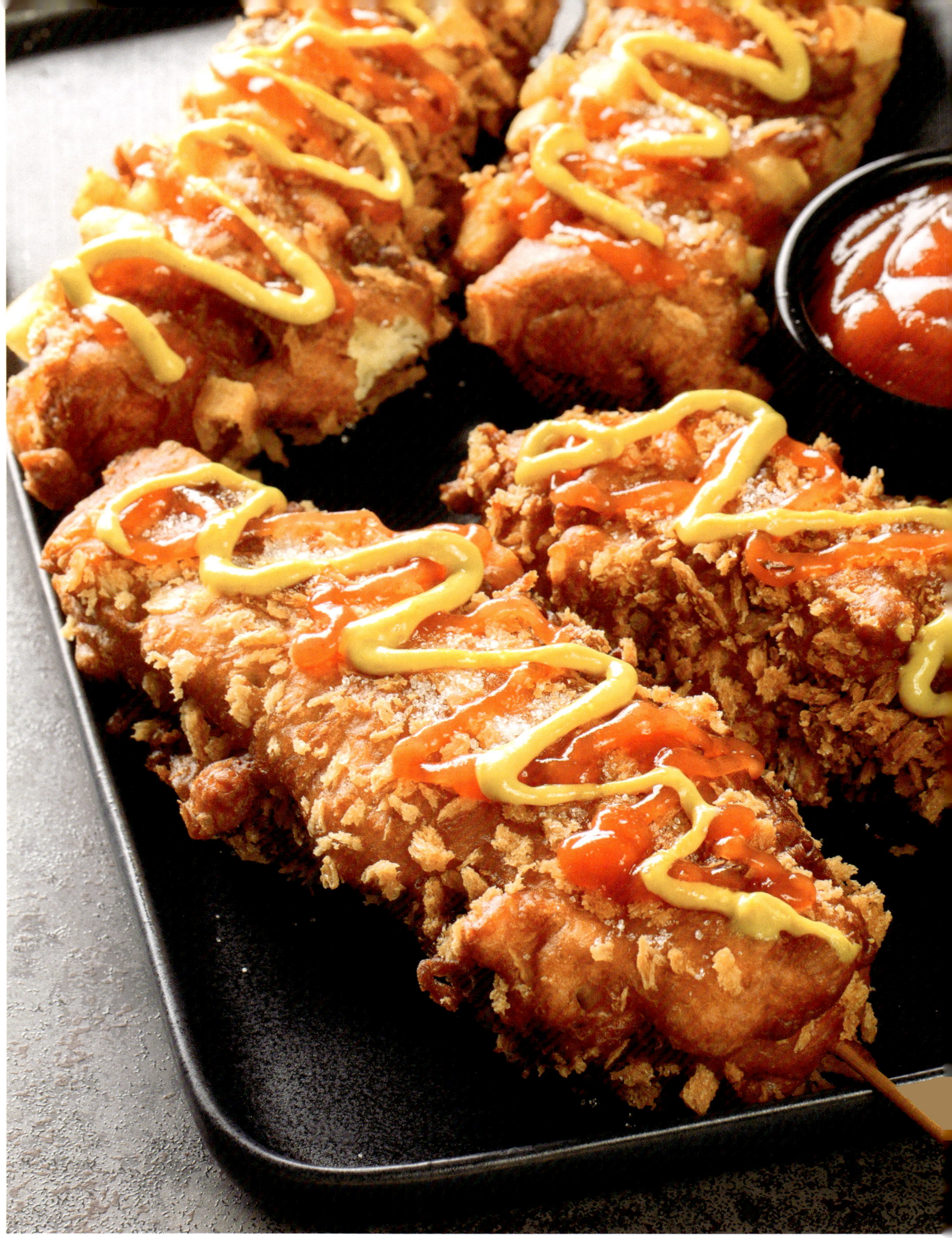

KOREAN HOT DOGS

3 hot dog sausages, cut in half

350g firm mozzarella cheese, cut into thick batons a similar size to the hot dog halves

1¼ cups (155g) plain flour

2 tbsps sugar + extra to finish

¼ tsp salt

2 tsps baking powder

1 large egg

¾ cup (185ml) milk

2 cups (250g) panko breadcrumbs

Oil for deep frying

Mustard and tomato sauce to serve

STEPS

1. Thread the hot dog sausages and cheese onto skewers with hot dogs on the bottom and cheese on top. Place in the fridge to until ready to cook.
2. In a bowl, whisk together the flour, sugar, salt and baking powder. Mix in the egg and milk until thick and smooth. Pour into a tall cup and place into the fridge until ready to cook.
3. Pour the panko breadcrumbs onto a shallow dish.
4. Heat 5-10cm oil in a deep fryer or a deep, wide pot over medium-high heat until it reaches 175°C. When the oil is almost at temp, take the skewers from the fridge and dip them into the batter, making sure they are completely coated. Roll in panko breadcrumbs, pressing gently with your hands to ensure even coating.
5. Carefully add coated hot dogs to the hot oil and fry for 3-4 minutes or until golden and crispy, turning as needed. Transfer to a wire rack, sprinkle with sugar and drizzle with mustard and tomato sauce.

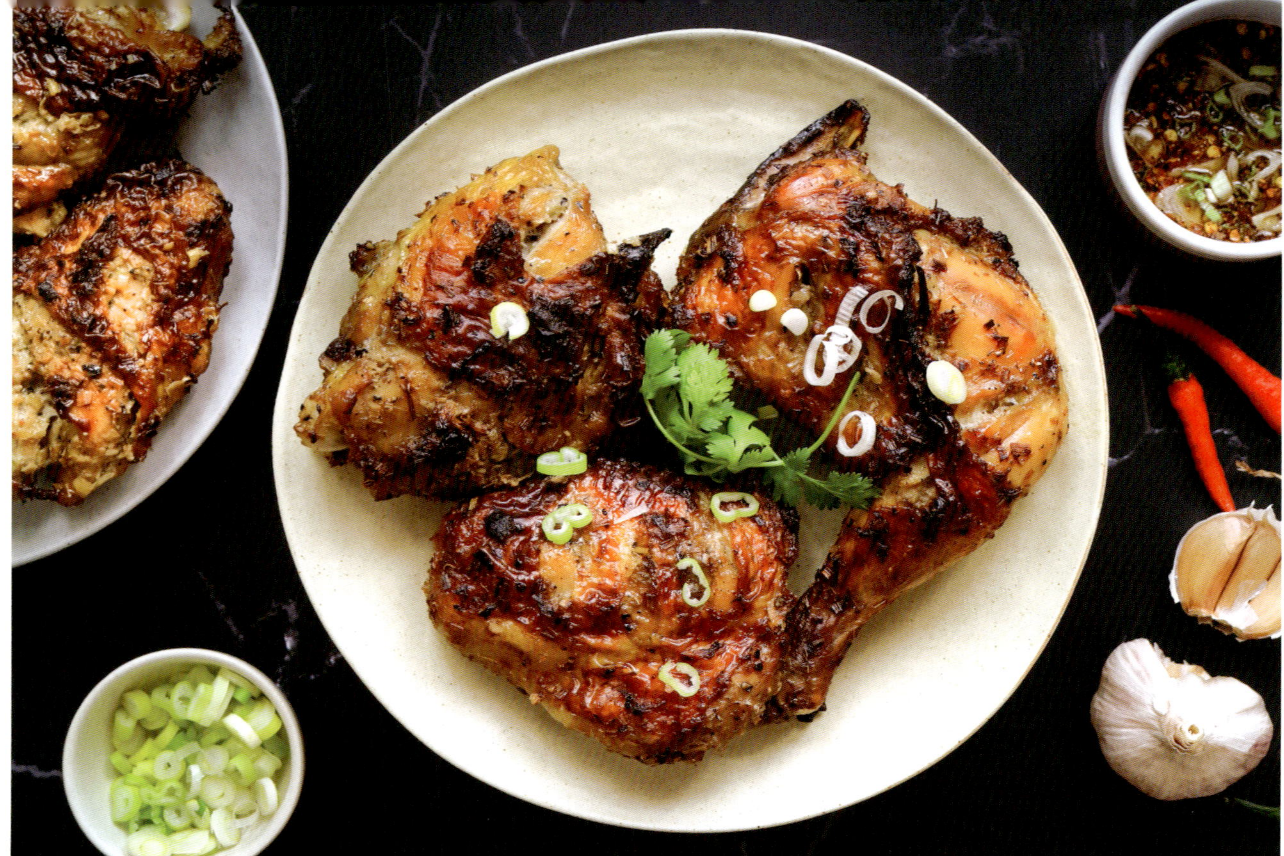

THAI ROAST CHICKEN

- 5 tbsps peanut oil
- 3 tbsps fish sauce
- 2 tbsps oyster sauce
- 1 tsp dried chilli flakes
- 1 tbsp sugar
- 2 Asian shallots, peeled
- 3 cloves garlic, peeled
- 2 stalks fresh lemongrass, cut into pieces
- 1 lime, zested
- 8 bone-in chicken pieces, thighs or drumsticks
- Chopped spring onion and coriander leaves to serve

STEPS

1. Add 3 tablespoons oil, fish sauce, oyster sauce, chilli flakes, sugar, shallots, garlic, lemongrass and lime zest to a food processor. Process until smooth.
2. Transfer paste to a bowl, along with the chicken. Toss to coat the chicken in the marinade. Cover, transfer to the fridge, and marinate for 1-4 hours.
3. Preheat the oven to 175°C. Heat the remaining oil in a large ovenproof frying pan over medium-high heat.
4. Reserving the marinade, add chicken to the pan skin-side down. Cook for 4 minutes. Turn the chicken, add the reserved marinade to the pan, and transfer to the oven. Roast for 25-30 minutes, until the chicken is cooked through.
5. Scatter with chopped spring onion and coriander leaves to serve,.

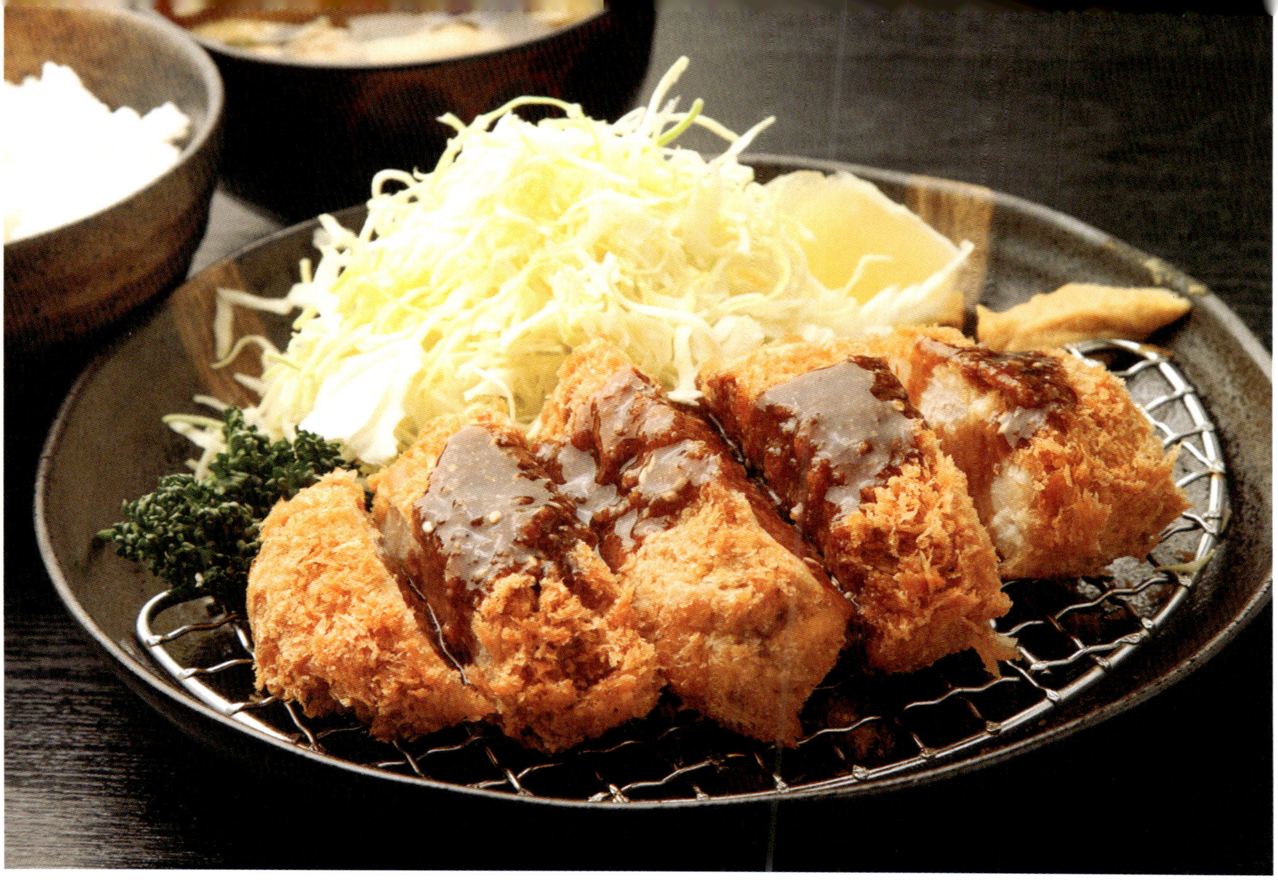

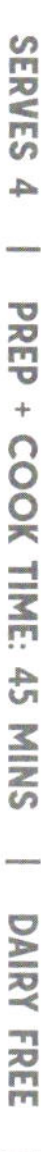

PORK TONKATSU

SAUCE

¼ cup (60ml) tomato ketchup

3 tbsps Worcestershire sauce

2 tbsps oyster sauce

4 tsps sugar

1 tsp salt

1 tsp Dijon mustard

PORK

4 boneless pork loin chops

½ cup (60g) plain flour

1 egg, beaten

1½ cups (185g) panko breadcrumbs

Oil for frying

STEPS

1. Combine sauce ingredients in a small bowl and whisk together. Set aside.
2. Between two sheets of plastic wrap, pound the chops with a rolling pin to about ½ cm thick. Sprinkle with salt and pepper.
3. Toss pork chops in flour, dip in the beaten egg, then immediately coat both sides in panko breadcrumbs. Press breadcrumbs onto the meat, then set aside for a few minutes.
4. Heat about 2cm of oil in a large frying pan over medium-high heat. When shimmering, carefully add the pork chops. Fry in batches for 3 minutes each side or until deep golden brown, then turn and fry the other side. Drain on paper towels.
5. Serve the pork with the sauce and your choice of vegetables.

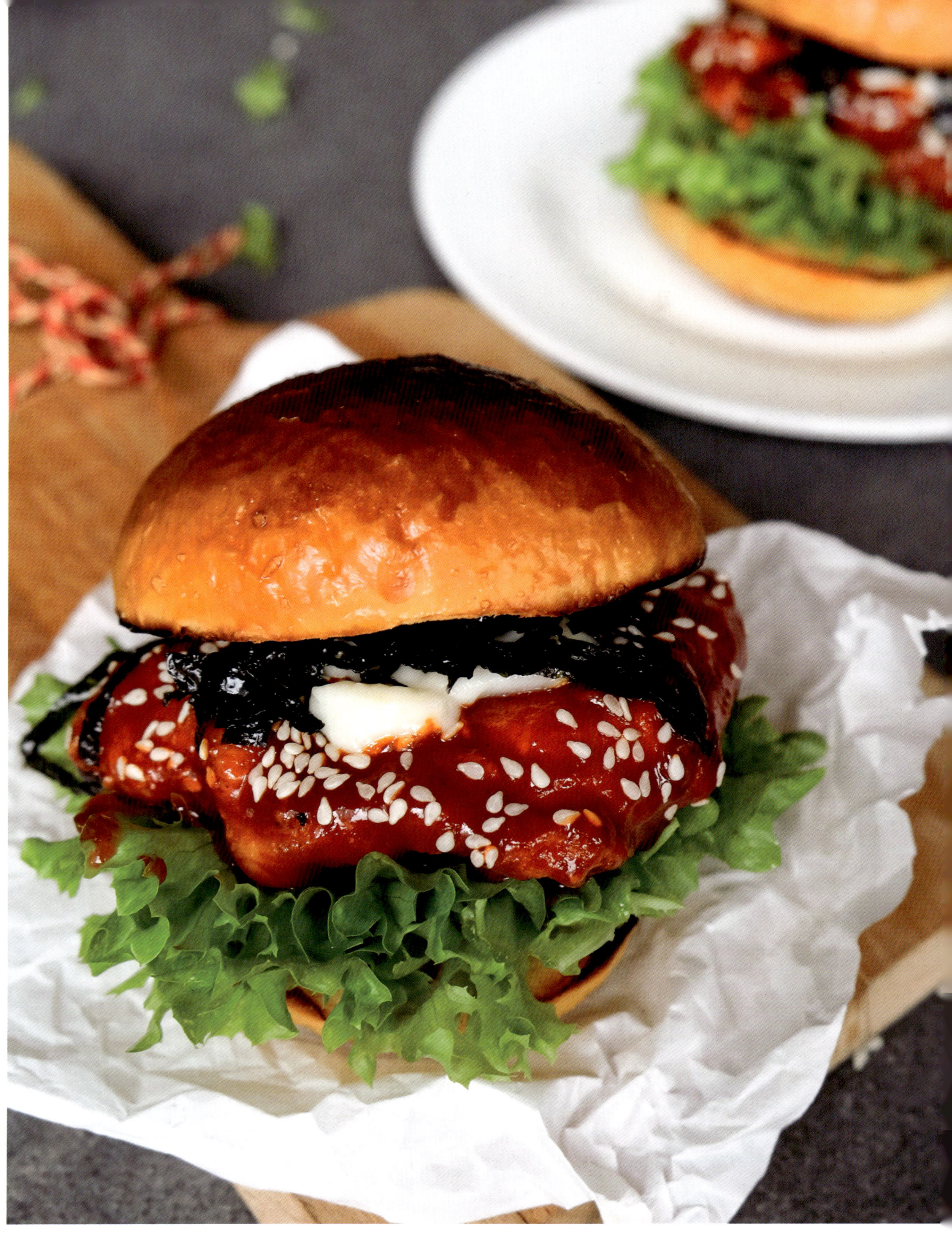

KOREAN CHICKEN BURGERS

SERVES 4 | PREP + COOK TIME: 45 MINS | DAIRY FREE |

SAUCE

6 tbsps dark brown sugar

2 tbsps gochujang (Korean chilli paste)

2 tbsps soy sauce

3 cloves garlic, crushed

Small piece ginger, grated

2 tsps sesame oil

BURGERS

4 skinless, boneless chicken thigh fillets

Salt and pepper to taste

Large piece of ginger, finely grated

⅔ cup (100g) cornflour

Vegetable oil for frying

4 lettuce leaves, torn

4 brioche buns, toasted

2 tbsps mayonnaise

2 nori sheets, cut into thin strips

2 tsps sesame seeds

STEPS

1. To make the sauce, put all the ingredients in a saucepan and simmer gently until syrupy. Take off the heat and set aside.
2. Season chicken with salt and pepper, rub with grated ginger then place chicken in a bowl with cornflour and toss to coat.
3. Heat about 2cm of vegetable oil in a large frying pan to 180°C. Fry the chicken thighs for 4-5 minutes each side until crisp. Remove from the oil onto paper towel and leave to cool for a couple of minutes.
4. Return the chicken to the hot oil and re-fry until ultra-crisp and you can hear it crackle. Remove to paper towel to drain.
5. Build your burgers by placing some lettuce on the base of a bun, top with the crispy chicken and drizzle over the sticky sauce, spoon over mayonnaise and scatter with nori and sesame seeds.

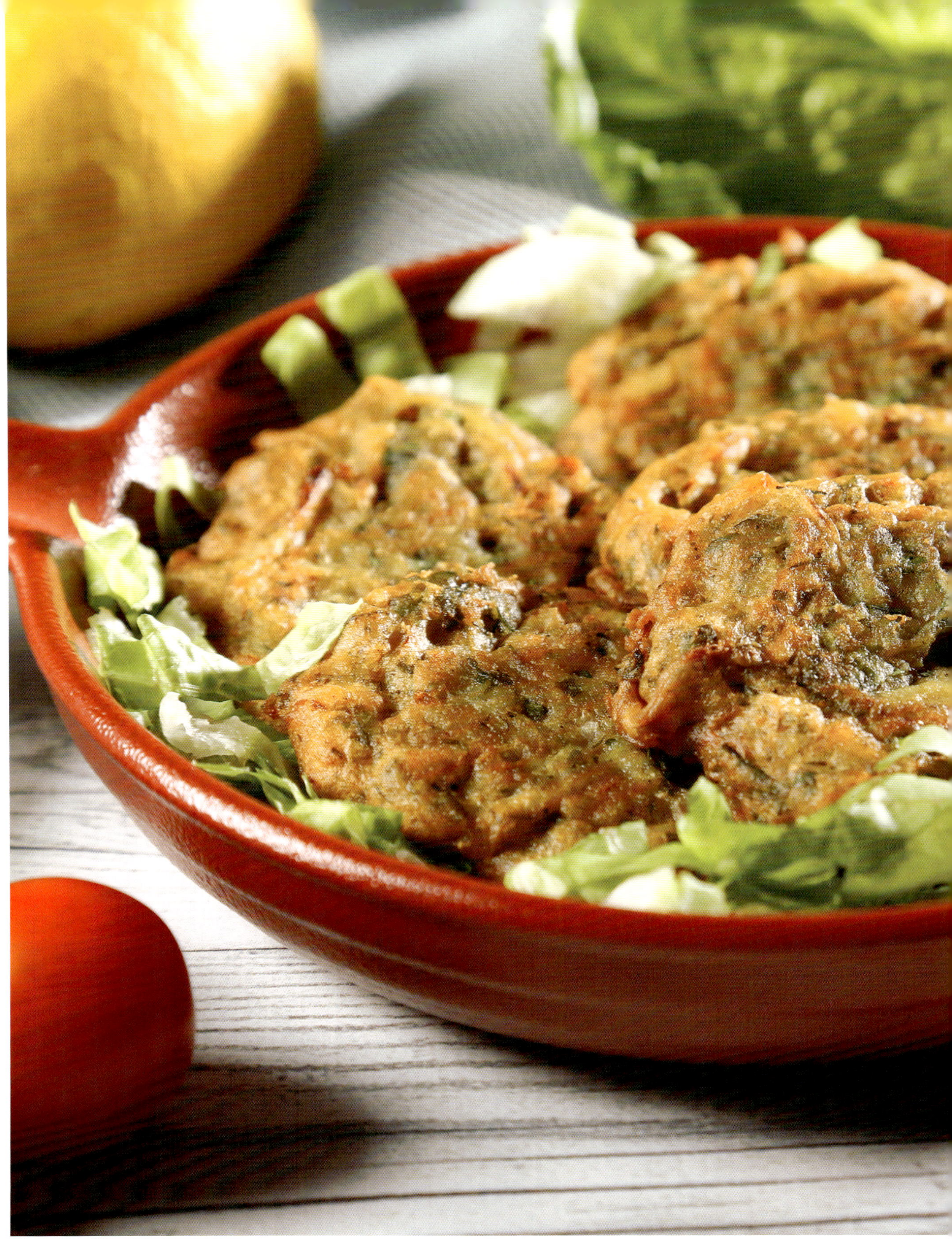

CURRIED CAULIFLOWER FRITTERS

1 head cauliflower, cut into florets
2 tbsps olive oil
4 Asian shallots, chopped
2 tbsps Greek yoghurt
1 lemon, juiced
Salt to taste
½ cup (60g) dry breadcrumbs
2 eggs
2 tbsps flour
1 clove garlic, grated
1½ tsps curry powder
1 tsp ground cumin
½ tsp ground turmeric
¼ tsp cinnamon
Vegetable oil for frying

STEPS

Preheat oven to 200°C.

1. Place the cauliflower on a lined baking tray and drizzle with 1 tablespoon olive oil. Place in the oven for 20 minutes, turning once midway through.
2. Heat 1 tablespoon oil in a small saucepan on a medium-low heat. Add in the shallots and saute until soft, approximately 6 minutes. Place the cooked shallots, yoghurt, lemon juice and salt in a bowl and stir to combine. Set aside.
3. Transfer the cauliflower to a food processor and pulse until coarsely ground. Place the cauliflower in a large bowl and add the shallot mix along with breadcrumbs, eggs, flour, garlic, spices and salt. Mix thoroughly until combined. Cover the bowl and transfer to the fridge to chill for up to 3 hours.
4. Take spoonfuls of the mixture and use your hands to form into patties.
5. Place a frying pan over medium-high heat, and pour in vegetable oil until it reaches 1cm up the sides. Add the fritters, cooking two or three at once. Cook for 2-3 minutes until golden brown. Gently flip and cook on the other side for 1-2 minutes. Transfer to paper towels to drain. Repeat to cook the rest of the fritters. Serve hot.

SERVES 6 | PREP+ COOK TIME 55 MINS + CHILLING | VEG |

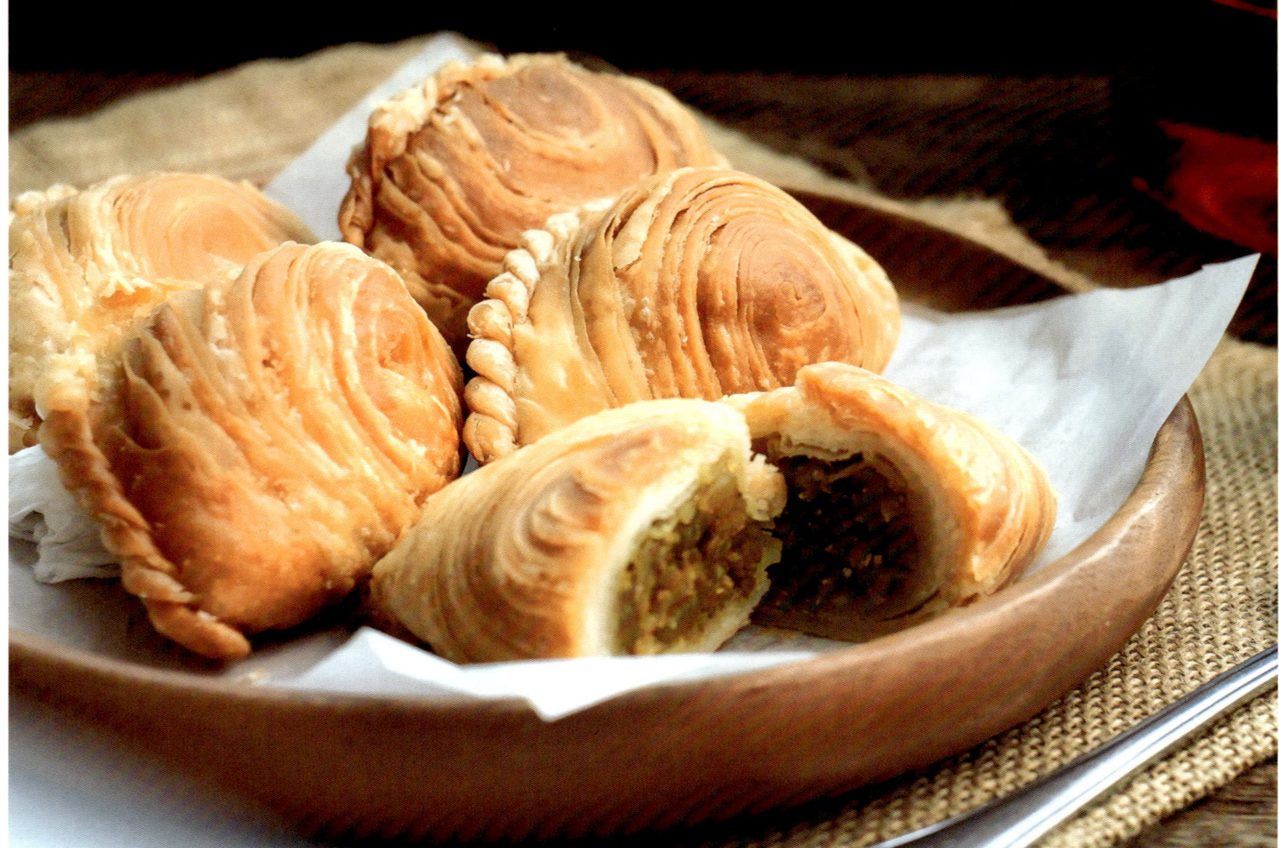

SPICY CURRY PATTIES

1 tbsp peanut oil

1 onion, chopped

2 tbsps curry powder

1 clove garlic, minced

300g lean beef mince

1 large potato, diced into 1½ cm cubes

½ tsp salt

2 sheets frozen puff pastry, thawed

1 egg, beaten

STEPS

1. Heat oil in a pan over medium-high heat. Add onion and fry for 3-5 minutes until soft and translucent. Add curry powder and garlic and cook for 30 seconds until fragrant. Add beef and cook, breaking up with a spoon, for 3-4 minutes until browned.

2. Add potatoes and salt into the pan. Reduce heat to medium-low and simmer for 20 minutes until the potatoes are cooked through. Remove from heat and let cool for at least 20-25 minutes.

3. Cut out 12cm circles of puff pastry. Fill each circle with a spoonful of filling. Fold over and twist edges to seal.

4. Brush with beaten egg and bake at 200°C for 20 minutes until golden brown.

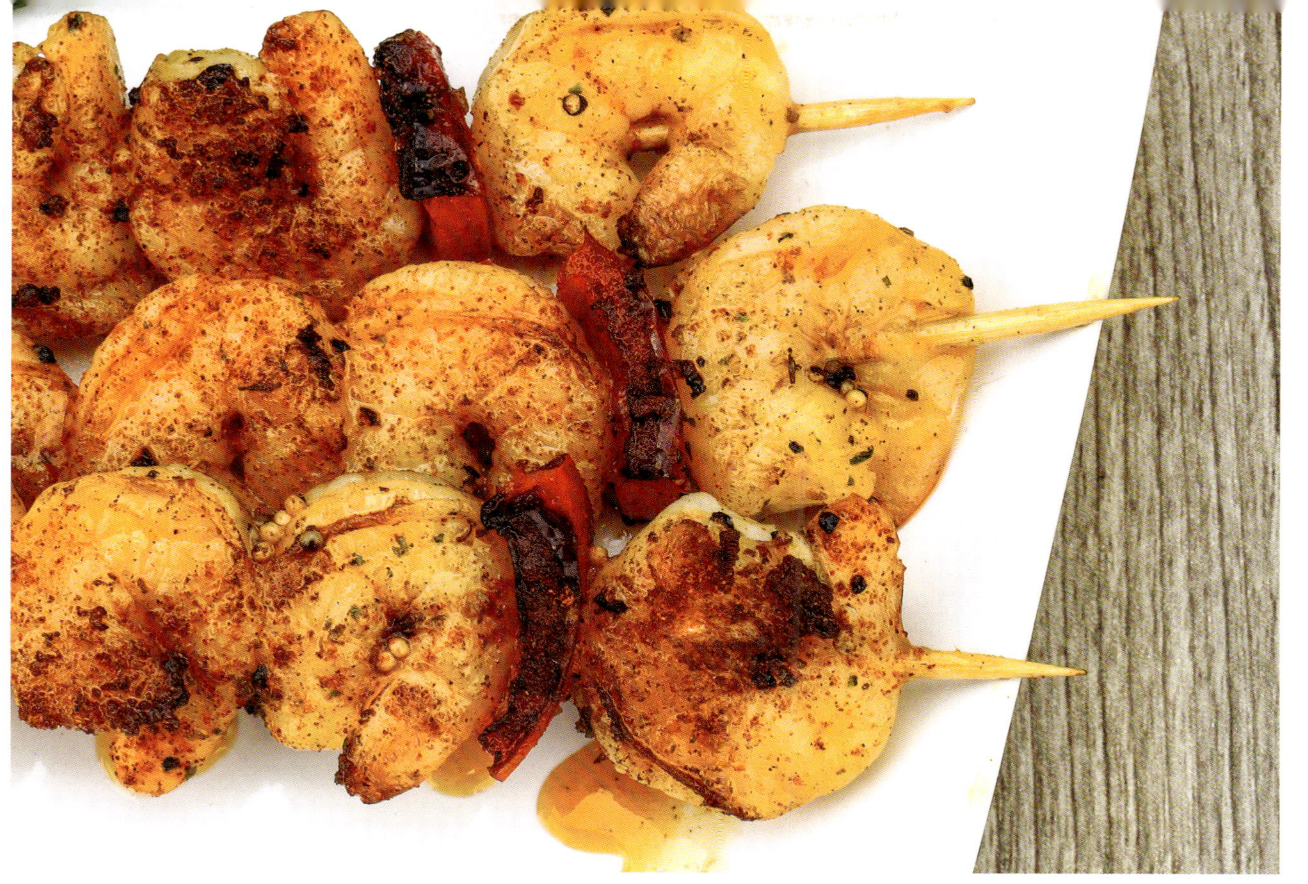

CURRIED PRAWN KEBABS

3 tbsps fresh lemon juice

1 tbsp soy sauce

1 tbsp Dijon mustard

2 cloves garlic, finely chopped

1 tbsp dark brown sugar

2 tsps Thai red curry paste

500g medium raw prawns, peeled and deveined

1 capsicum, sliced

STEPS

1. In a shallow dish, mix together the lemon juice, soy sauce, mustard, garlic, sugar and curry paste. Add prawns, stir to coat and cover. Marinate in the fridge for 1 hour.
2. Preheat barbecue to a high heat. Lightly oil the cooking grate. Thread the prawns and capsicum on to soaked skewers.
3. Transfer the marinade to a saucepan and boil for 2-3 minutes. Remove from the heat and transfer to the barbecue area.
4. Barbecue prawns for 3 minutes each side, or until opaque, basting occasionally with the marinade. Serve immediately.

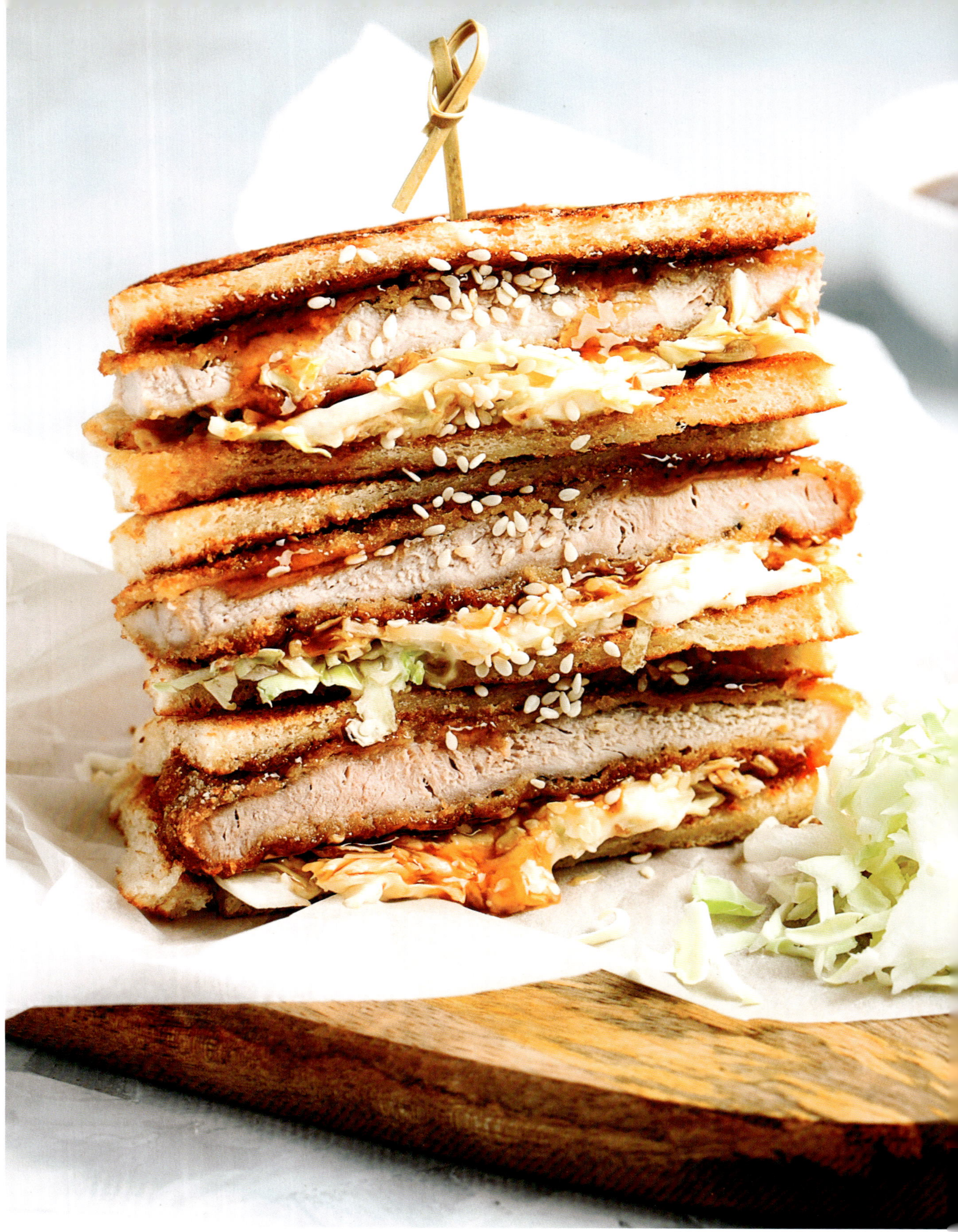

KATSU SANDWICH

SERVES 2 | PREP + COOK TIME: 30 MINS | DAIRY FREE |

SAUCE

4 tbsps tomato sauce

3 tsps Worcestershire sauce

1½ tsps soy sauce

¼ tsp garlic powder

¼ tsp English mustard powder

TONKATSU

2 boneless pork chops

Salt and pepper to taste

2 tbsps plain flour

1 egg

¾ cup (100g) panko breadcrumbs

Vegetable oil, for frying

SANDWICHES

½ small white cabbage

4 thick slices white bread

2 tbsps Japanese mustard, or Dijon mustard

2 tbsps Kewpie mayonnaise

Sesame seeds to serve

STEPS

1. Mix together all the ingredients for the sauce and set aside.

2. Season the pork chops with salt and pepper then coat them in the flour. Beat the egg in a shallow bowl and spread the panko breadcrumbs out on a plate. Dip the chops first into the egg, then into the breadcrumbs, making sure they are well coated.

3. In a deep-fryer or large, heavy-bottomed pan, heat 3cm of oil to 160°C. Fry the coated chops one at a time, flipping every few minutes to ensure even browning. Cook for 6-8 minutes depending on the size of the chops. The chops should be 65°C in the centre when measured with a meat thermometer. Let the chops rest on a wire rack for 5 minutes.

4. While the pork is cooking finely shred the white cabbage and toast the bread.

5. Spread two slices of toast with a thin layer of mustard, followed by a generous layer of mayonnaise. Place a chop on top of each and top with the sauce followed by some cabbage. Top with the remaining slices of toast, then cut each sandwich in half. Serve sprinkled with sesame seeds.

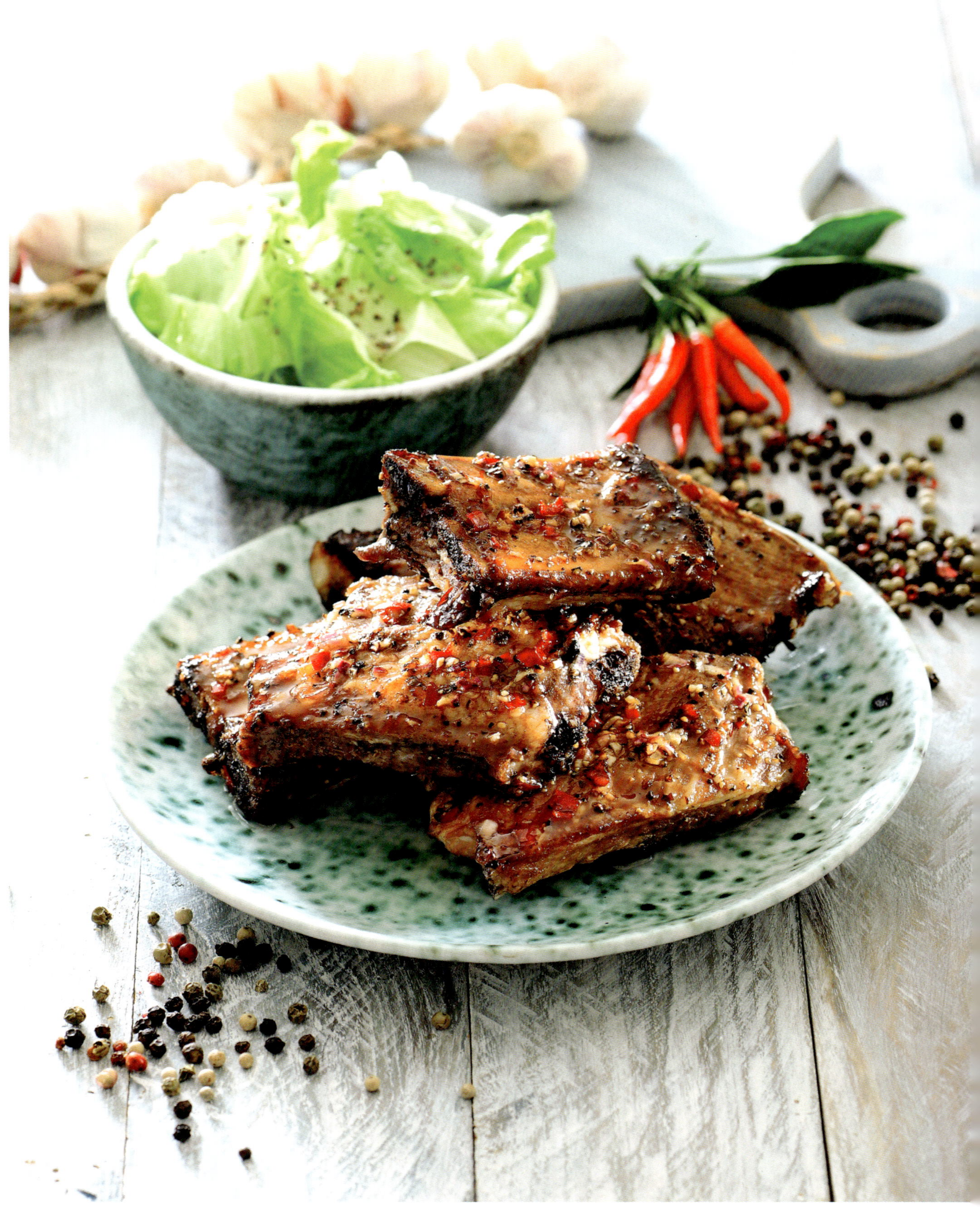

THAI GLAZED SPARE RIBS

GLAZE

2 tbsps fish sauce

2 tbsps tamarind paste

3 tbsps brown sugar

1 tbsp lime juice

2 bird's-eye chillies, finely chopped

2 cloves garlic, minced

1 tbsp toasted rice powder (found in Asian markets or see the recipe on page 46 to make your own)

1 tsp finely minced coriander stems

2 tomatoes, grated

RIBS

2kg pork ribs, cut into 2- or 3-rib sections

¼ cup (60ml) light soy sauce

1 tbsp garlic powder

½ tsp ground white pepper

Vegetable oil for deep-frying

STEPS

1. In a small bowl, whisk together the fish sauce, tamarind paste, brown sugar, lime juice, chillies, garlic, rice powder and coriander stems until the sugar dissolves. Add the grated tomatoes and stir together. Refrigerate until ready to use.

2. Place the ribs in a large bowl and add the soy sauce, garlic powder and white pepper. Toss to coat. Let stand at room temperature for 10-20 minutes.

3. Fill a wok or large, heavy-bottomed pan with at least 5cm of oil. Heat the oil over medium heat to 190°C. (You can test the oil by adding a little piece of bread to the oil; if it sizzles immediately but doesn't burn, the oil is ready.) Fry the ribs in batches for about 4 minutes, turning occasionally with a slotted spoon, until they're just cooked and well browned on all sides.

4. Transfer the ribs to a plate lined with paper towel to drain. Then, place the warm ribs in a large bowl, spoon over the glaze and toss to coat.

5. Transfer to a plate and serve immediately.

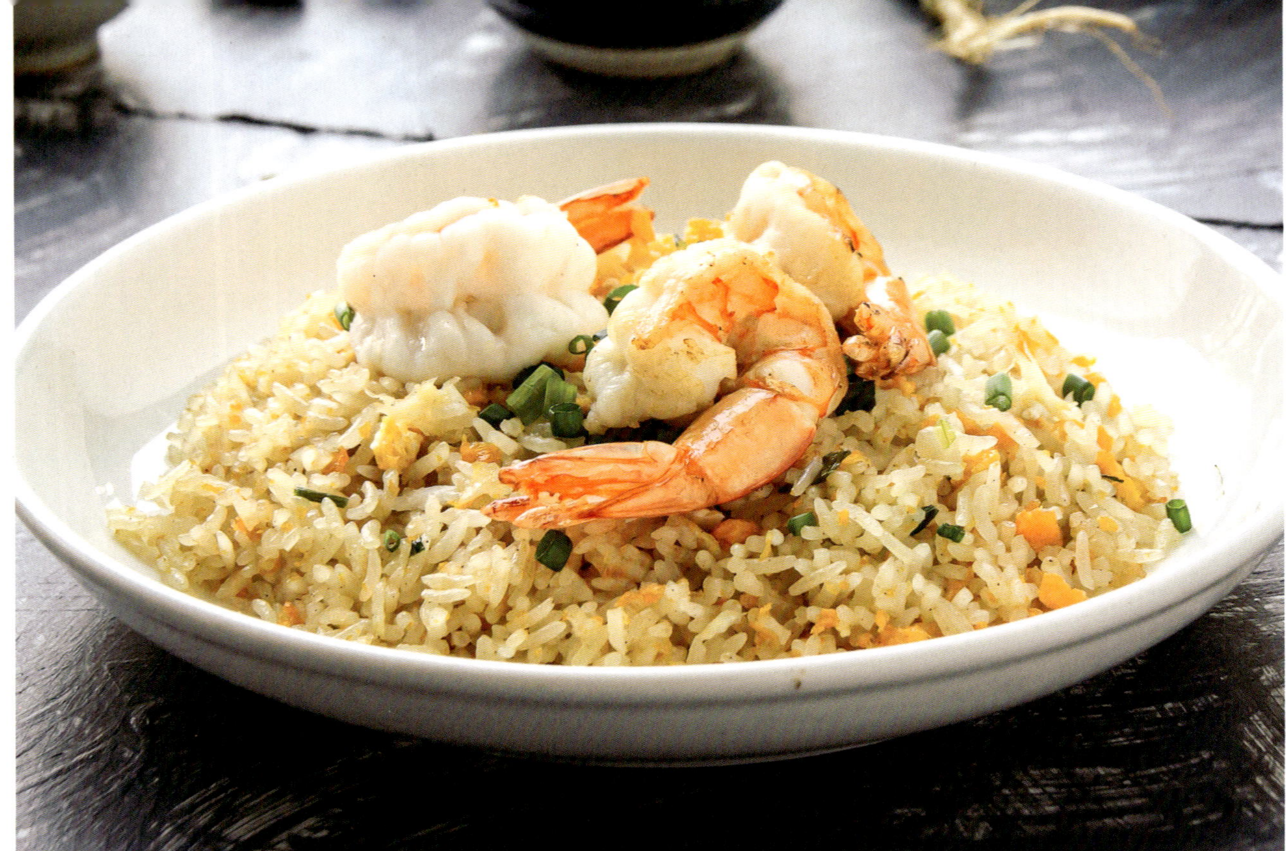

PRAWN FRIED RICE

2 tbsps + 2 tsps sunflower oil
2 small red chillies, chopped
2 cloves garlic, finely chopped
400g peeled green prawns, tails intact
3 eggs, lightly beaten
1¼ cups (200g) white rice, cooked
⅓ cup (80ml) soy sauce
1 tsp sesame oil
2 tbsps sweet chilli sauce
3 spring onions, finely chopped, to serve

STEPS

1. Heat 2 tablespoons sunflower oil in a frying pan over a medium-high heat. Cook chilli and garlic, stirring, for 1 minute or until fragrant. Add prawns and cook for 3-4 minutes until opaque. Set aside.

2. Heat 2 teaspoons sunflower oil in a wok or large frying pan over medium-high heat. Add the egg and cook, stirring, for 1-2 minutes until softly scrambled. Add the cooked rice, soy sauce, sesame oil and sweet chilli sauce then cook, stirring, for 2-3 minutes to warm through.

3. Top the rice with the prawns and garnish with spring onions to serve.

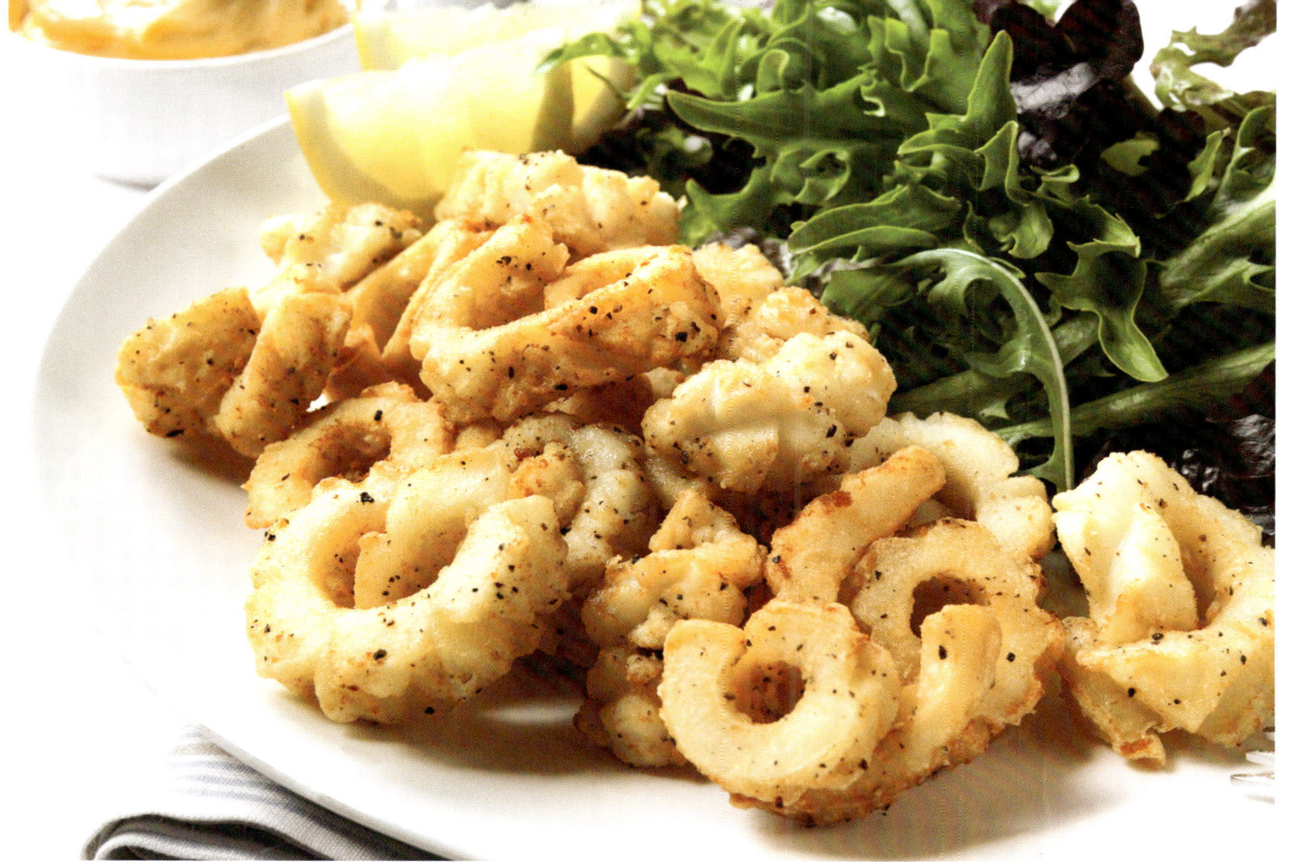

SALT & PEPPER SQUID

800g squid tubes, cleaned

½ cup (80g) rice flour

1½ tbsps pepper

1 tbsp salt

1 tsp chilli flakes (optional)

Oil for frying

Green salad to serve

STEPS

Preheat oven to 160°C.

1. Prepare each squid tube by scoring a criss-cross pattern with a sharp knife and removing excess moisture by patting dry with a paper towel. Cut squid into pieces.
2. Combine flour, pepper, salt and chilli flakes, if using, in a shallow bowl. Lightly coat squid in flour mixture.
3. In a saucepan, heat 3cm oil over medium-high heat. Add squid a few pieces at a time and fry, turning occasionally, for 2 minutes or until light golden. Transfer to a baking tray.
4. Place in oven to keep warm while cooking remaining squid.
5. Serve with green salad.

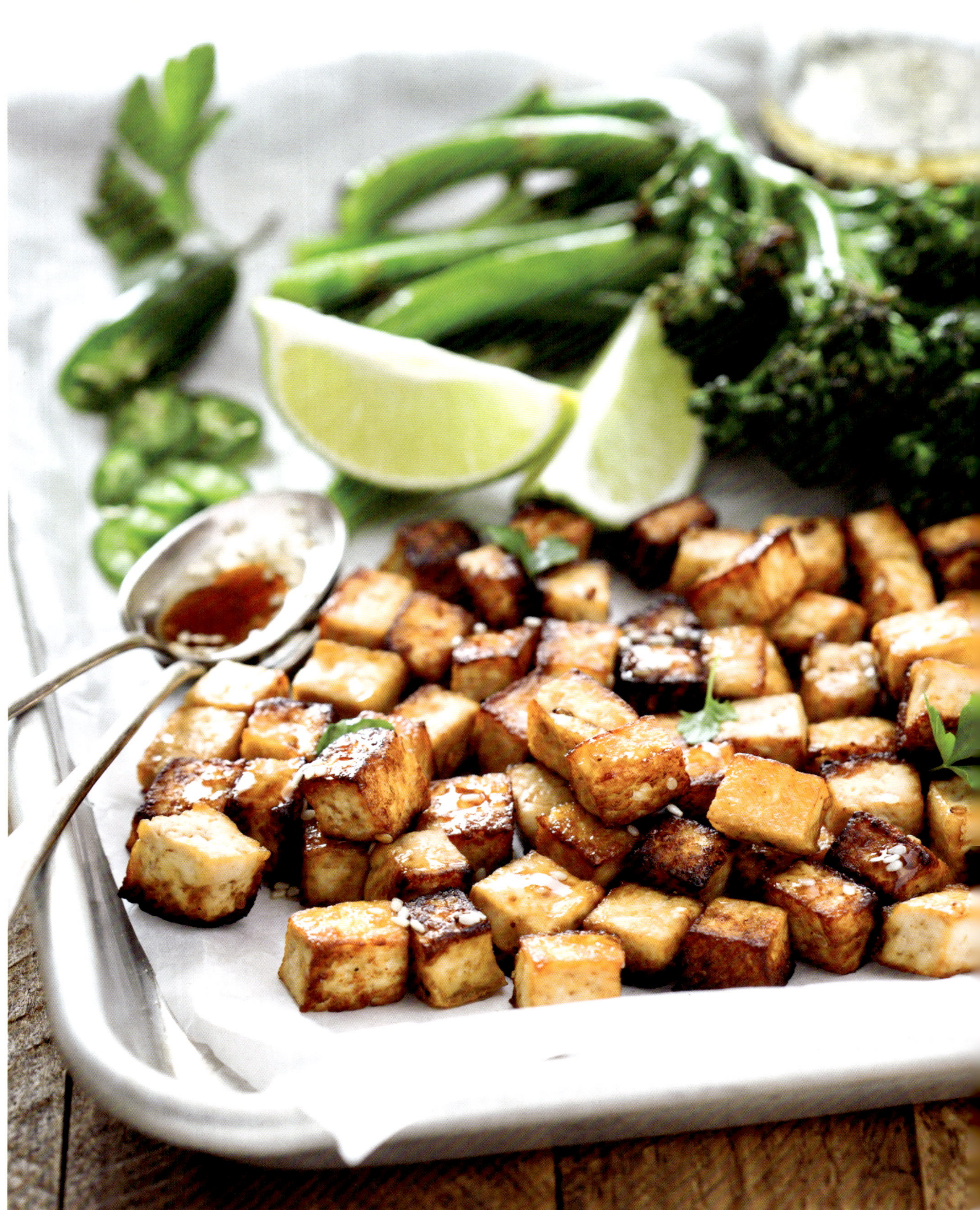

BAKED SWEET GARLIC TOFU

450g extra-firm tofu

1 tbsp sesame oil

4 dried chillies, halved (optional)

Sesame seeds and chopped fresh parsley to garnish

Steamed broccolini to serve

SAUCE

¼ cup (60ml) soy sauce

2 tbsps rice wine vinegar

2 tbsps maple syrup

2 tbsps water

4 cloves garlic, minced

2 tsps cornflour

STEPS

1. Slice the tofu and then place it flat on a baking tray or chopping board covered in paper towels. Place a plate on top. Press for 5 minutes. Allow the water to absorb and replace towels if needed. Pat dry and chop into small cubes.
2. Meanwhile, place the sauce ingredients together in a small bowl and whisk to combine. Set aside.
3. Heat sesame oil in a large frying pan over medium heat. Add tofu cubes in a single layer. Cook for 10 minutes, turning occasionally during cooking to brown all sides. Add chillies, if using, halfway through cooking.
4. Garnish with sesame seeds and chopped parsley and serve with broccolini.

SERVES 4 | PREP + COOK TIME: 30 MINS | VEG | DAIRY FREE |

CHICKEN & BROCCOLI STIR-FRY

½ cup (125ml) chicken stock

¼ cup (60ml) oyster sauce

1 tbsp rice wine vinegar

Medium piece ginger, grated

3 cloves garlic, minced

1 tsp Sriracha (optional)

500g boneless, skinless chicken thighs, cut into bite-size pieces

½ tsp salt

¼ tsp pepper

2 tbsps cornflour

1 tbsp peanut oil

1 tbsp sesame oil

3 cups (225g) broccoli florets

½ tsp toasted sesame seeds

¼ tsp dried chilli flakes

2 spring onions, green parts only, chopped

STEPS

1. In a small bowl, whisk together chicken stock, oyster sauce, vinegar, ginger, garlic and Sriracha, if using; set aside.
2. Season chicken with ½ teaspoon salt and ¼ teaspoon pepper. Add to a bowl with the cornflour and toss to coat.
3. Heat peanut oil and sesame oil in a large frying pan or wok over medium-high heat. Working in batches, add chicken to the pan in a single layer and cook for about 7-8 minutes until golden brown. Stir in broccoli and sauce. Cook for 3-4 minutes until broccoli is just tender.
4. Scatter with sesame seeds, chilli flakes and spring onion tops to serve.

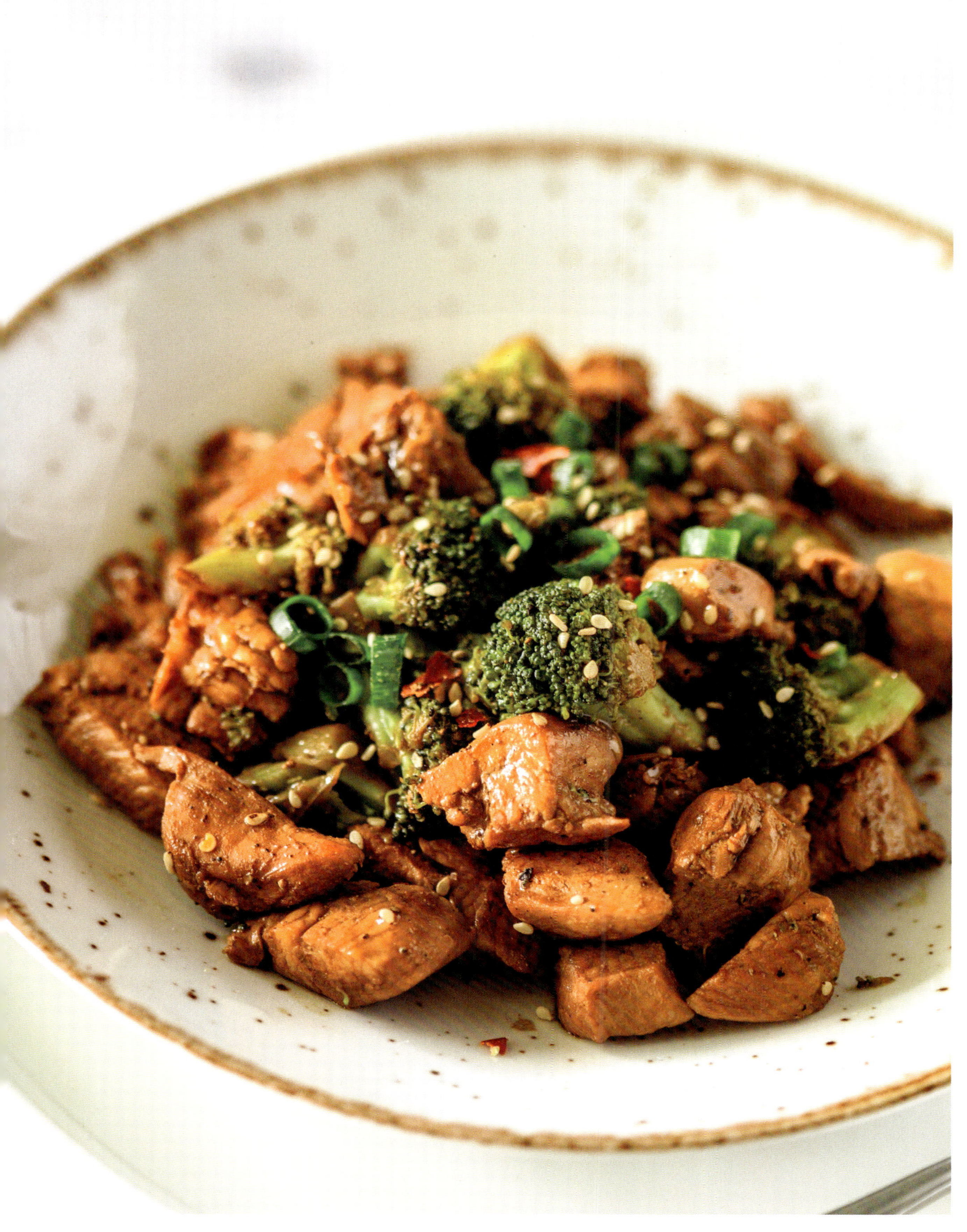

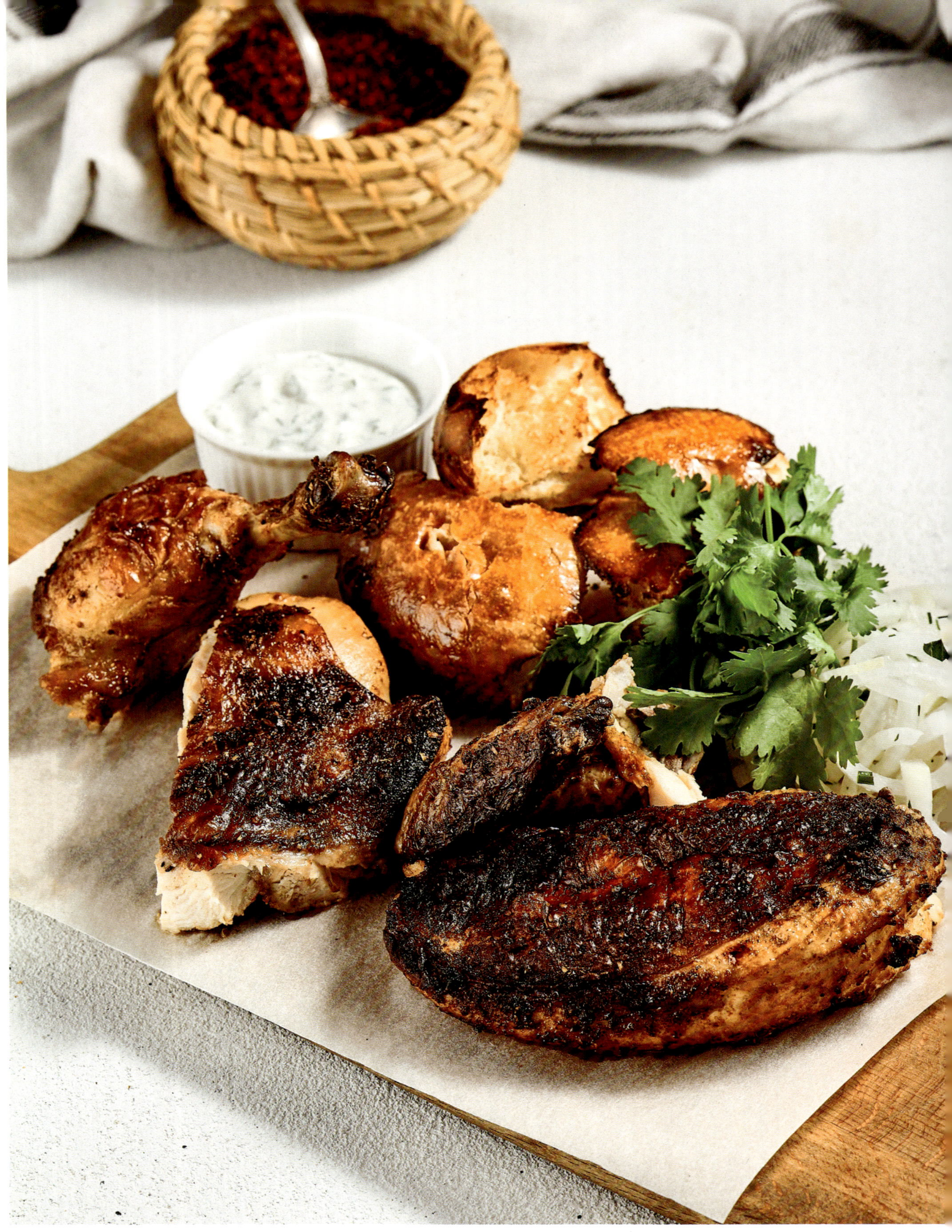

CHICKEN TABAKA

1kg whole chicken

1 tsp ground coriander

1 tsp ground paprika

1 tsp chilli powder

1 tsp dried mint

1 tsp dried basil

Salt to taste

YOGHURT SAUCE

1 cup (250ml) Greek yoghurt

1 clove garlic, minced

¼ cup (10g) chopped mint leaves

1 tbsp lemon juice

½ Lebanese cucumber, grated and lightly squeezed

Salt to taste

TO SERVE

4 toasted bread rolls

Handful of fresh coriander leaves

½ white onion, thinly sliced and tossed with 1 tsp chopped mint leaves

STEPS

1. Slice the chicken lengthwise, between the breast fillets, and open out to get a 'butterfly' form. Wipe the inside and outside with a paper towel.
2. Combine all spices, herbs and salt in a small bowl. Rub the spice mix evenly over both sides of the chicken. Place chicken in a baking dish, cover and refrigerate for at least 1 hour, preferably overnight.
3. Preheat oven to 200°C. Line a baking tray with foil. Place the butterflied chicken skin-side down directly on the oven rack in the middle of the oven, over the foil-covered baking tray. Bake for 30 minutes then gently turn chicken over and bake for another 30-35 minutes, skin-side up, until a crisp crust forms.
4. To make the yoghurt sauce combine all the ingredients and mix well.
5. Cut chicken into pieces. Serve with yoghurt sauce, toasted bread rolls, fresh coriander and sliced white onion.

SERVES 4 | PREP + COOK TIME: 1 HOUR 20 MINS + MARINATING |

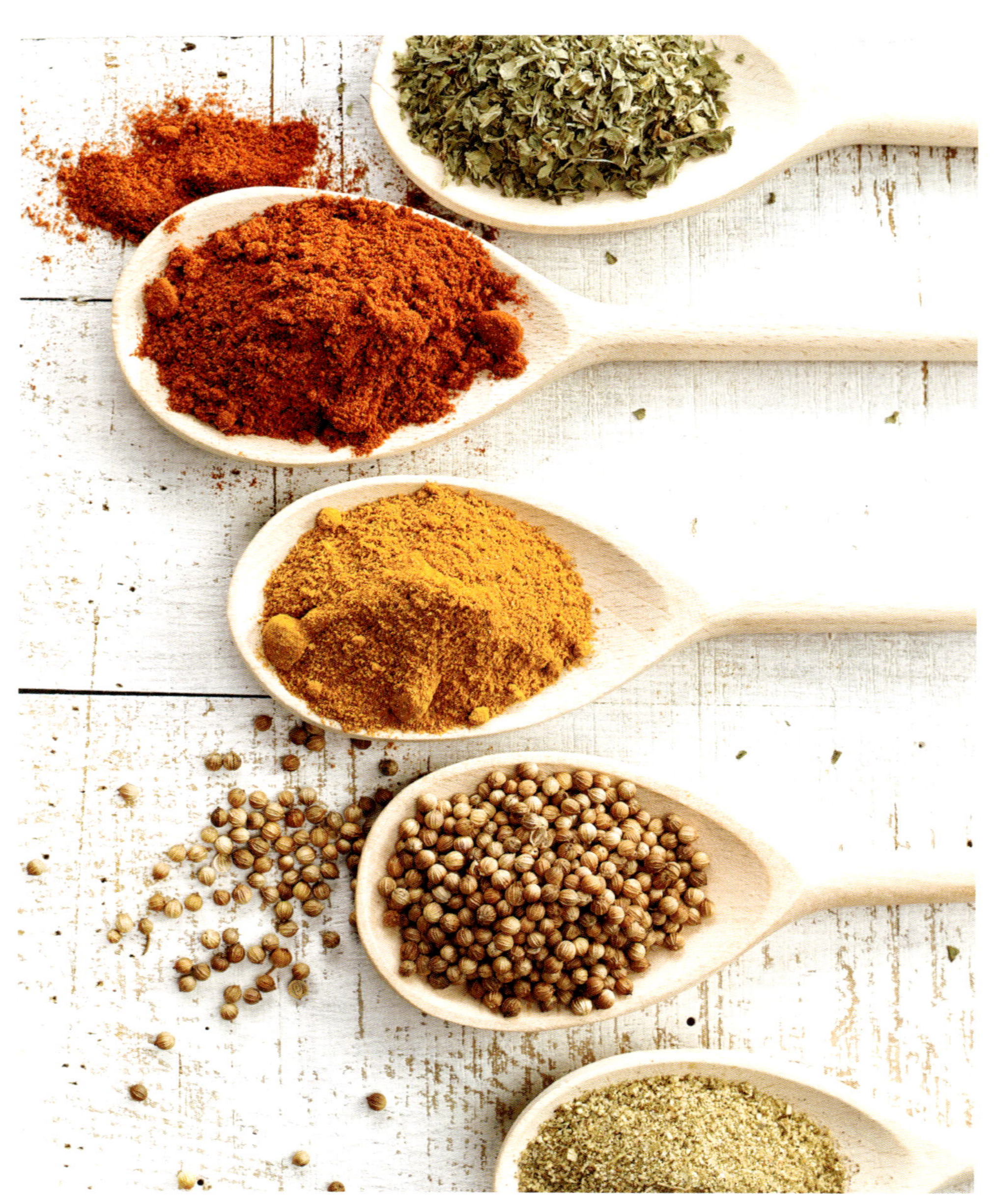

CURRIES & SOUPS

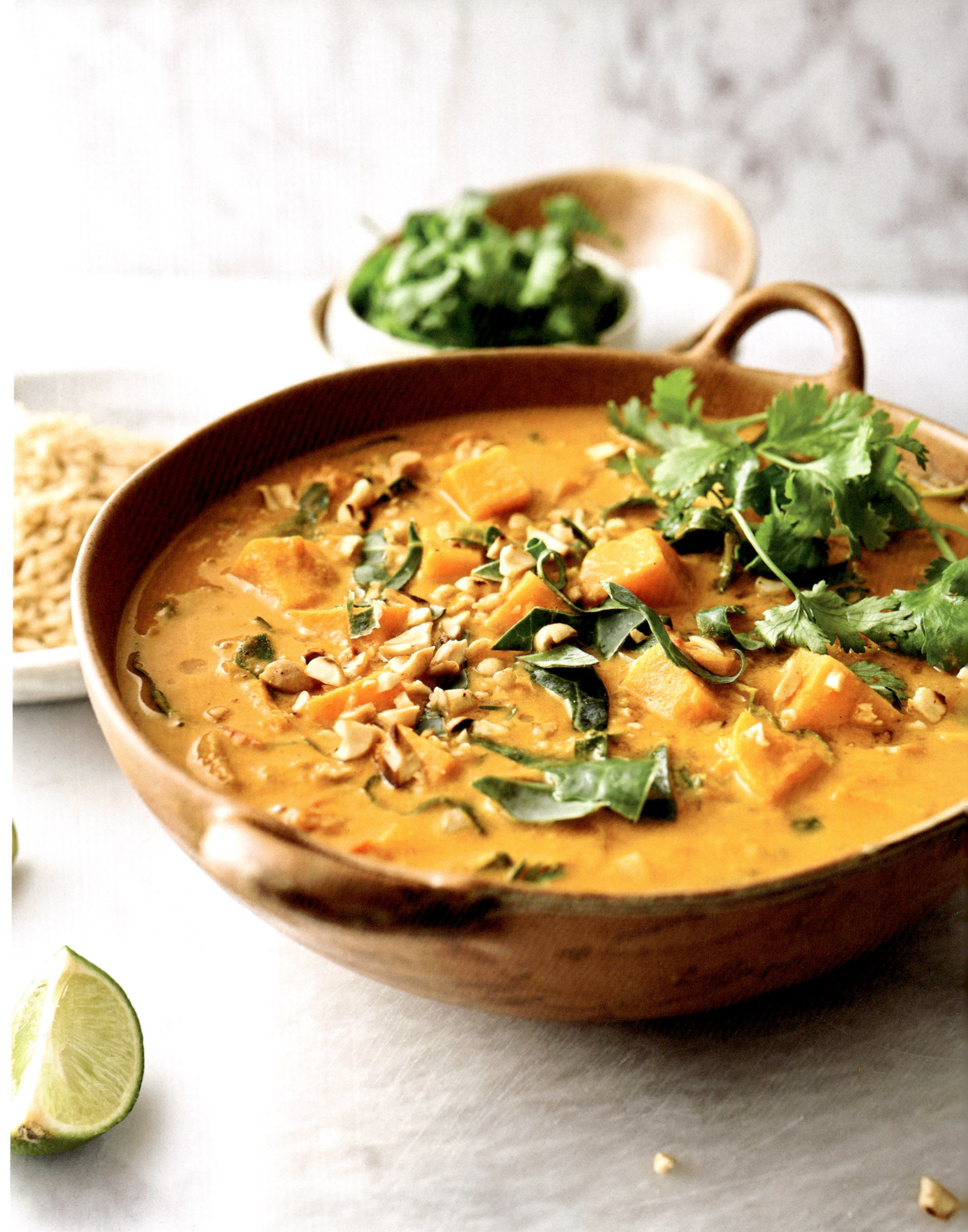

BUTTERNUT PUMPKIN CURRY

1 tbsp coconut oil
2 Asian shallots, chopped
750g butternut pumpkin, diced
Medium piece ginger, grated
3 tbsps red curry paste
½ tbsp curry powder
¾ cup (185ml) vegetable stock
1 x 400g can coconut milk
2 kaffir lime leaves
2 tsps fish sauce
2 tsps sugar
Crushed peanuts and fresh coriander to serve

STEPS

1. Heat the oil in a large, deep frying pan over medium-high heat. Add the shallots and saute for 5-6 minutes or until golden. Add the butternut pumpkin and grated ginger. Stir to coat.

2. Add the red curry paste and curry powder and stir to coat the pumpkin. Continue to cook the curry 2-3 minutes until pumpkin is fragrant.

3. Add the stock, coconut milk, kaffir lime, fish sauce and sugar. Bring to a simmer, then cover and reduce heat. Simmer gently for 12-18 minutes until pumpkin is cooked through.

4. Topped with crushed nuts and fresh coriander.

SERVES 4 | PREP + COOK TIME: 30 MINS | GLUTEN FREE | DAIRY FREE |

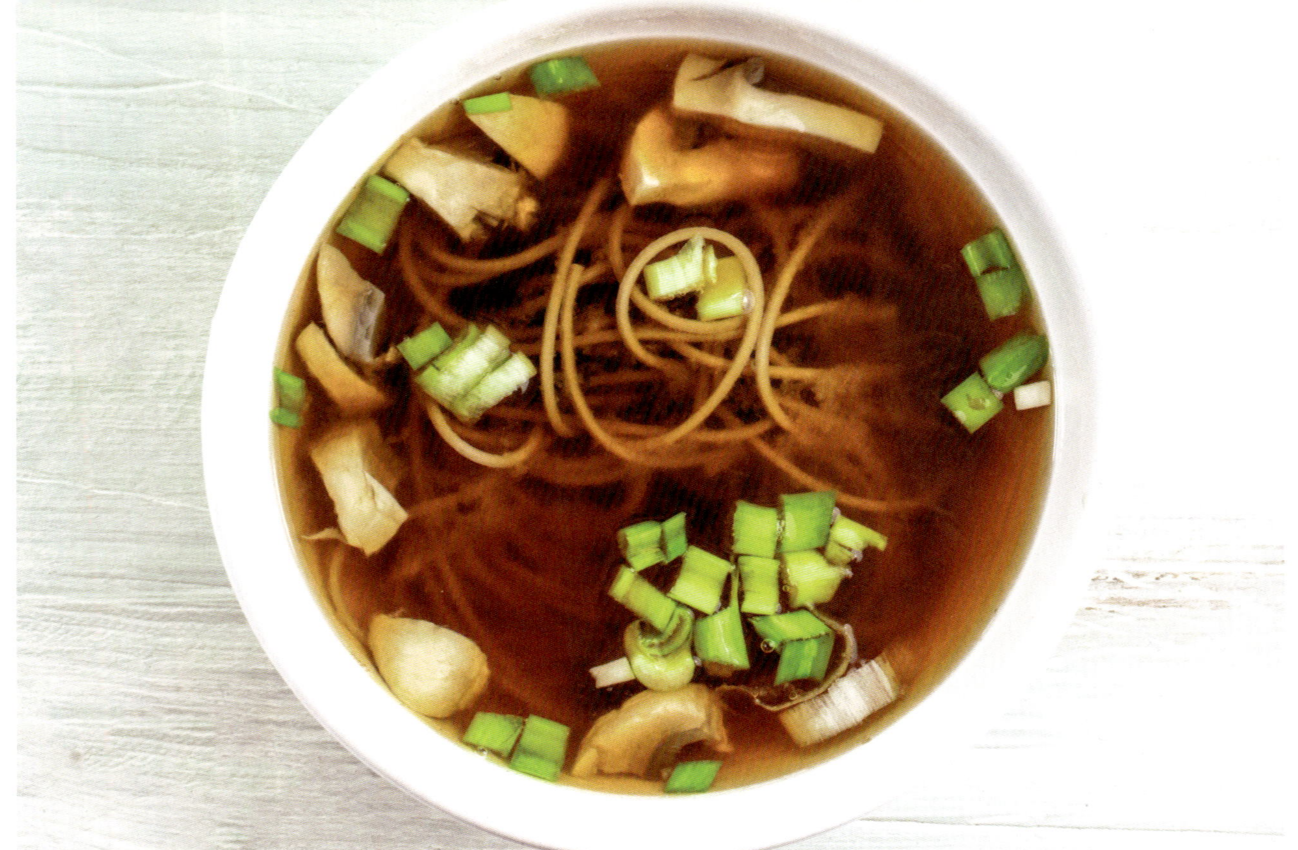

MISO WITH SOBA NOODLES

- 180g soba noodles
- 4½ cups (1.125L) dashi stock
- 3-4 tbsps white miso
- 1 tsp grated ginger
- 2 spring onions, chopped
- ½ cup (40g) thickly sliced mushrooms
- Tamari or soy sauce to taste

STEPS

1. Cook the soba noodles according to the packet directions. Drain and run under cold water.
2. Gently heat the dashi stock in a saucepan until hot.
3. In a small bowl, stir the miso paste together with a little of the hot dashi stock until smooth. Add the miso paste to the pan and stir to incorporate.
4. Add the ginger, spring onion and mushrooms. Simmer gently for 10 minutes.
5. Add the cooked soba noodles and heat through. Season with tamari or soy sauce to serve.

NOTE: Dashi stock can be purchased in granule or sachet form from most major supermarkets.

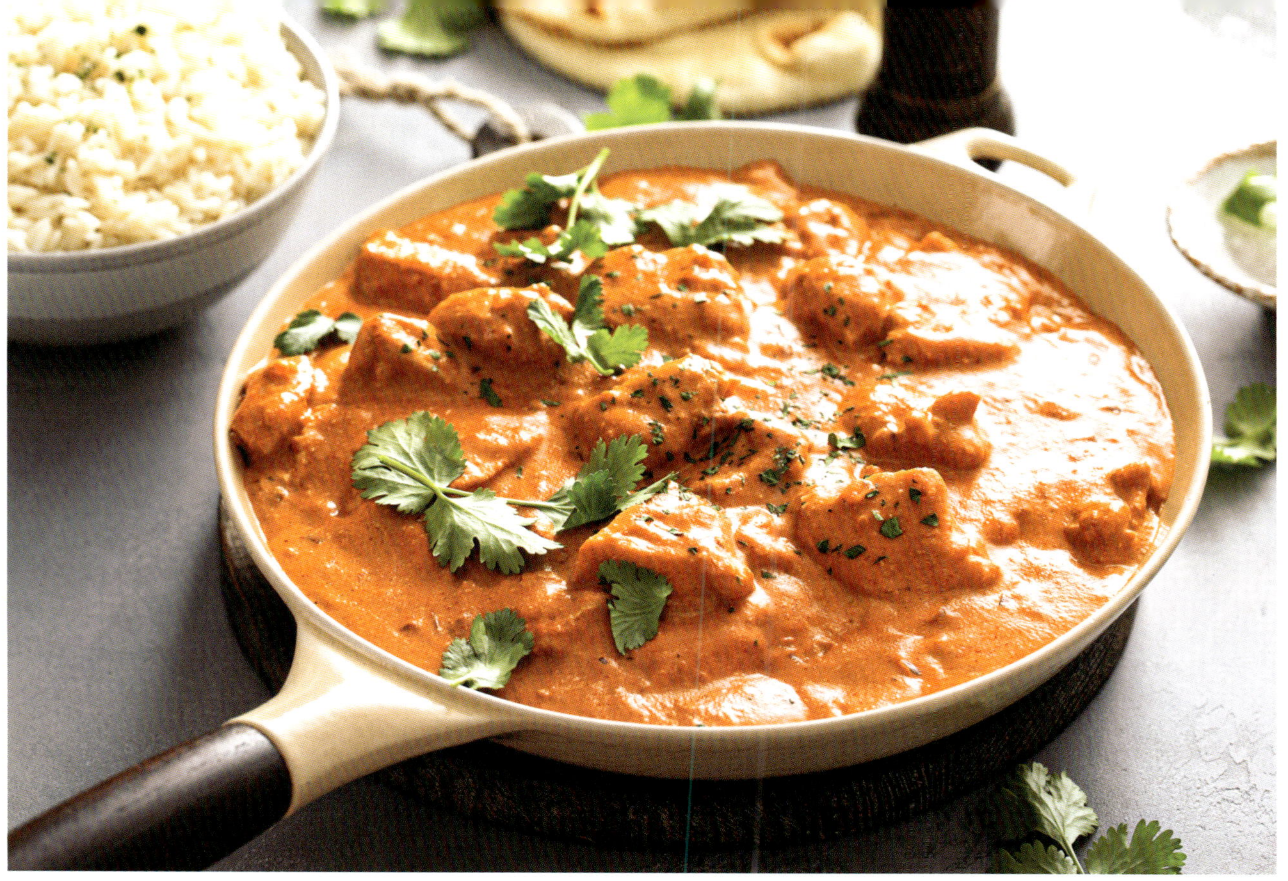

SERVES 4 | PREP + COOK TIME: 50 MINS + MARINATING | GLUTEN FREE |

CHICKEN TIKKA MASALA

6-8 boneless chicken thigh fillets, cut into chunks

⅓ cup (100ml) plain yoghurt

4 tbsps tikka masala paste

Salt and pepper to taste

2 tbsps peanut oil

1 onion, finely chopped

½ fresh green chilli, deseeded and finely chopped

3 cloves garlic, crushed

Large piece ginger, finely grated

1 bay leaf

1 cinnamon stick

¾ cup (185ml) chicken stock

1 x 400g can chopped tomatoes

1 tsp tomato paste

½ cup (125ml) thickened cream

1 tbsp fresh lemon juice

Handful of fresh coriander leaves to serve

STEPS

1. Combine chicken, yoghurt and half the masala paste in a bowl. Season with salt and pepper and stir to coat. Cover and refrigerate for 3 hours.

2. Heat 1 tablespoon oil in a saucepan over medium heat. Add onion, chilli, garlic and ginger and stir for 5 minutes until onion is soft. Add remaining curry paste and cook for 2 minutes, stirring.

3. Add bay leaf, cinnamon, stock, tomatoes and tomato paste. Bring to a boil and then reduce heat to low. Simmer for 15 minutes until sauce thickens.

4. Heat 1 tablespoon oil in a large frying pan over medium heat. Cook chicken for 5 minutes until lightly browned. Add chicken to sauce and simmer for 15 minutes or until cooked through. Add cream and lemon juice and stir well to combine. Cook for 5 more minutes.

5. Scatter with coriander leaves to serve.

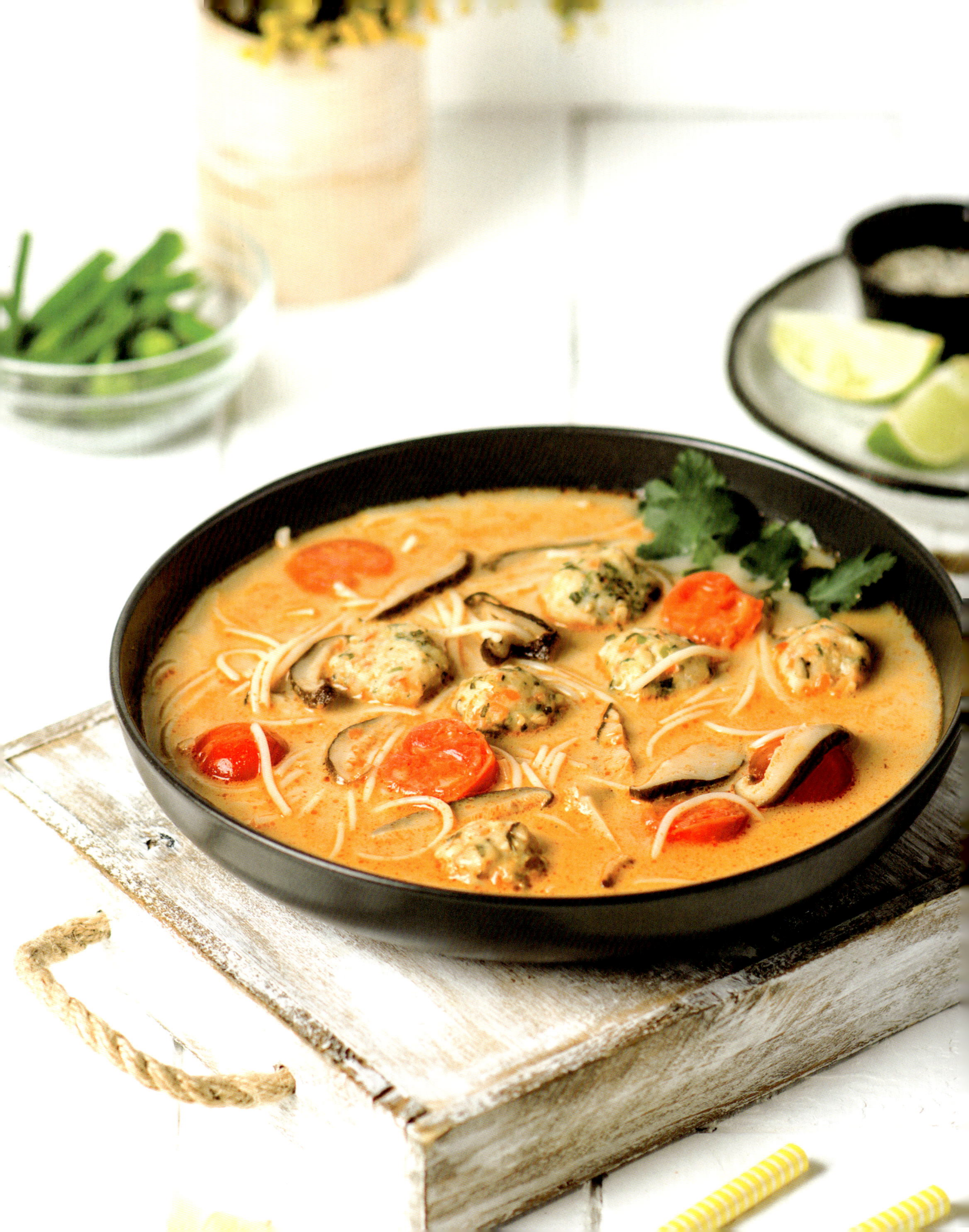

THAI CHICKEN MEATBALL SOUP

500g chicken mince

2 spring onions, finely chopped

2 tbsps coriander leaves, chopped + extra leaves to garnish

3 cloves garlic, minced

Medium piece ginger, grated

2 tbsps soy sauce

1 tbsp coconut oil

2 Asian shallots, thinly sliced

150g shiitake mushrooms, sliced

3 tbsps Thai red curry paste

1 x 400g can coconut milk

4 cups (1L) chicken stock

½ cup (100g) cherry tomatoes, halved

Juice of 1 lime

Cooked rice noodles

STEPS

Preheat the oven to 200°C.

1. In a mixing bowl, combine chicken, spring onions, chopped coriander, garlic, ginger and 1 tablespoon of soy sauce. With oiled hands, form the mixture into 4cm balls and place on a lined baking tray. Bake for 15 minutes or until just cooked.
2. Heat oil in a large saucepan over medium-high heat. Add the shallots and saute for 3-5 minutes until soft and translucent. Add the mushrooms and cook for another 2-3 minutes, until tender. Stir in the red curry paste. Cook for 1 minute until fragrant. Add the coconut milk, chicken stock and remaining 1 tablespoon of soy sauce.
3. Place the baked meatballs into the pan along with the cherry tomato halves and bring to a gentle simmer. Reduce the heat and continue simmering for 5-10 minutes or until the meatballs are cooked through. Stir in the lime juice.
4. Divide the noodles between bowls and spoon over the soup. Scatter with coriander leaves to serve.

SERVES 4 | PREP + COOK TIME: 45 MINS | DAIRY FREE |

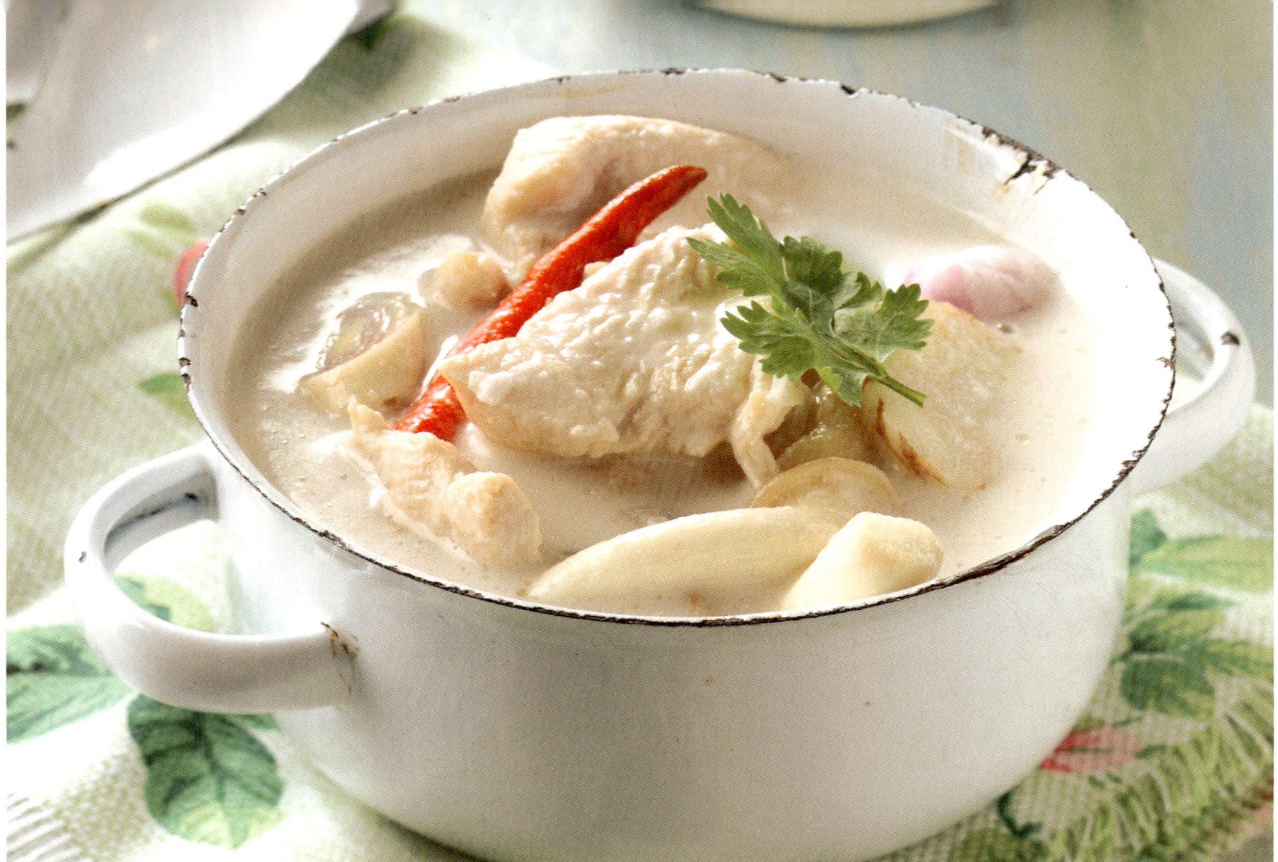

TOM KHA GAI

1 tbsp coconut oil

2 Asian shallots, quartered

2 cloves garlic, chopped

Medium piece galangal or ginger, sliced

1 stalk lemongrass, cut into 3cm lengths

2 tsps Thai red curry paste

3 cups (750ml) chicken stock

4 whole red chillies

1 x 400ml can coconut milk

450g chicken breasts or thigh fillets, cut into bite-size pieces

1 cup (75g) shimeji, oyster or sliced button mushrooms

1 tbsp coconut sugar

1 tbsp fish sauce + more to taste

2 tbsps fresh lime juice

Fresh coriander leaves to garnish

STEPS

1. Heat coconut oil in a large pan over medium heat. Add shallot, garlic, galangal or ginger, lemongrass and curry paste. Cook, stirring frequently, for 5 minutes, or until onions are soft. Add stock and chillies and bring to a boil. Reduce heat and simmer uncovered for 30 minutes.

2. Use a slotted spoon to remove ginger and lemongrass. Discard.

3. Add in coconut milk, chicken and mushrooms. Simmer for 10 minutes until the chicken is just cooked through. Add sugar, fish sauce and lime juice.

4. Cook for 2 minutes, then ladle into serving bowls and top with fresh coriander.

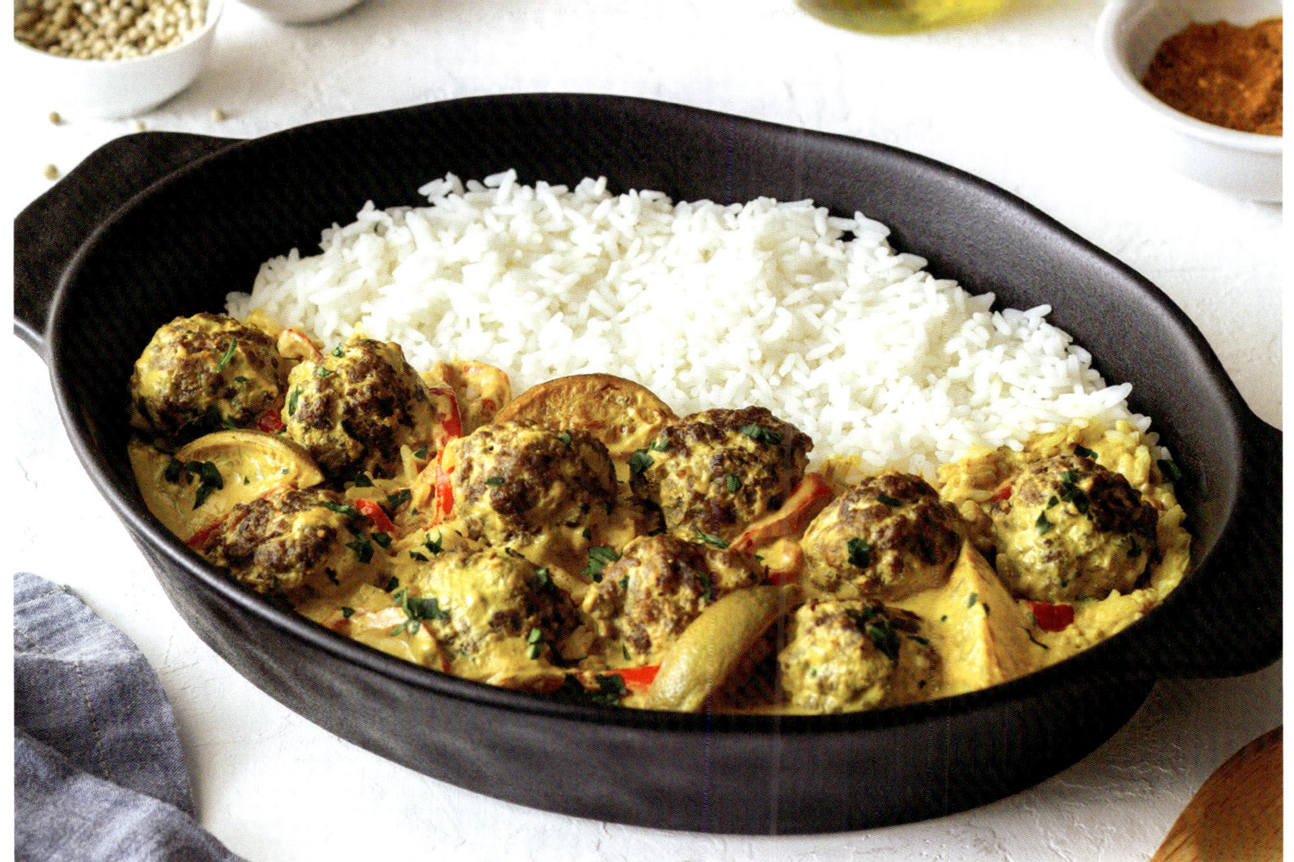

MEATBALL COCONUT CURRY

MEATBALLS

1kg beef mince

2 cloves garlic, grated

Small piece ginger, grated

2 tbsps breadcrumbs

¼ cup (10g) finely chopped coriander leaves

½ tsp salt

Pepper to taste

CURRY

2 tbsps peanut oil or ghee

1½ tbsps Thai red curry paste

1 x 400ml can coconut milk

¾ cup (200ml) water

1 x 225g can bamboo shoots, drained

1 lime, cut into wedges

TO SERVE

1 red chilli, finely sliced

2 tbsps chopped coriander leaves

Boiled white rice

STEPS

1. Combine meatball ingredients in a bowl then form into small meatballs.
2. Heat the oil in a large frying pan over medium-high heat. Brown the meatballs for 5 minutes then transfer to a plate.
3. Add the curry paste to the pan, fry for 1 minute, then pour in the coconut milk and water. Bring back to the boil and stir until smooth.
4. Return the meatballs to the pan, along with the bamboo shoots and lime wedges. Simmer for 10 minutes until meatballs are cooked through and the sauce is thickened.
5. Scatter with sliced chilli and chopped coriander and serve with rice.

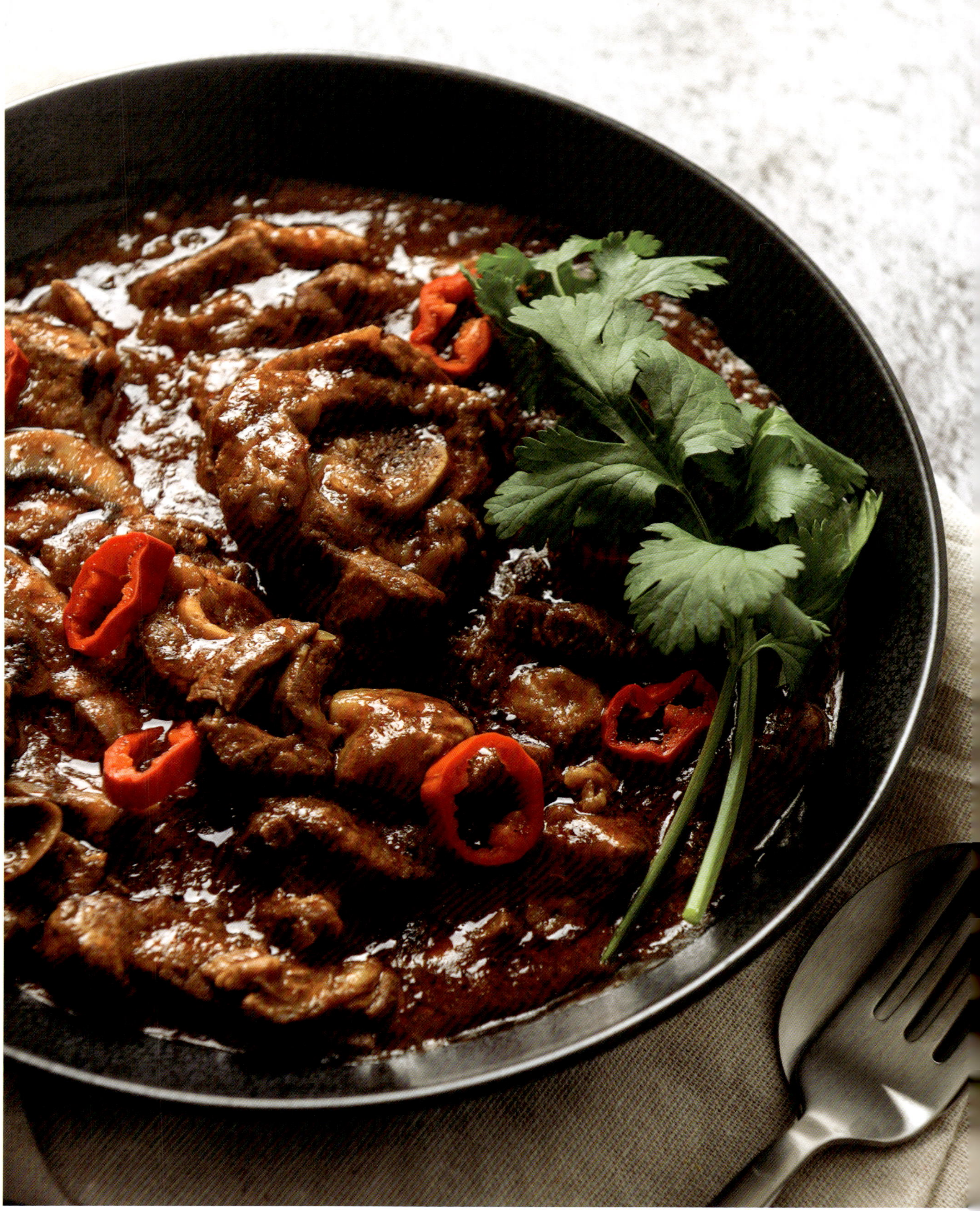

SERVES 4 | PREP + COOK TIME: 1 HOUR 20 MINS | GLUTEN FREE |

LAMB ROGAN JOSH

Medium piece ginger, coarsely chopped
6 cloves garlic, peeled
3 tbsps + ¾ cup (185ml) water
3 tbsps vegetable oil or ghee
750g diced lamb
7 cardamon pods
2 bay leaves
4 whole cloves
6 peppercorns
1 cinnamon stick
3 medium onions, finely chopped
1 tsp ground coriander
1½ tsps ground cumin
1 tbsp paprika
¾ tsp cayenne pepper
¾ tsp salt
3 tbsps plain yoghurt
2 x 400g cans chopped tomatoes
1 red chilli, sliced
Handful of fresh coriander leaves to serve

STEPS

1. Place the ginger, garlic and 3 tablespoons water into a blender. Blend to a smooth paste.

2. Heat oil or ghee in a heavy pan over medium-high heat. Brown the meat in several batches and set aside.

3. Using the same pan, add the cardamon, bay leaves, cloves, peppercorns and cinnamon to the hot oil. Stir once and leave to cook for 1 minute, then add the onions. Stir-fry for 5 minutes until onions are soft and golden. Add the ginger and garlic paste and stir for 30 seconds until fragrant. Then add the ground coriander, cumin, paprika, cayenne pepper and salt. Stir-fry for 30 seconds before returning the meat to the pan. Cook for another 30 seconds.

4. Reduce heat to low then add 1 tablespoon of the yoghurt and stir until well combined. Add the remaining yoghurt a tablespoon at a time in the same way. Cook, stirring occasionally, for another 3 minutes.

5. Add ¾ cup water and canned tomatoes. Bring to the boil, scraping all the browned spices off the bottom of the pot. Cover and cook on a low heat, stirring occasionally, for 1 hour or until lamb is tender. Add more water during cooking if mixture starts to dry out. Scatter with sliced chilli and fresh coriander leaves to serve.

NOTE: The flavours in this curry are amazing but you can choose to use a rogan josh curry paste to make this recipe really easy.

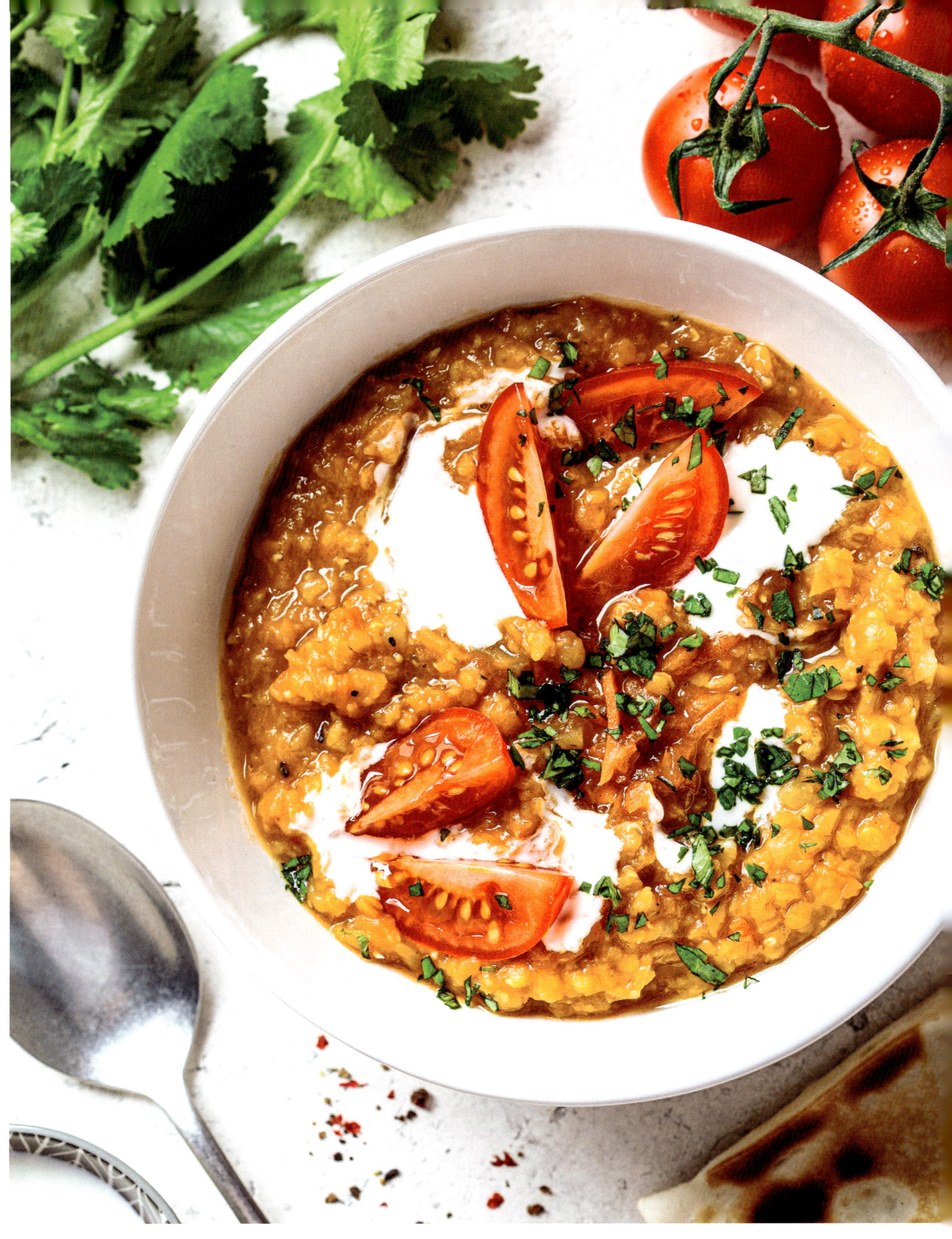

RED LENTIL CURRY BOWL

1 tbsp coconut oil

1 onion, finely chopped

6 cloves garlic, crushed

1 tsp brown mustard seeds

1 tsp ground turmeric

½ tsp ground coriander

1 tsp curry powder

1 tsp ground cumin

1¼ tsps salt

1 x 400ml can coconut milk

⅔ cup (150g) tomato paste

3 cups (750ml) boiling water

1 cup (200g) dried red lentils

TO SERVE

2 tomatoes, quartered

¼ cup (60ml) yoghurt

2 tbsps chopped coriander

STEPS

1. Heat oil in a saucepan on low-medium heat. Add onion and cook for 5 minutes, stirring occasionally, until golden. Add garlic and fry for 1 minute until fragrant. Add the brown mustard seeds and cook for 30 seconds until seeds start to pop. Add turmeric, coriander, curry powder, cumin and salt and cook for a further 30 seconds, stirring constantly.

2. Pour in the coconut milk, tomato paste, boiling water and lentils and stir to combine. Bring to a boil, cover and cook on a low heat for 45 minutes. Remove from heat and let stand for 5 minutes.

3. Top the curry with tomato pieces, yoghurt and chopped coriander.

SERVES 4 | PREP + COOK TIME: 1 HOUR | VEG | GLUTEN FREE |

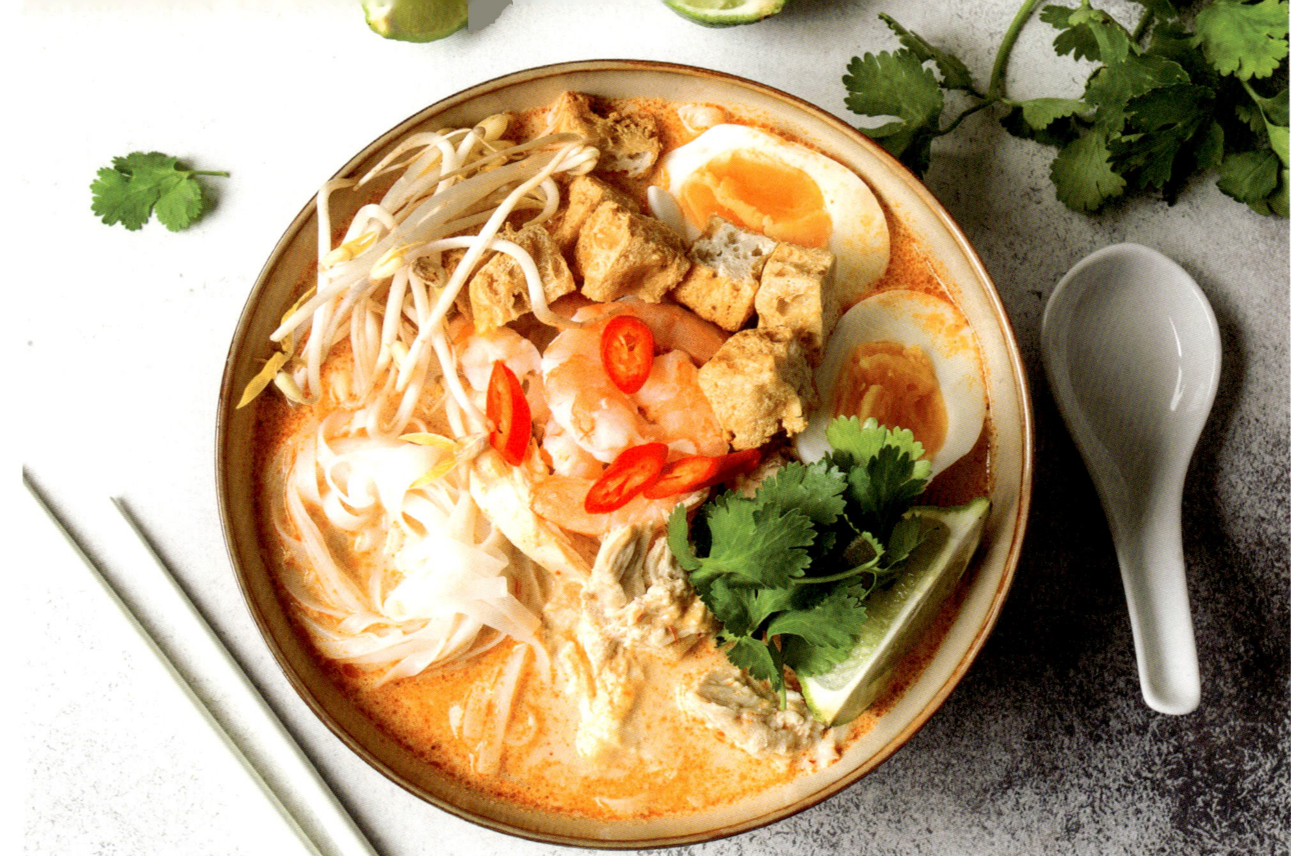

CHICKEN & PRAWN LAKSA

300g rice stick noodles

2 tbsps coconut oil

½ cup (150g) laksa paste

1 x 400ml can coconut milk

2 cups (500ml) chicken stock

½ large barbecued chicken, skin and bones removed, meat shredded

350g raw prawns

1 cup (110g) bean sprouts to serve

1 cup (100g) tofu puffs

4 eggs, soft boiled

½ cup (10g) coriander leaves

1 red chilli, sliced

4 lime wedges to serve

STEPS

1. Cook noodles according to the packet directions. Drain and set aside.
2. Heat coconut oil in wok or large frying pan over medium heat. Add laksa paste. Stir-fry for 1 minute until fragrant. Add coconut milk and stock. Bring to the boil.
3. Add chicken and reduce heat to low. Simmer for 2-3 minutes until chicken is heated through.
4. Steam the prawns over a pan of simmering water for 3-4 minutes until cooked.
5. Divide noodles between bowls. Spoon over laksa. Top with prawns, bean sprouts, tofu puffs, eggs, coriander leaves, sliced chilli and lime wedges.

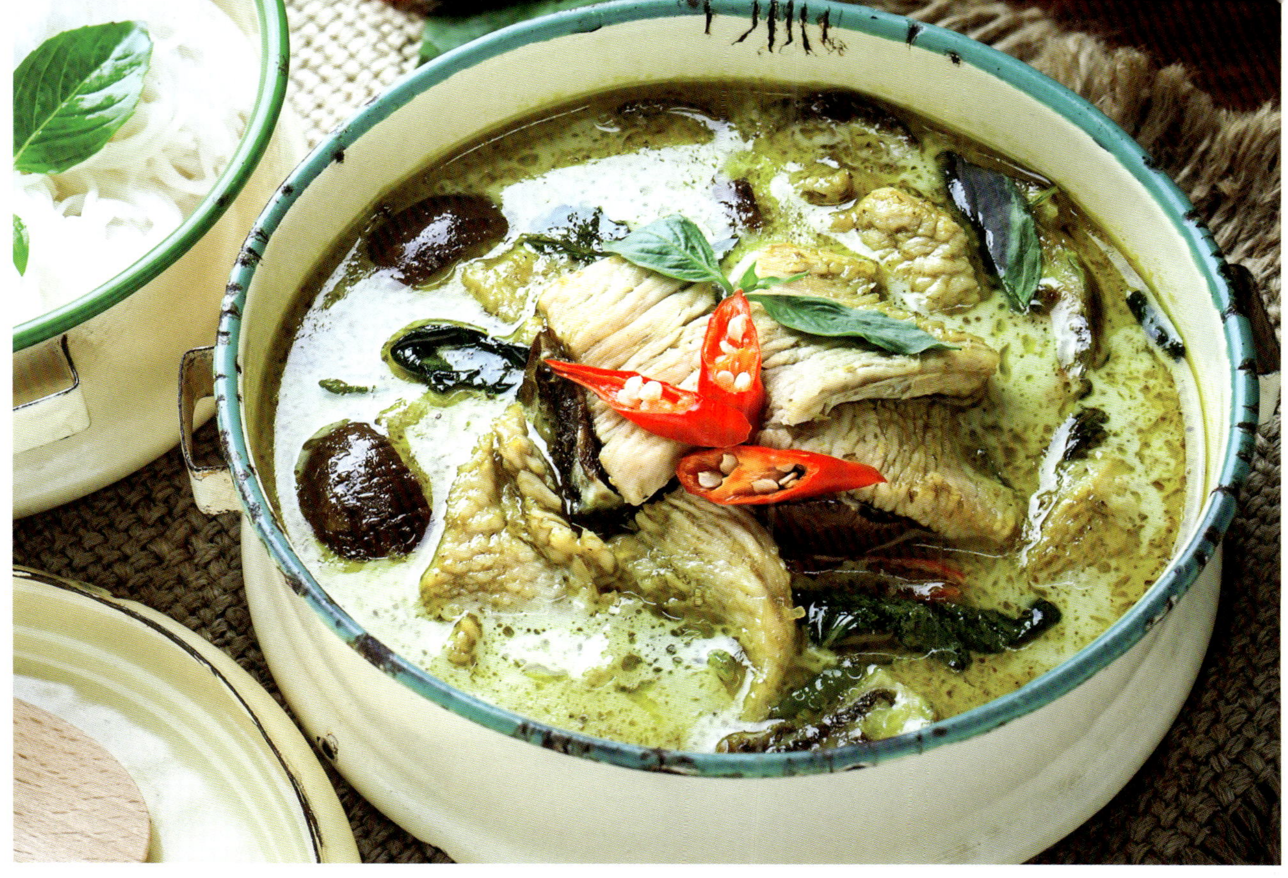

GREEN CHICKEN CURRY

- 1 tbsp oil
- 1½ tbsps green curry paste
- 1 x 210ml can coconut cream
- 8 chicken thigh fillets, cut into pieces
- 4-6 Thai eggplants, quartered or 1 medium eggplant, cut into bite-size pieces
- 6-8 kaffir lime leaves, torn into strips
- 1 x 400ml can coconut milk
- 1 bunch bok choy, leaves separated
- 1 tbsp fish sauce
- 1 tbsp palm sugar, finely chopped
- ½ cup (10g) fresh Thai basil leaves
- Sliced red chilli to serve
- Noodles or rice to serve

STEPS

1. Heat oil in a large frying pan or saucepan over medium-low heat. Add curry paste and cook, stirring, for 10 minutes until fragrant. Do not allow the paste to burn.
2. Pour in the coconut cream. Bring to a boil and then reduce heat. Simmer for 5 minutes.
3. Add the chicken, eggplant, kaffir lime leaves and coconut milk and stir. Reduce to a low heat for 10 minutes, stirring occasionally, until the chicken is cooked through. Add the bok choy and cook, stirring occasionally, for 2 minutes or until tender. Remove from heat. Add the fish sauce, palm sugar and half the basil to the curry mixture and stir.
4. Spoon the curry into bowls and top with the remaining basil and sliced red chilli. Serve with noodles or rice.

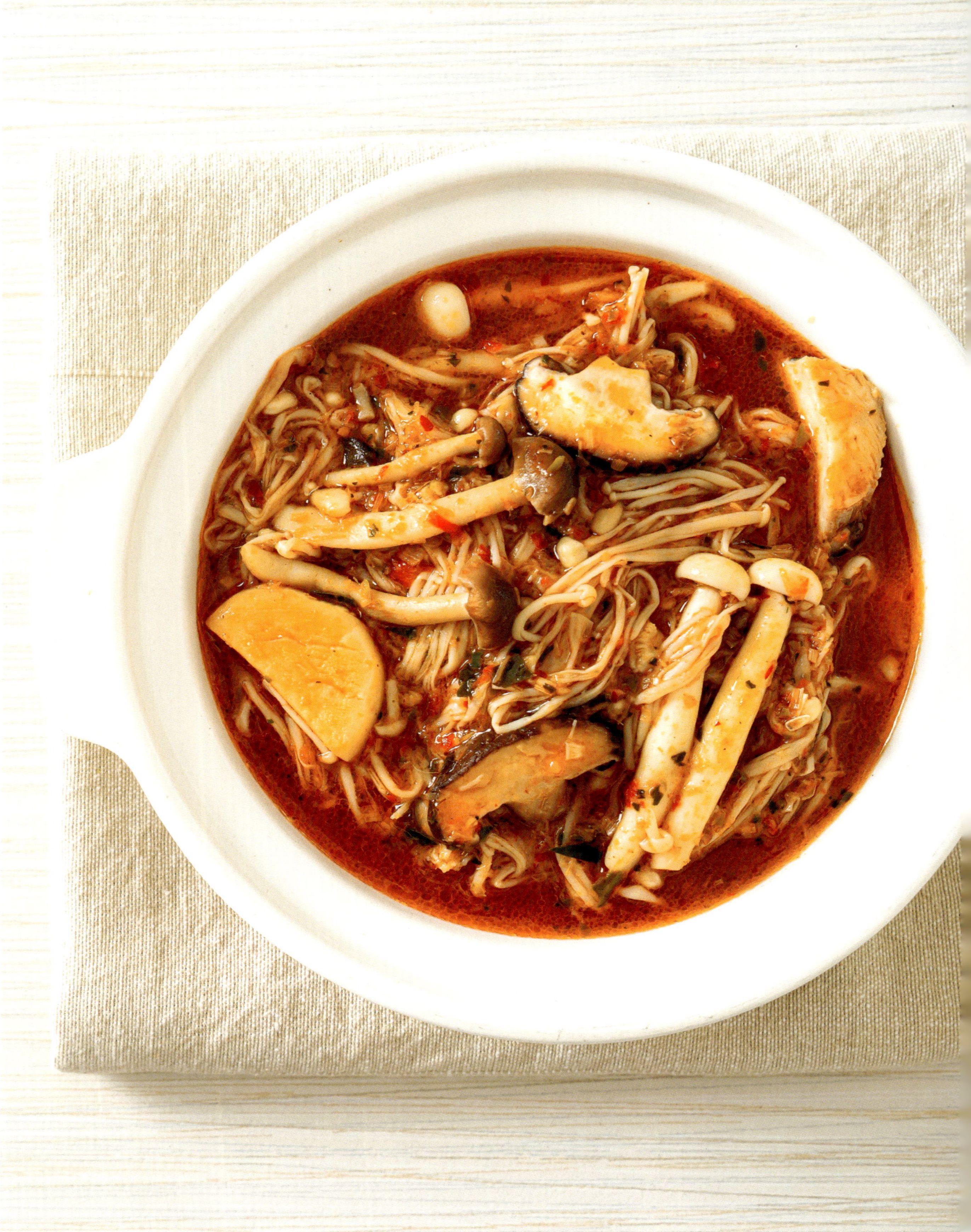

MUSHROOM TOM YUM SOUP

1 stalk lemongrass

Medium piece galangal

3-4 kaffir lime leaves

8 cups (2L) vegetable stock

1 cup (75g) shiitake mushrooms, sliced

1 cup (70g) enoki mushrooms

1 cup (75g) shimeji mushrooms

4 king oyster mushrooms, cut into bite-size pieces

1 Thai red chilli, finely chopped

1 cup (225g) cherry tomatoes, halved

1 tbsp Thai chilli paste (nam prik pao)

2 tbsps fish sauce

1 tsp brown sugar or palm sugar

3 tbsps lime juice or to taste

¼ cup (5g) fresh coriander leaves, chopped

STEPS

1. Crush the lemongrass stalk, galangal and kaffir lime leaves. Place in a large saucepan with the stock and bring to a simmer. Simmer for 10-15 minutes over medium heat.

2. Remove the lemongrass, galangal and kaffir lime leaves from the stock and discard.

3. Add mushrooms, chilli, tomatoes, chilli paste, fish sauce and sugar. Mix and cover the pan. Cook for another 5 minutes.

4. Stir in the lime juice and chopped coriander before serving.

NOTE: You can buy a pack of exotic mushrooms from major supermarkets that will work well in this recipe.

SERVES 4 | PREP + COOK TIME: 25 MINS | GLUTEN FREE | DAIRY FREE |

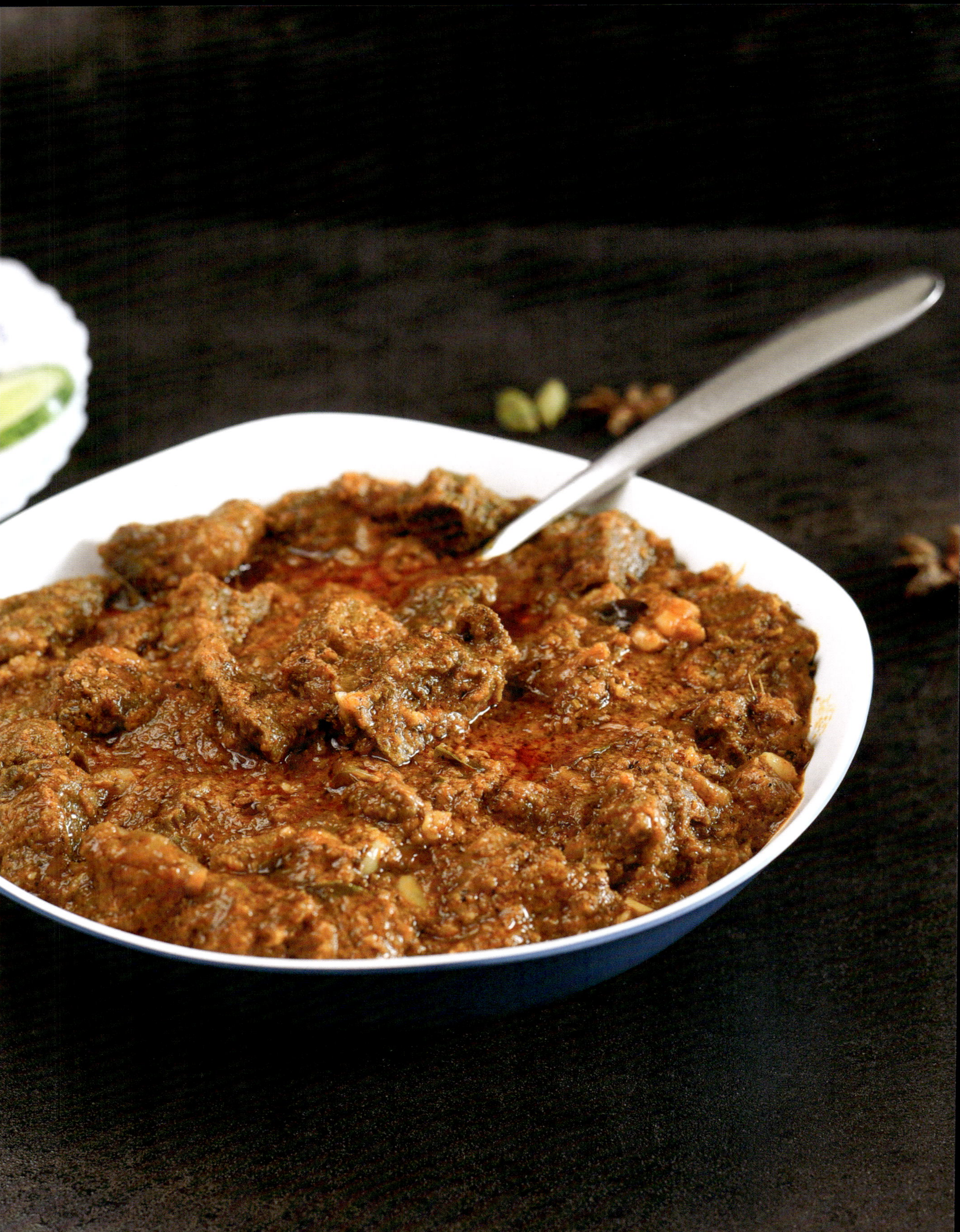

KERALAN BEEF CURRY

4 tbsps ghee or oil

2 onions, sliced

Small piece ginger, finely chopped

2 green chillies, split lengthwise

3-4 sprigs curry leaves

1kg chuck steak or braising steak, cut into 2½ cm cubes

1 cup (250ml) water, or as required

2 tomatoes, diced

Salt to taste

CURRY PASTE

Small piece ginger, chopped

5 cloves garlic, chopped

3 tsps Kashmiri chilli powder

¼ tsp ground turmeric

1 tsp ground coriander

½ tsp fennel seeds

1 cinnamon stick

2 cloves

2 cardamon pods

1 star anise

½ tsp whole black peppercorns

STEPS

1. Combine the paste ingredients in a spice grinder or high-speed blender and grind into a paste.
2. Heat ghee or oil in a large pan over medium-high heat. Add sliced onion, ginger, green chillies and curry leaves. Saute for 3-5 minutes until onion turns translucent.
3. Add the curry paste and fry until oil starts to separate.
4. Add beef and stir to coat. Add water, tomatoes and salt to taste, cover and simmer very gently for 1 hour 30 minutes, until beef is tender, adding more water as needed.

SERVES 4 | PREP + COOK TIME: 1 HOUR 50 MINS | GLUTEN FREE |

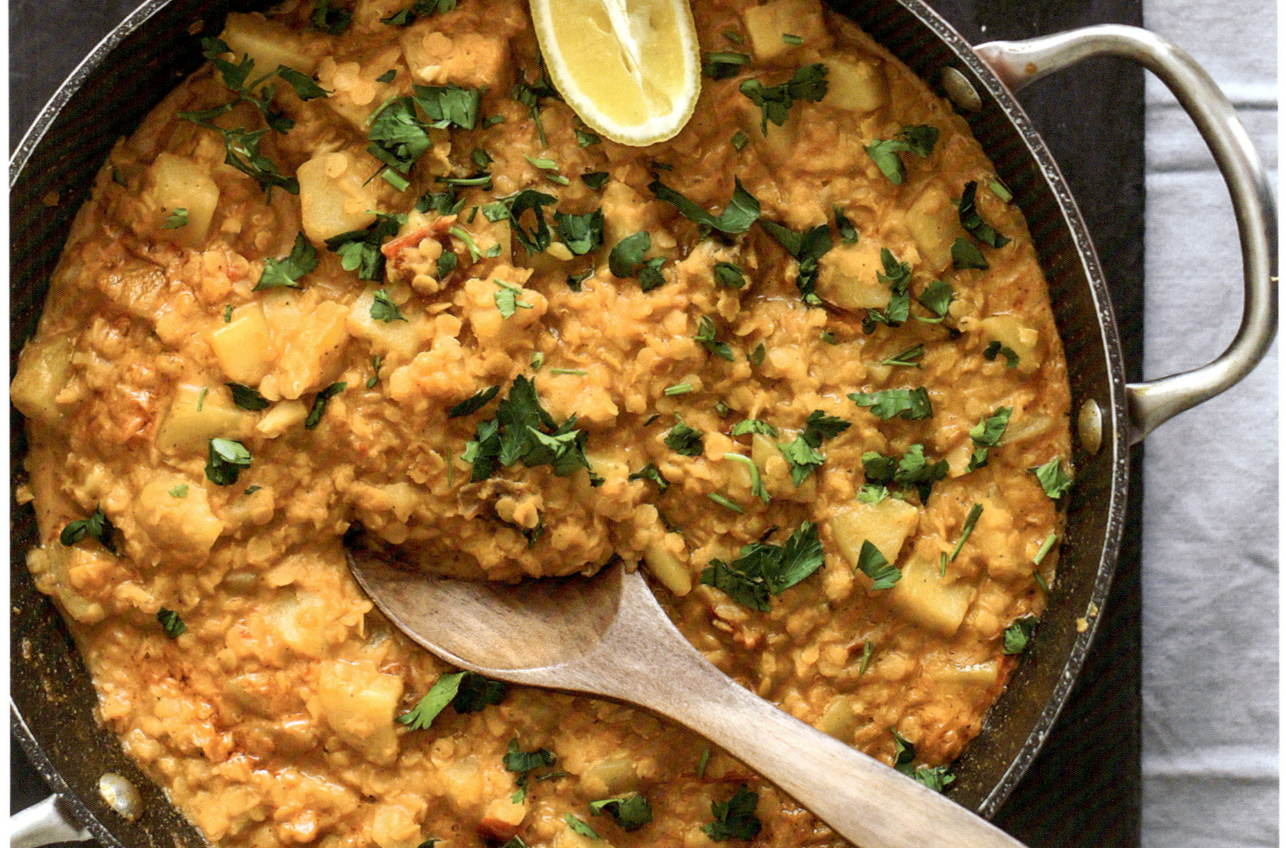

POTATO & LENTIL CURRY

3 tbsps olive oil
1 onion, chopped
2 cloves garlic, minced
2 tsps minced fresh ginger
1¼ cups (250g) dried red lentils
1⅔ cups (400ml) vegetable stock
1 x 400g can diced tomatoes
1 x 400ml can coconut milk
2 potatoes, cubed
½ tsp salt
1 tbsp garam masala
1 tsp ground cumin
1 tsp ground turmeric
¼ tsp dried chilli flakes
¼ cup (10g) chopped fresh coriander
Juice of ½ lemon
Steamed rice to serve

STEPS

1. Heat oil in a large frying pan over medium-high heat and cook onion, stirring regularly, for 3-5 minutes until soft and translucent. Add garlic and ginger and cook for 1 minute until fragrant.
2. Add lentils, stock, tomatoes, coconut milk and potato. Bring to a boil, reduce heat to low and simmer for about 20 minutes, until tender.
3. Add salt and spices and cook for 5 minutes more.
4. Stir through chopped coriander and squeeze over lemon juice.
5. Serve with steamed rice.

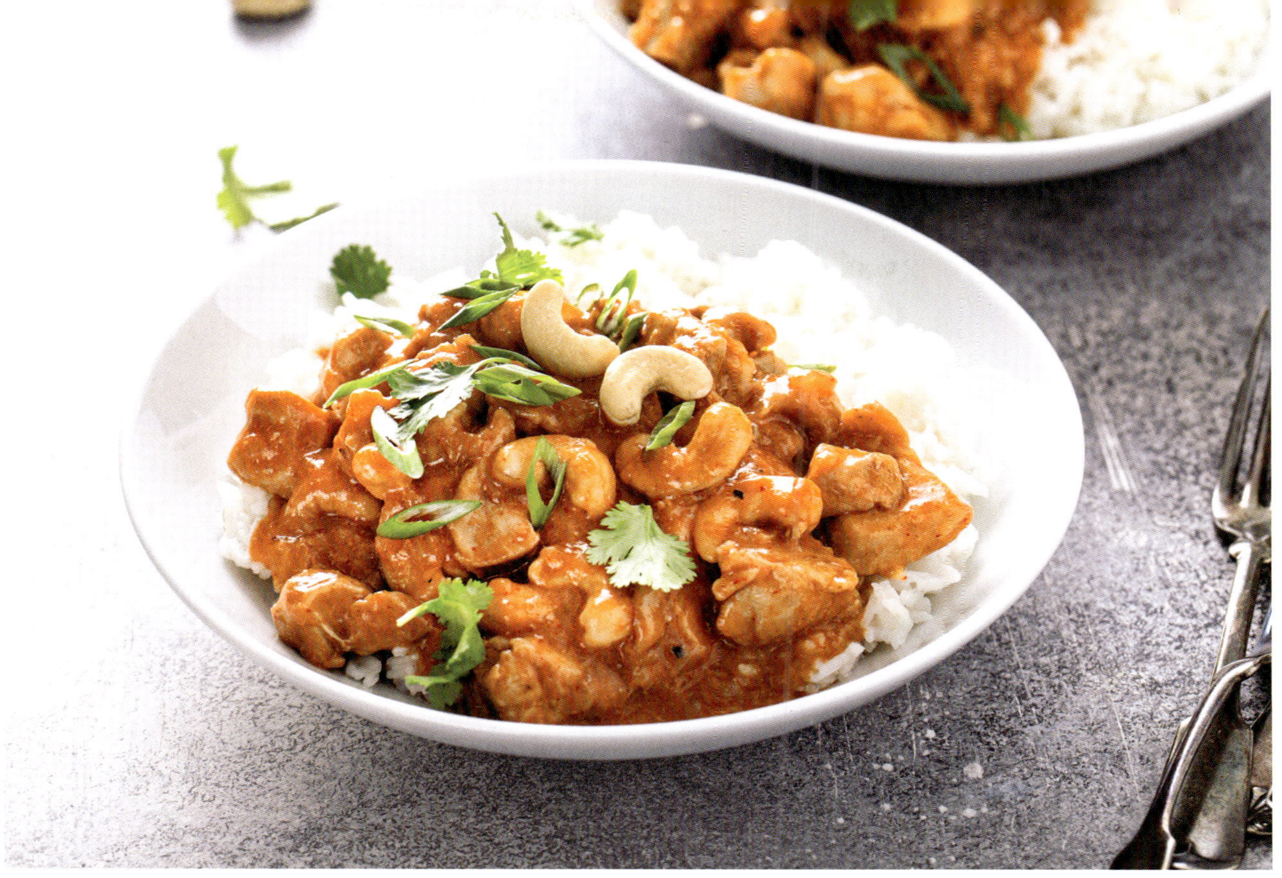

EASY RED CHICKEN CURRY

8 chicken thigh fillets, cubed

1½ tbsps Thai red curry paste

1½ tbsps vegetable oil

1 x 400ml can coconut milk

2 tbsps fish sauce

3 tsps brown sugar

2 large dried chillies, roughly chopped

½ cup (60g) cashews

Cooked rice to serve

Coriander leaves and chopped spring onions, to garnish

STEPS

1. Put the chicken and curry paste in a mixing bowl, and toss to coat. Cover the bowl and if time allows place in the fridge for 1 hour.
2. Heat oil in a wok over medium heat. Fry the chicken for 2-3 minutes or until lightly browned. Pour in the coconut milk and reduce heat to a low simmer. Cook, stirring occasionally, for 5 minutes or until chicken is tender.
3. Stir in fish sauce and sugar. Cook for a further minute. Add chillies and cashews. Cook for 3 minutes more.
4. Serve with rice and top with chopped coriander and chopped spring onions.

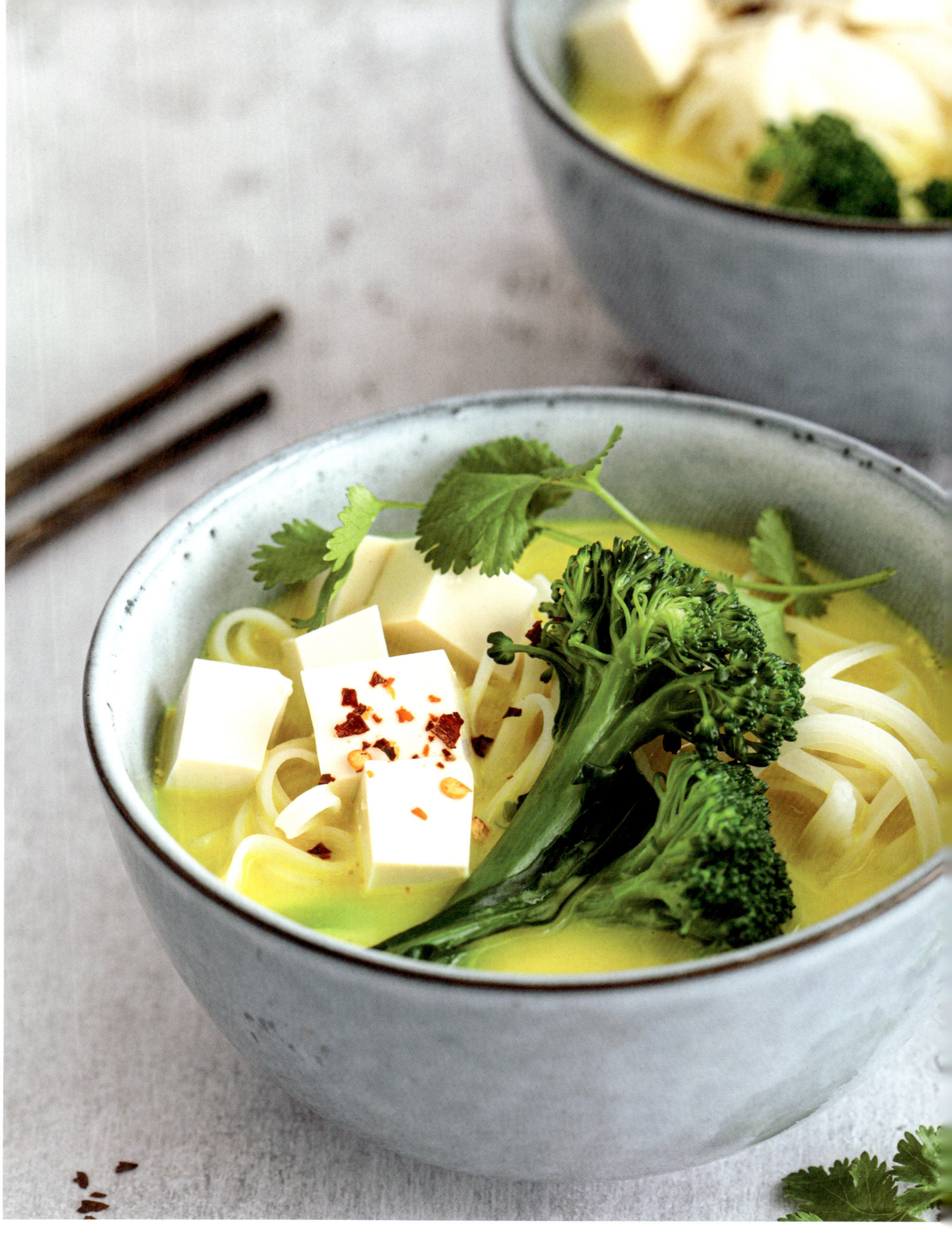

VEGAN LAKSA

2 tbsps peanut or other neutral-flavoured oil
3-4 tbsps vegan Thai red curry paste
1 tsp ground turmeric
1 tsp ground coriander
½ tsp ground cumin
5 cups (1.25L) vegetable stock
1 tsp salt or to taste
1 stalk lemongrass, crushed
1 x 400ml can coconut milk
Juice of ½ lime
1½ tsps sugar

TO SERVE

200g flat rice noodles, cooked
8-12 broccoli florets, steamed
250g silken tofu, cubed
1 tsp dried chilli flakes
Fresh coriander, chopped

STEPS

1. Heat oil in a heavy-bottomed frying pan over low heat. Add the curry paste and fry for 15 minutes, stirring occasionally. Add dry spices and continue to fry for 5 minutes, stirring regularly.
2. Add in stock, salt and lemongrass. Cover and bring to a gentle simmer. Simmer for 30 minutes.
3. Remove and discard lemongrass. Stir in coconut milk and bring to a simmer. Season with lime juice and sugar.
4. Divide the noodles between four bowls. Pour over the laksa and top with steamed broccoli, tofu, dried chilli flakes and fresh coriander.

SERVES 4 | PREP + COOK TIME: 1 HOUR | VEG | GLUTEN FREE | DAIRY FREE |

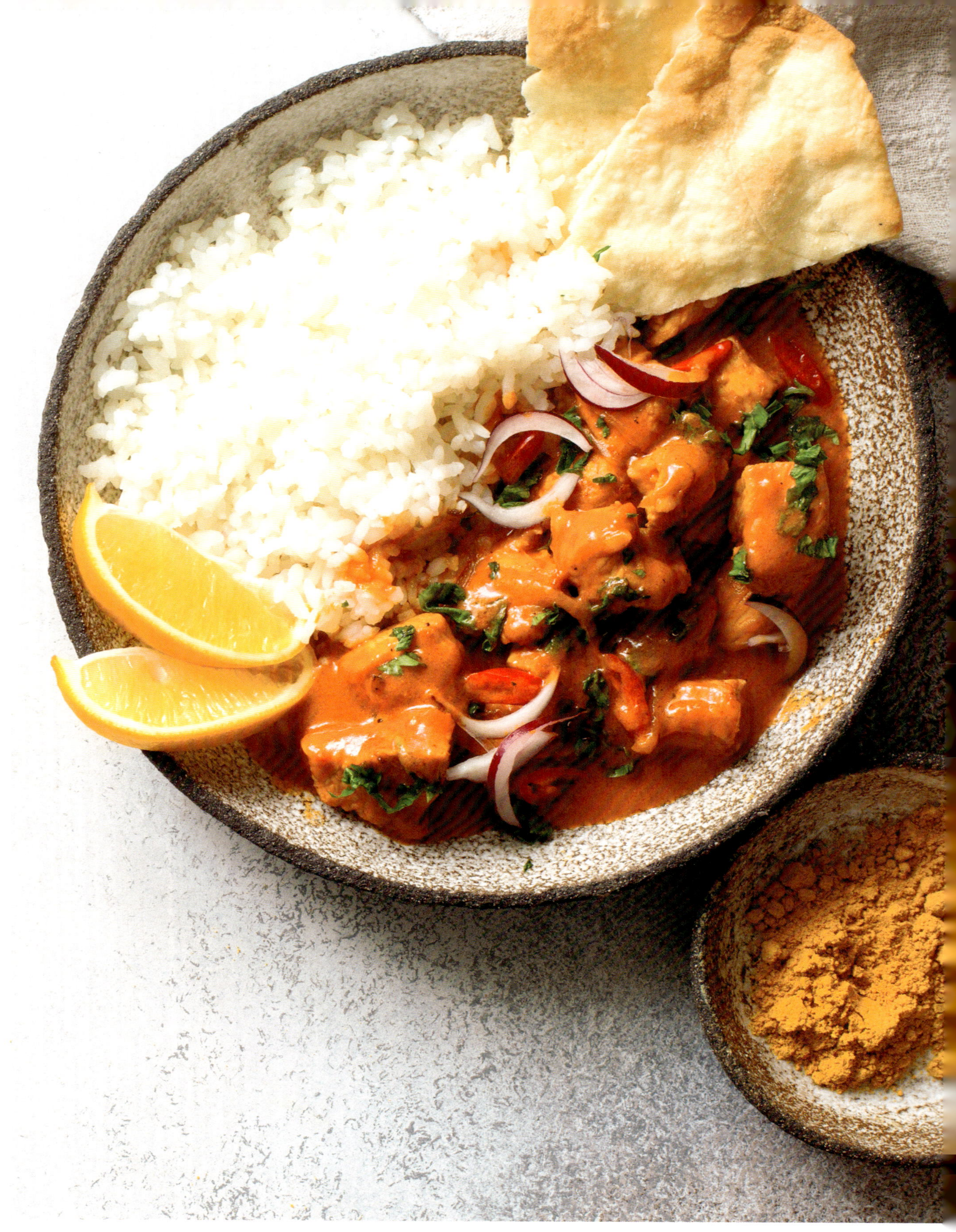

CHICKEN BHUNA

SERVES 6 | PREP + COOK TIME: 1 HOUR 5 MINS | GLUTEN FREE

3 medium onions; 2 finely chopped, 1 roughly chopped

⅓ cup (100ml) vegetable oil

Medium piece ginger, minced

3 cloves garlic, minced

1 tbsp mild curry powder

1 tsp ground turmeric

1 tsp chilli powder

¼ cup (60ml) water

800g chicken thighs, diced

⅓ cup (100ml) plain yoghurt

4 tbsps tomato paste

1¼ cups (300ml) water

2 tsps garam masala

TO SERVE

Sliced red onion and sliced red chilli, (optional)

Chopped coriander leaves

Cooked rice

Naan bread or roti (omit for gluten-free)

STEPS

1. Bring a small pan of water to the boil and add half the roughly chopped onion. Boil for 10 minutes until soft, drain and puree with a stick blender.

2. Heat oil in a large saucepan over medium-high heat. Add the finely chopped onions and reduce to a low heat. Cook the onions, stirring regularly, for 10 minutes, until golden brown. Add ginger and garlic, curry powder, turmeric, chilli powder and water. Fry for 2 minutes. Add the diced chicken and stir in well.

3. In a jug mix together the onion puree with yoghurt, tomato paste and water. Pour into the saucepan and mix well. Bring to a boil, then reduce heat and simmer for 15-20 minutes, stirring occasionally.

4. Add garam masala, stir and cook for a further 2 minutes.

5. Scatter with sliced red onions, chillies and coriander leaves if desired. Serve with rice and naan or roti.

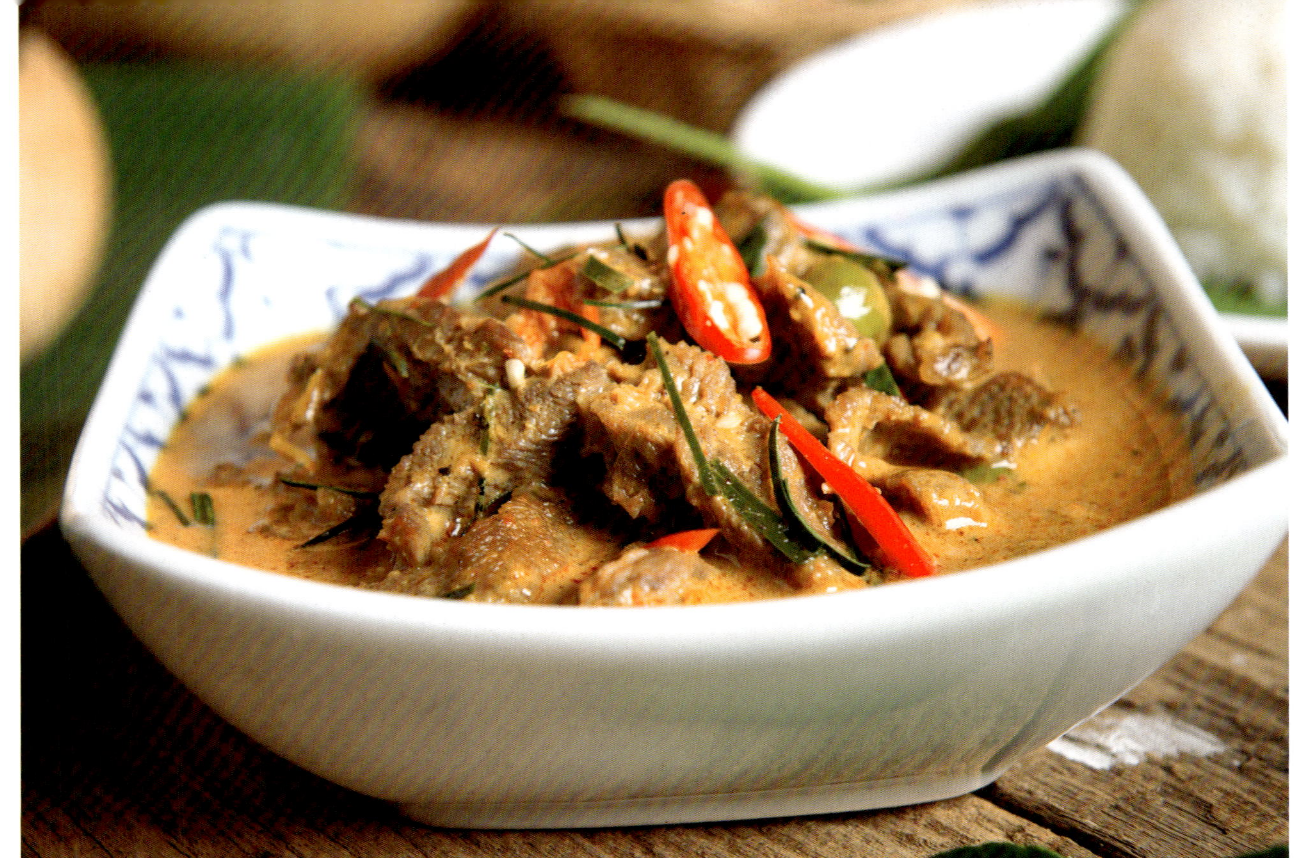

BEEF PANANG CURRY

¾ cup (100g) unsalted peanuts

1 tbsp peanut oil

⅓ cup (100g) panang curry paste

1 x 400ml can coconut milk

4 dried kaffir lime leaves, thinly shredded

½ cup (120g) pea eggplants or diced eggplant

2 tbsps palm sugar or light muscovado sugar

2-3 tbsps fish sauce, to taste

500g sirloin steak, trimmed of obvious fat and finely sliced

1 lime, juiced

1 red chilli, finely sliced

STEPS

1. Put the peanuts in a dry frying pan and toast over a low heat for a few minutes, shaking the pan often, until golden and fragrant. Roughly chop peanuts and set aside.

2. Heat the oil in a wok or large, deep-sided frying pan over medium-low heat. Add the panang paste and cook, stirring often, for 5 minutes until fragrant and sizzling. Add the coconut milk and lime leaves and increase the heat. Bubble for 2-3 minutes until slightly thickened. Add eggplant and stir in sugar and 2 tablespoons fish sauce. Continue to simmer for 5 minutes to reduce.

3. Add the steak and cook for 2-3 minutes until it is no longer pink. Add the lime juice, then taste the curry and add more fish sauce if needed.

4. Remove from the heat and scatter with the peanuts and sliced chilli. Serve hot.

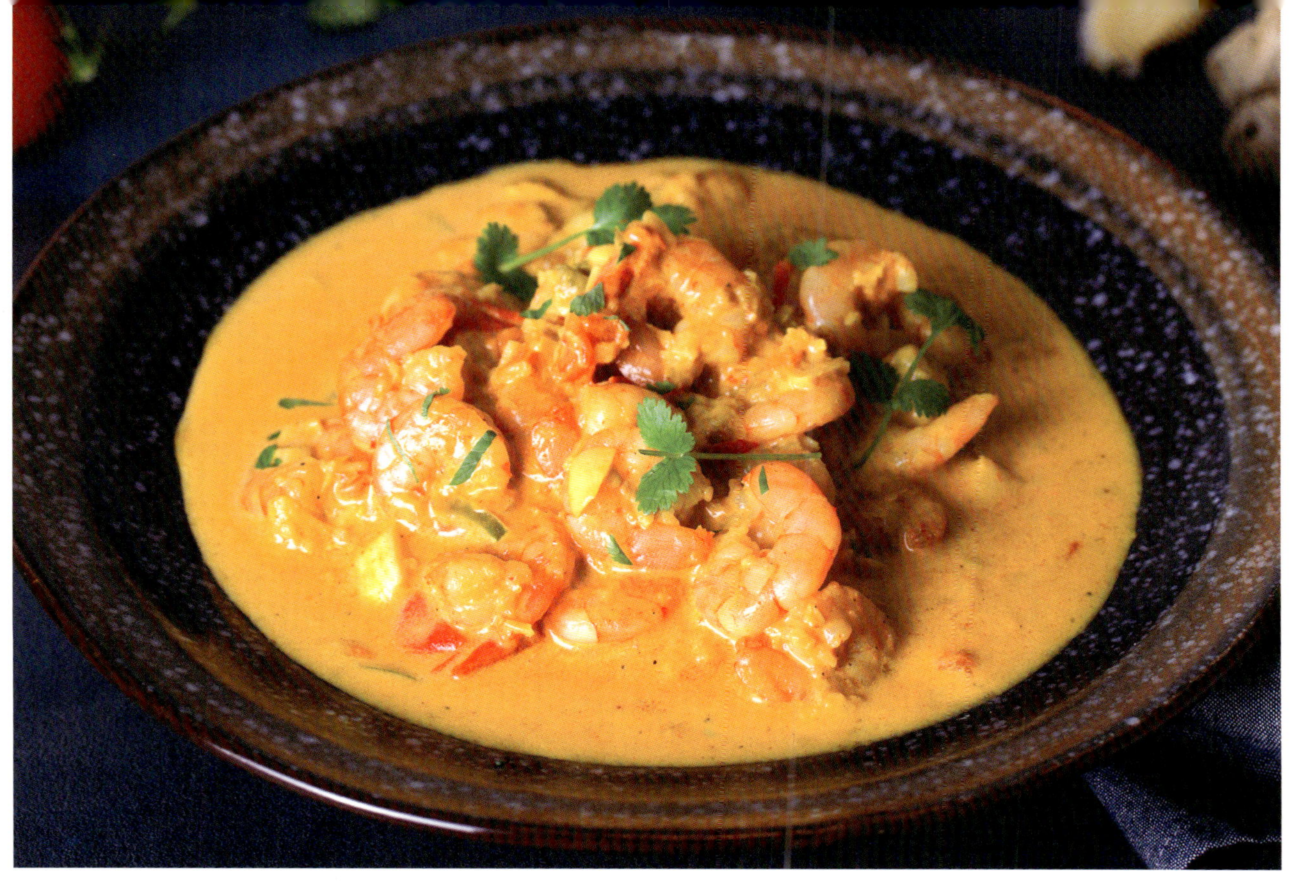

THAI PRAWN CURRY

1 tbsp peanut oil

⅓ cup (100g) Thai yellow curry paste

1 long red chilli, chopped (optional)

1 cup (250ml) chicken stock

1 x 400ml can coconut cream

750g green king prawns, peeled and deveined

1 tbsp palm sugar or brown sugar

2 tbsps fish sauce

1 tbsp lime juice

⅓ cup (5g) fresh coriander leaves, chopped

STEPS

1. Heat the oil in a wok over medium heat. Add curry paste and chilli. Cook, stirring, for 2 minutes or until fragrant.
2. Gradually add stock and coconut cream. Bring to the boil. Reduce heat to medium-low. Simmer for 10 minutes or until mixture slightly thickens.
3. Bring to the boil once more. Add prawns. Cook for 2-3 minutes or until prawns turn pink.
4. Stir in sugar, fish sauce, lime juice and coriander leaves. Serve immediately.

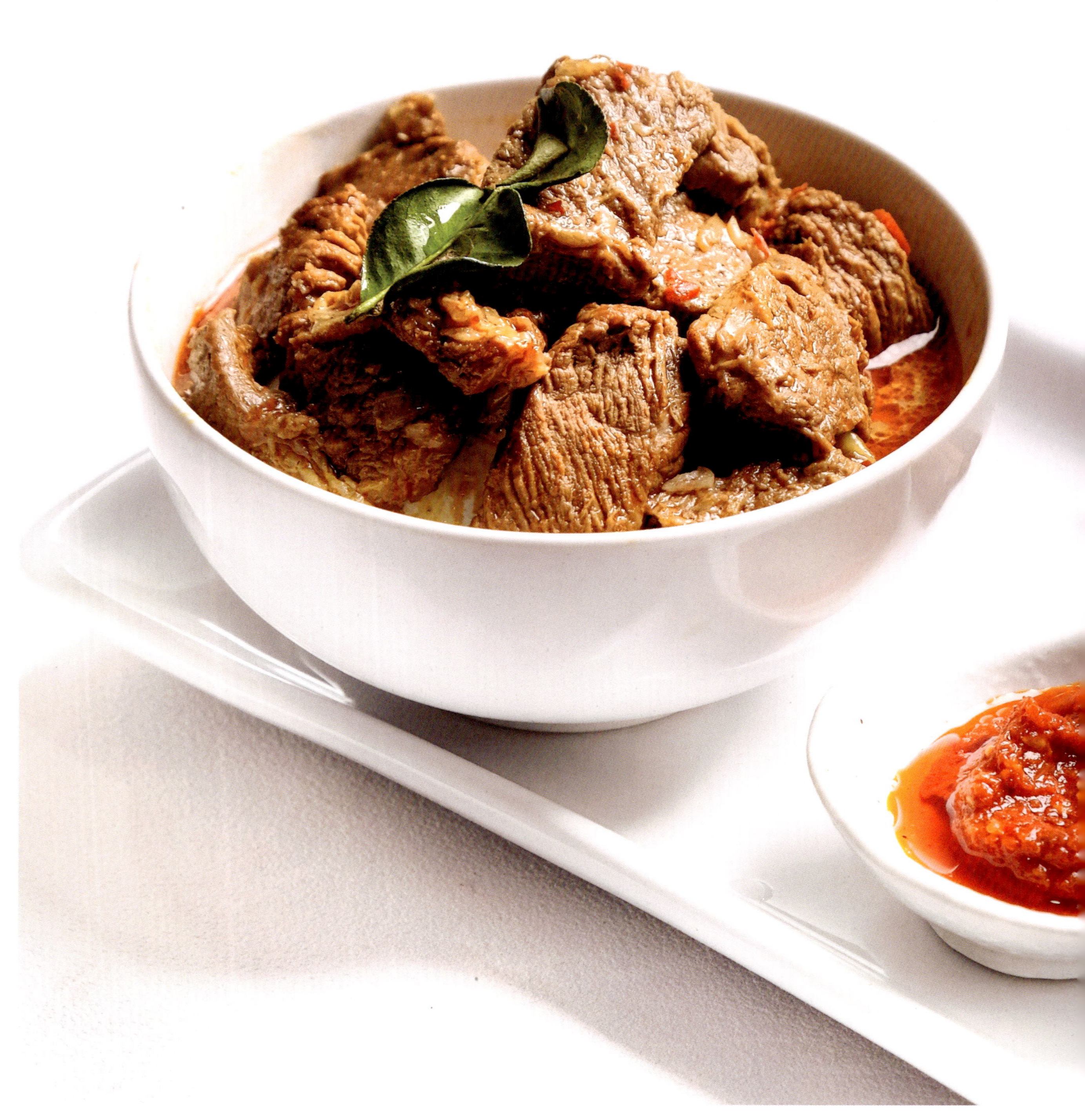

BEEF RENDANG

500g beef shank or chuck

3 bay leaves

4 cups (1L) water

3 tbsps oil

2 tsps tamarind paste

2 stalks lemongrass, bruised and knotted

2 cardamon pods

1 star anise

1 cinnamon stick

¾ cup (200ml) coconut cream

SPICE PASTE

10 Asian shallots, roughly chopped

10 red chillies

6 cloves garlic

Medium piece ginger

Medium piece galangal

Medium piece turmeric or 2 tsps ground turmeric

½ tsp ground white pepper

½ tsp ground nutmeg

½ tsp coriander seeds

¼ tsp cumin seeds

2 tsps salt

1 tsp sugar

STEPS

1. Place beef, bay leaves and water in a pot and bring to a boil. Reduce heat and simmer for about 1 hour until the meat is tender. Remove the beef and cut into 3cm pieces Reserve the beef stock.
2. Place all the ingredients for the spice paste into a blender and blitz into a paste. Add a little water if needed.
3. Heat the oil in a large saucepan over medium heat and saute spice paste, tamarind paste, lemongrass, cardamon, star anise and cinnamon stick for about 3 minutes until fragrant.
4. Pour the reserved beef stock into the pan and bring to a boil. Pour in the coconut milk and bring to a boil.
5. Return the beef to the pan, reduce heat and simmer for 30-60 minutes until the liquid is slightly reduced and thickened. Turn off heat and serve immediately.

SERVES 4 | PREP + COOK TIME: 2 HOURS 30 MINS | GLUTEN FREE | DAIRY FREE |

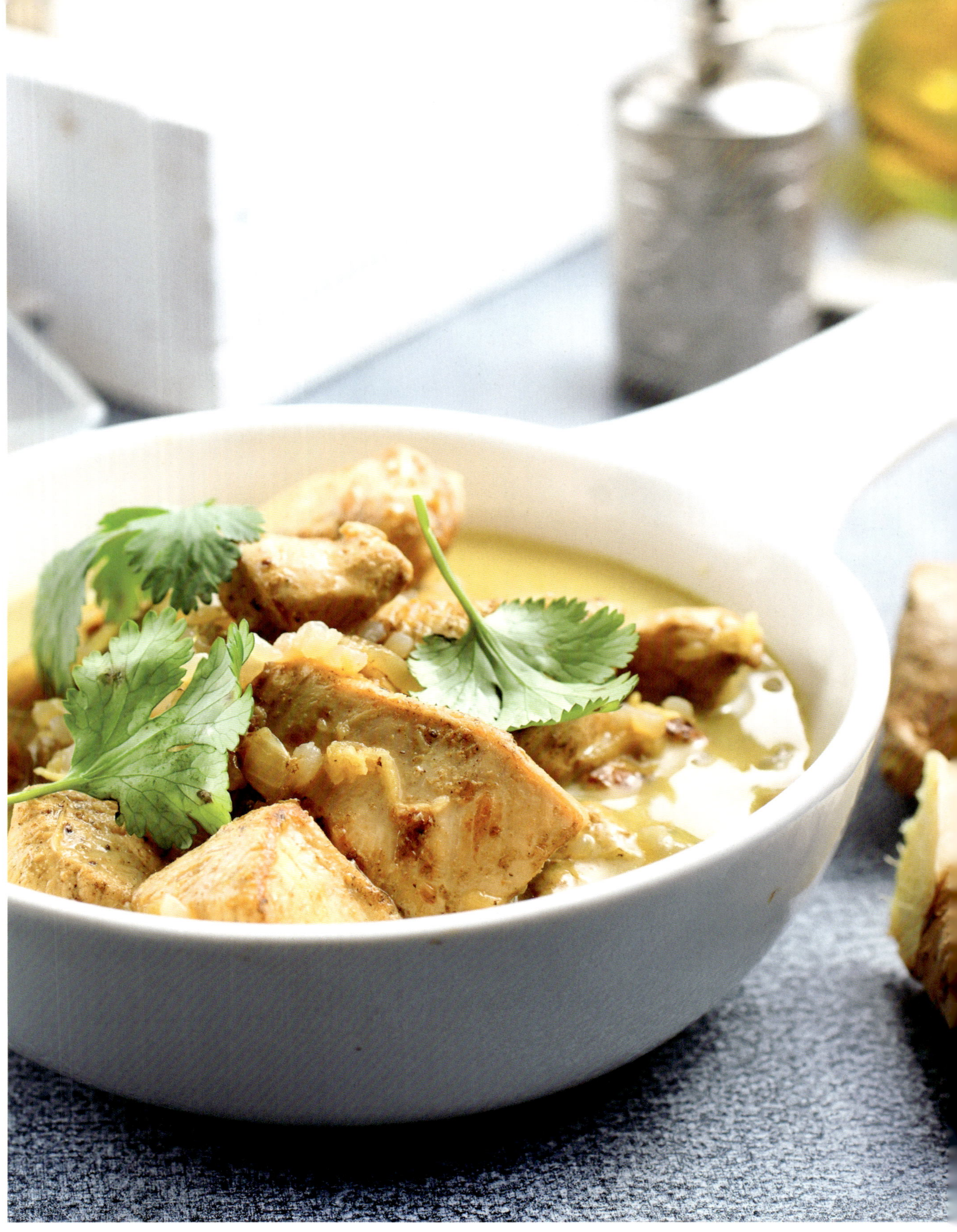

THAI YELLOW CHICKEN CURRY

1 tbsp coconut oil

500g boneless, skinless chicken thighs, cut into bite-size pieces

1 large onion, chopped

2 carrots, thickly sliced

4 tbsps yellow curry paste

2 medium potatoes, diced into 2cm pieces

1 tsp ground turmeric

2 x 400g cans coconut milk

2 kaffir lime leaves

2 tbsps freshly squeezed lime juice

2 tbsps peanut butter

1 tbsp fish sauce

Handful of fresh coriander leaves to serve

STEPS

1. Heat the oil in a large Dutch oven over medium-high heat. Add chicken and saute for 4-5 minutes until browned. Remove the chicken from the pan and set aside.
2. Add the onion and carrots to the pan and cook for 6-8 minutes until tender-crisp.
3. Add the curry paste, potatoes and turmeric. Cook, stirring, for 2 minutes, then add coconut milk and lime leaves. Bring to a boil, reduce the heat and simmer for 10-15 minutes until the curry thickens and the vegetables are tender.
4. Add the chicken back to the pan along with the lime juice, peanut butter and fish sauce.
5. Scatter with coriander leaves to serve.

SERVES 4 | PREP + COOK TIME: 40 MINS | GLUTEN FREE | DAIRY FREE |

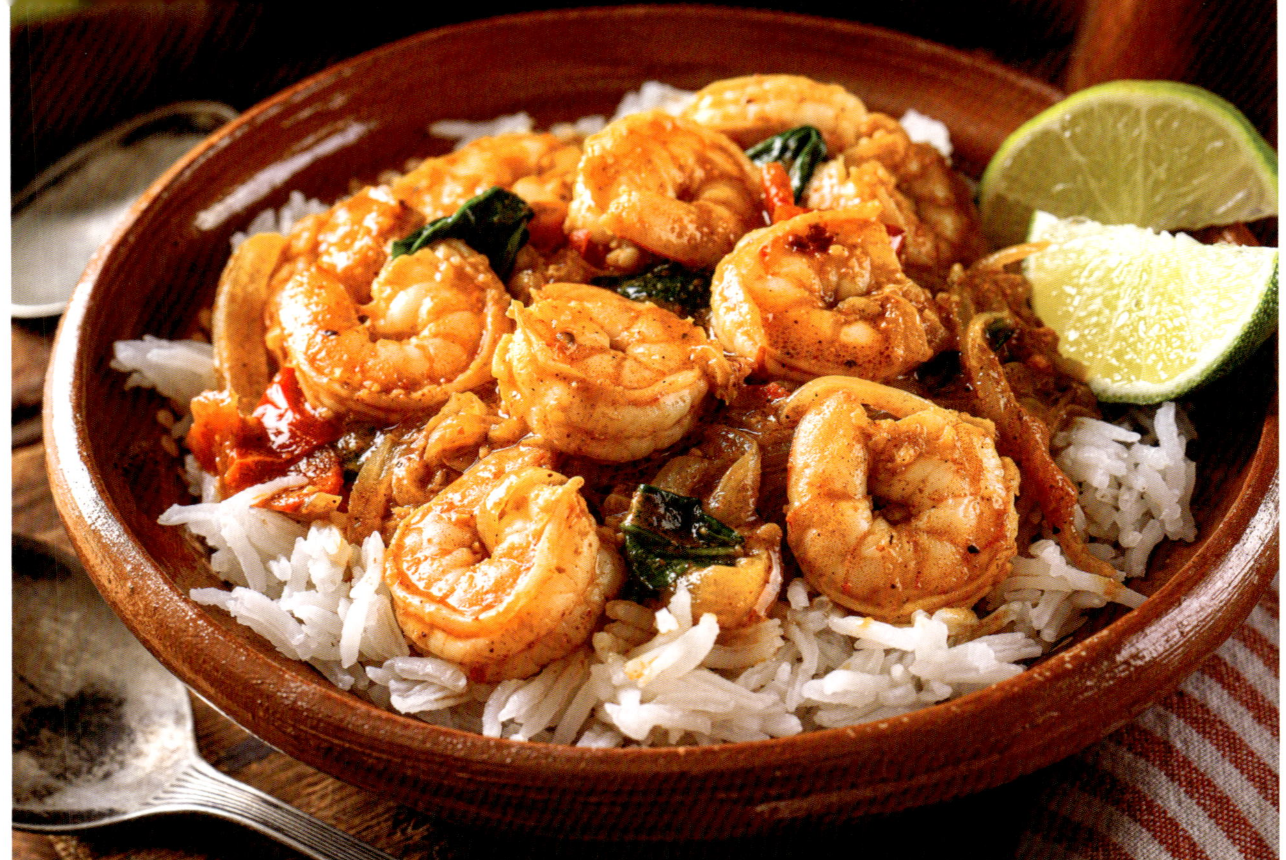

PRAWN TOMATO CURRY

1 tbsp ghee
1 onion, sliced
½ tsp salt
4 cloves garlic, minced
Large piece ginger, minced
1 green chilli, minced
1 tsp dried chilli flakes
1 tbsp garam masala
1½ tsps ground turmeric
400g ripe tomatoes, chopped
¼ cup (60ml) water
1 x 400g can coconut milk
400g king prawns, peeled and deveined
250g baby spinach
2 tbsps fresh coriander leaves, chopped
Cooked basmati rice to serve
1 lime, cut into wedges to serve

STEPS

1. Heat ghee in a large pan over medium-high heat. Add the onion and salt and cook, stirring regularly, for 3-5 minutes until soft. Add garlic, ginger, chilli, chilli flakes, garam masala and turmeric. Fry for 1 minute until fragrant.
2. Add tomatoes and water and cook for 5-10 minutes until the tomatoes start to break down.
3. Add coconut milk. Stir well and simmer for 15 minutes.
4. Add the prawns and cook for 3 minutes until just turning pink.
5. Stir through spinach and coriander and cook for 2 minutes until wilted. Serve with rice and lime wedges.

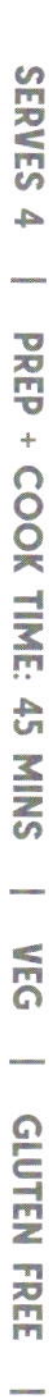

VEGETABLE KORMA

1 tbsp ghee or vegetable oil

1 large onion, chopped

Medium piece ginger, chopped

4 cloves garlic, minced

¼ cup (60g) tomato paste

1 tbsp each: curry powder and garam masala

1½ tsps each: cumin, coriander, turmeric, cardamon

½ tsp each: ground cloves, fennel

1 x 400ml can coconut milk

½ cup (60g) cashews

2 tbsps lemon juice

1¼ cups (310ml) water

½ head cauliflower, cut into florets

2 large carrots, cut into 2cm pieces

1 cup (170g) peas

1 cup (220g) baby corn

1 tbsp brown sugar

1-2 tsps salt

STEPS

1. Heat ghee in a deep frying pan over medium-high heat. Add onion. Cook, stirring, for 5 minutes until soft. Add ginger, garlic, tomato paste and spices. Stir and cook for 1 minute.
2. Add coconut milk, cashews, lemon juice and water. Cook for 5 minutes, then transfer to a food processor and blend until smooth.
3. Return to pan. Stir through vegetables, sugar and salt. Simmer for 30 minutes then serve.

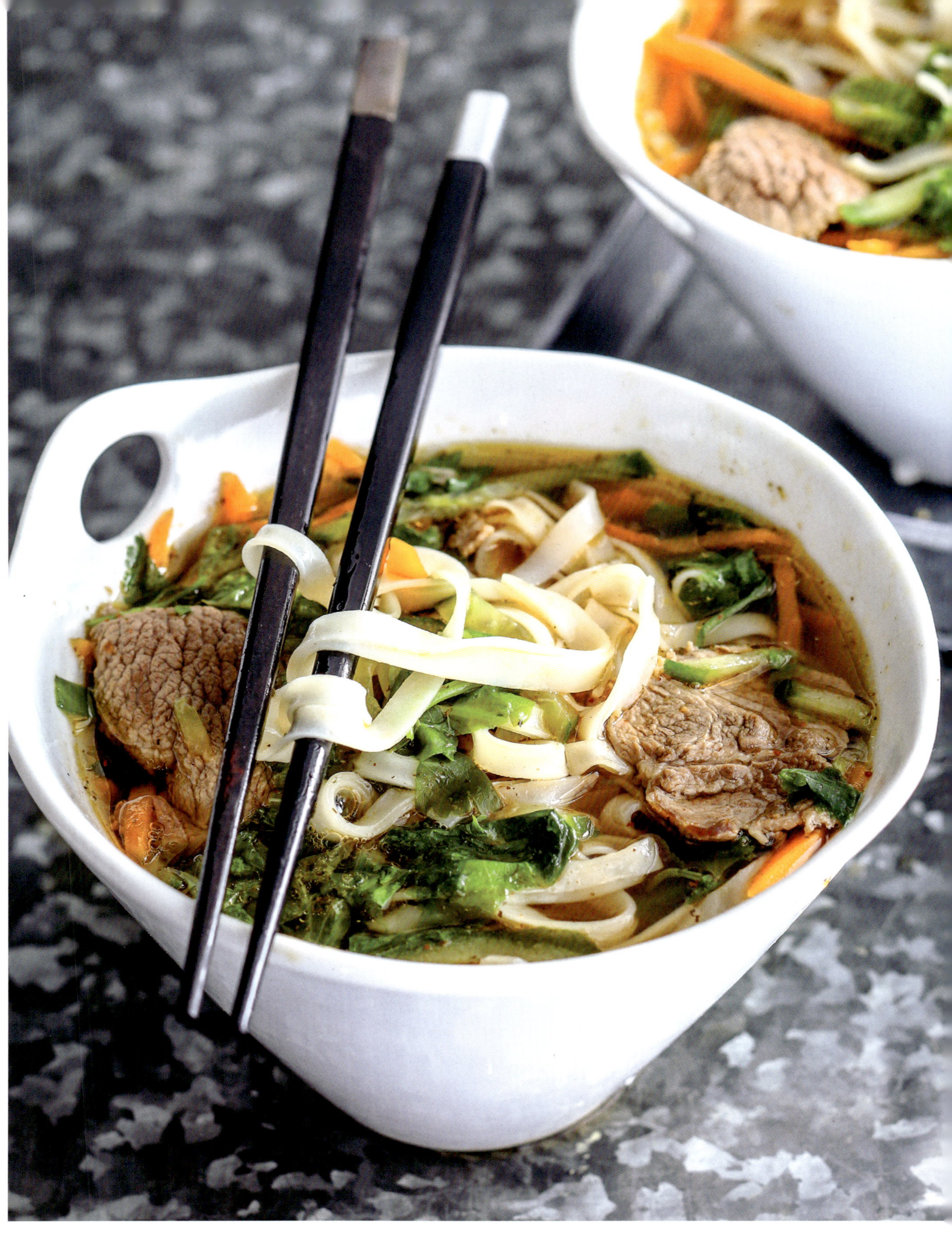

BEEF UDON SOUP

300g rice stick noodles
4 cups (1L) beef stock
1 tbsp sake
1 tbsp mirin
1 tbsp soy sauce
Small piece ginger, grated
Salt and pepper to taste
2 heads bok choy, roughly chopped
2 carrots, julienned
2 zucchinis, julienned
2 tbsps peanut oil
350g rump steak, very thinly sliced

STEPS

1. Cook the noodles according to the packet directions.
2. Place stock, sake, mirin, soy sauce and ginger in a saucepan, bring to the boil, then reduce heat to low and simmer for 10 minutes. Season with salt and pepper. Add bok choy, carrot and zucchini and simmer for 5 minutes more.
3. Heat oil in a wok over high heat, then when it is smoking, add beef and stir-fry for 1-2 minutes until just cooked.
4. Divide the noodles between serving bowls. Top with the beef and pour over the broth. Serve immediately.

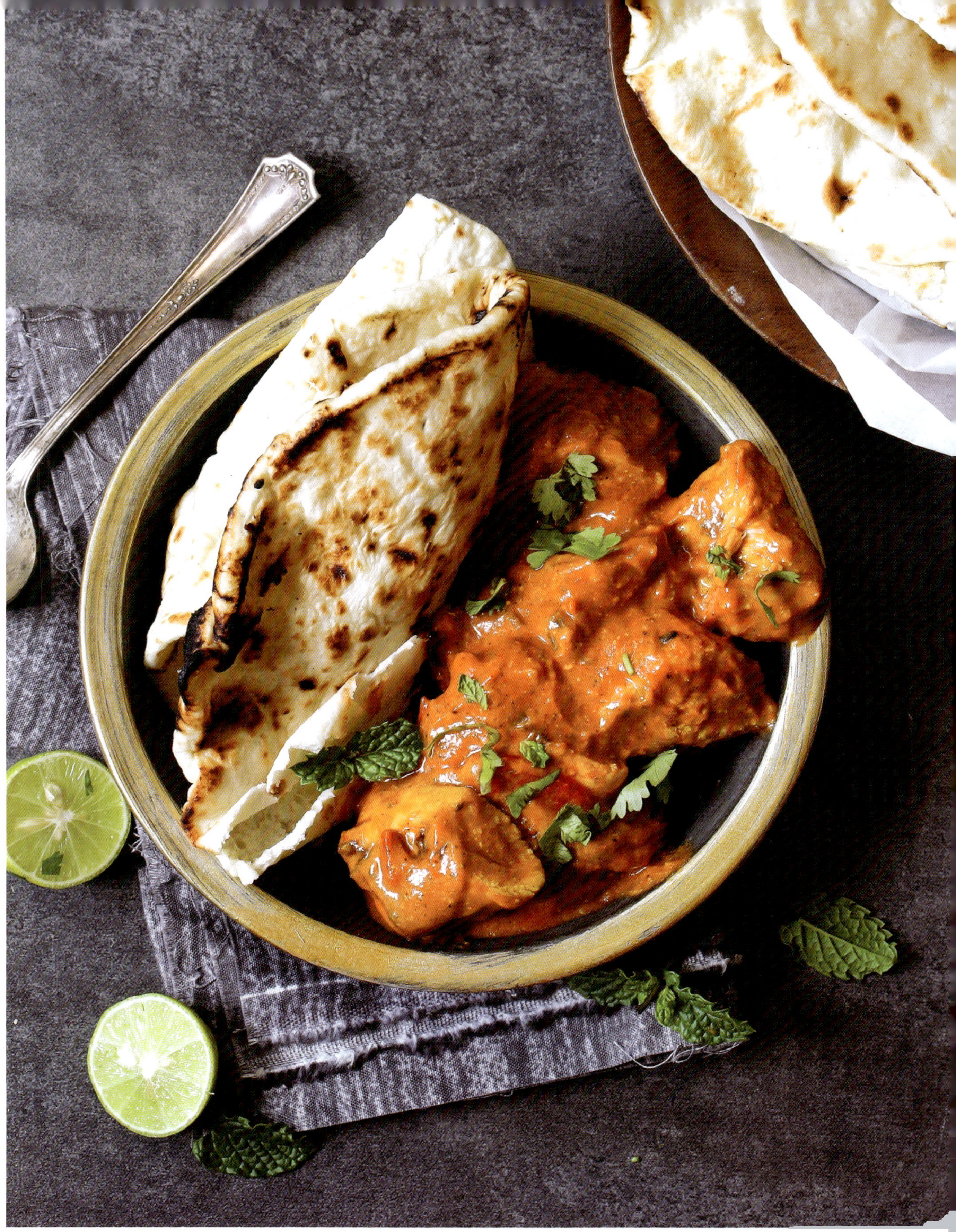

CLASSIC BUTTER CHICKEN

1 tbsp oil

1 tbsp butter

1 onion, diced

Small piece ginger, grated

3 cloves garlic, minced

750g boneless, skinless chicken breasts, cut into 2cm chunks

4 tbsps tomato paste

1 tbsp garam masala

1 tsp chilli powder or to taste

1 tsp ground fenugreek

1 tsp cumin

1 tsp salt

¼ tsp pepper

1 cup (250ml) cream

2 tbsps chopped coriander leaves

Naan bread, warmed, to serve

STEPS

1. Heat the oil and butter in a large frying pan or medium saucepan over medium-high heat. Add the onion and cook for 3-5 minutes until soft and translucent. Add ginger and garlic and let cook for 30 seconds, until fragrant.
2. Add the chicken, tomato paste, and spices. Cook for 5-6 minutes, until chicken is cooked through.
3. Add the cream and simmer for 8-10 minutes, stirring occasionally.
4. Scatter with chopped coriander and serve with naan bread.

SERVES 4 | PREP + COOK TIME: 20 MINS |

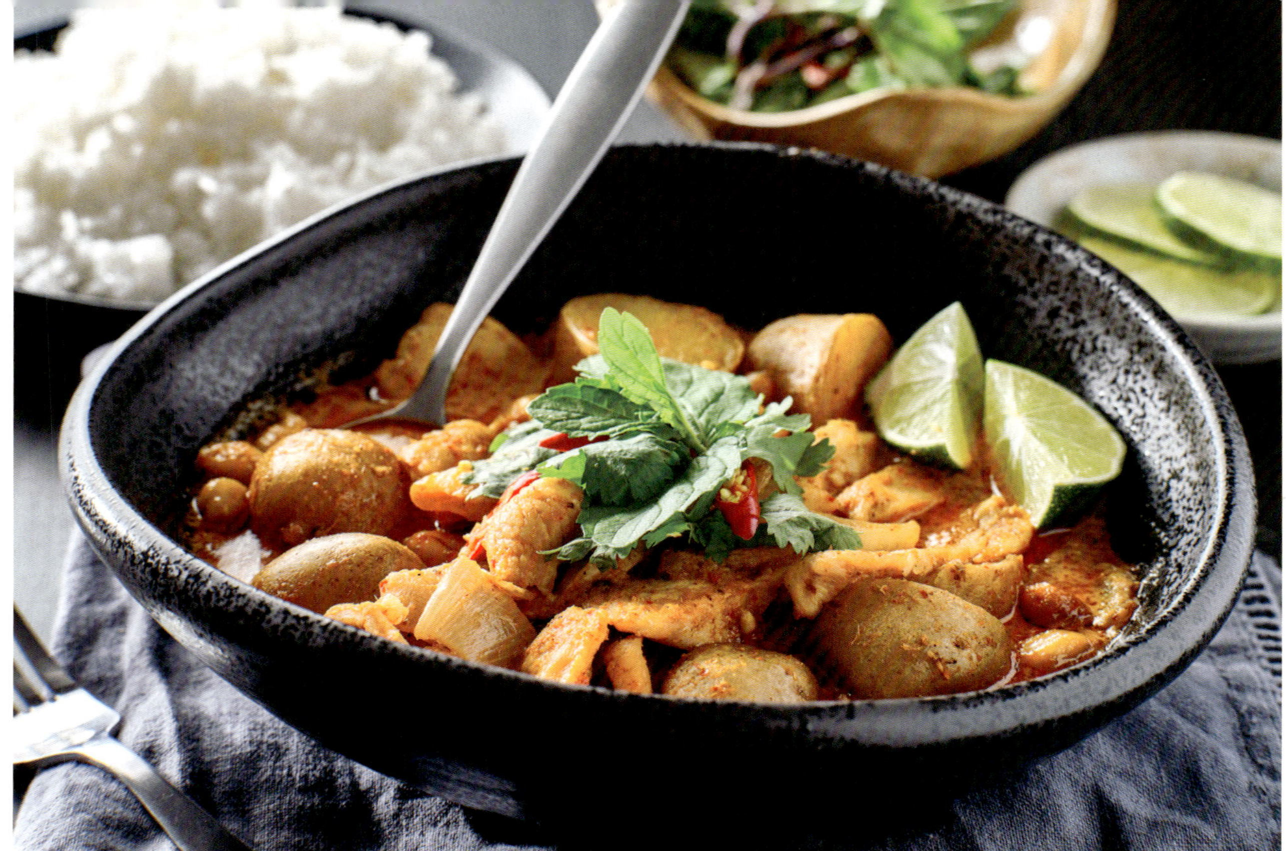

MASSAMAN CURRY

3 tbsps vegetable oil

½ cup (125g) massaman curry paste

2 x 400ml cans coconut milk

Small piece ginger, grated

2 tbsps chopped coriander

2 tbsps brown sugar

2 tbsps fish sauce

2 tbsps tamarind paste

1 tbsp lime juice

1 onion, sliced

500g chicken breasts, thinly sliced into bite-size pieces

8 new potatoes, halved

1 red chilli, sliced

1 tbsp peanut butter

½ cup (60g) peanuts

1 tbsp Sriracha or to taste

Lime wedges to serve

STEPS

1. Heat vegetable oil in a large, wide frying pan or saucepan over medium heat. Stir in curry paste; cook and stir for about 2-3 minutes.

2. Add one can coconut milk and stir to combine. Add ginger, coriander, sugar, fish sauce, tamarind and lime juice. Bring to a boil.

3. Add onion and chicken. Reduce to a simmer. Simmer for 5 minutes then add the second can of coconut milk and bring back to a boil.

4. Add potatoes, chilli, peanut butter, peanuts and Sriracha. Stir to combine. Cover and simmer for 15-20 minutes or until potatoes are tender. Serve with lime wedges.

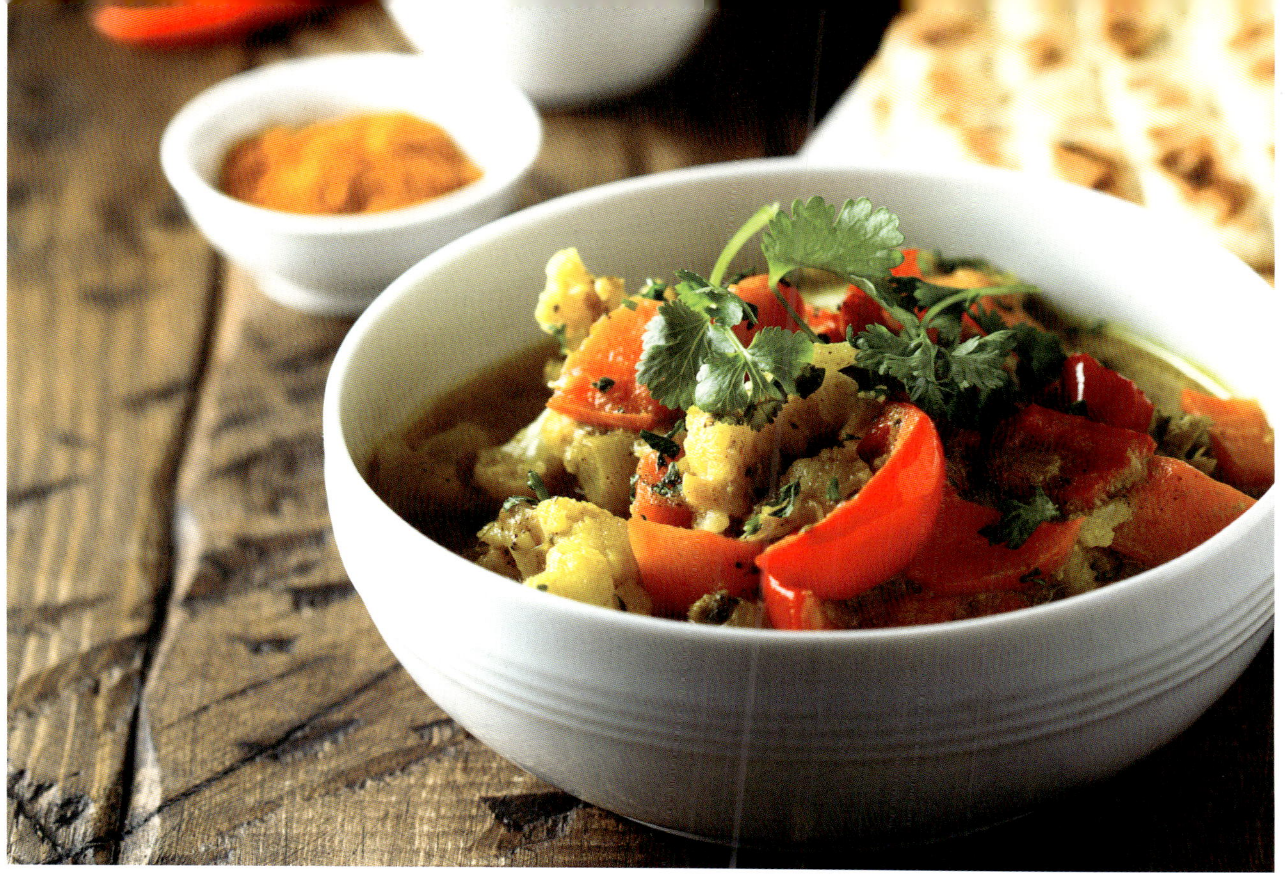

VEGETABLE CURRY

- 1 tbsp vegetable oil
- 1 onion, halved and thinly sliced
- 3 carrots, thickly sliced
- 2 potatoes, cut into 4cm pieces
- ½ head cauliflower, cut into florets
- 1 red capsicum, thickly sliced
- 1 tsp garam masala
- ¼ tsp ground turmeric
- 2 tsps fennel seeds
- ¼ tsp hot chilli powder
- 3 cloves garlic, finely chopped
- Small piece ginger, roughly chopped
- 1 x 400g can chopped tomatoes
- 2 ripe tomatoes, quartered
- 5 fresh curry leaves
- 1 cinnamon stick
- 1 cup (250ml) water
- Salt and pepper to taste
- Fresh coriander leaves to serve

STEPS

1. Heat oil in a large saucepan over medium heat. Add onion. Cook, stirring occasionally, for 5-7 minutes until soft. Add carrot and potato. Cook, stirring occasionally, for 5 minutes. Add cauliflower and capsicum. Cook for 1 minute.
2. Add garam masala, turmeric, fennel seeds, chilli, garlic and ginger. Cook, stirring, for 1 minute until fragrant.
3. Add chopped tomatoes and quartered tomatoes, curry leaves, cinnamon and water. Bring to a gentle boil. Reduce heat to low. Simmer, covered, for 20 minutes. Remove lid. Simmer for 15 minutes or until vegetables are tender.
4. Season. Sprinkle with coriander leaves to serve.

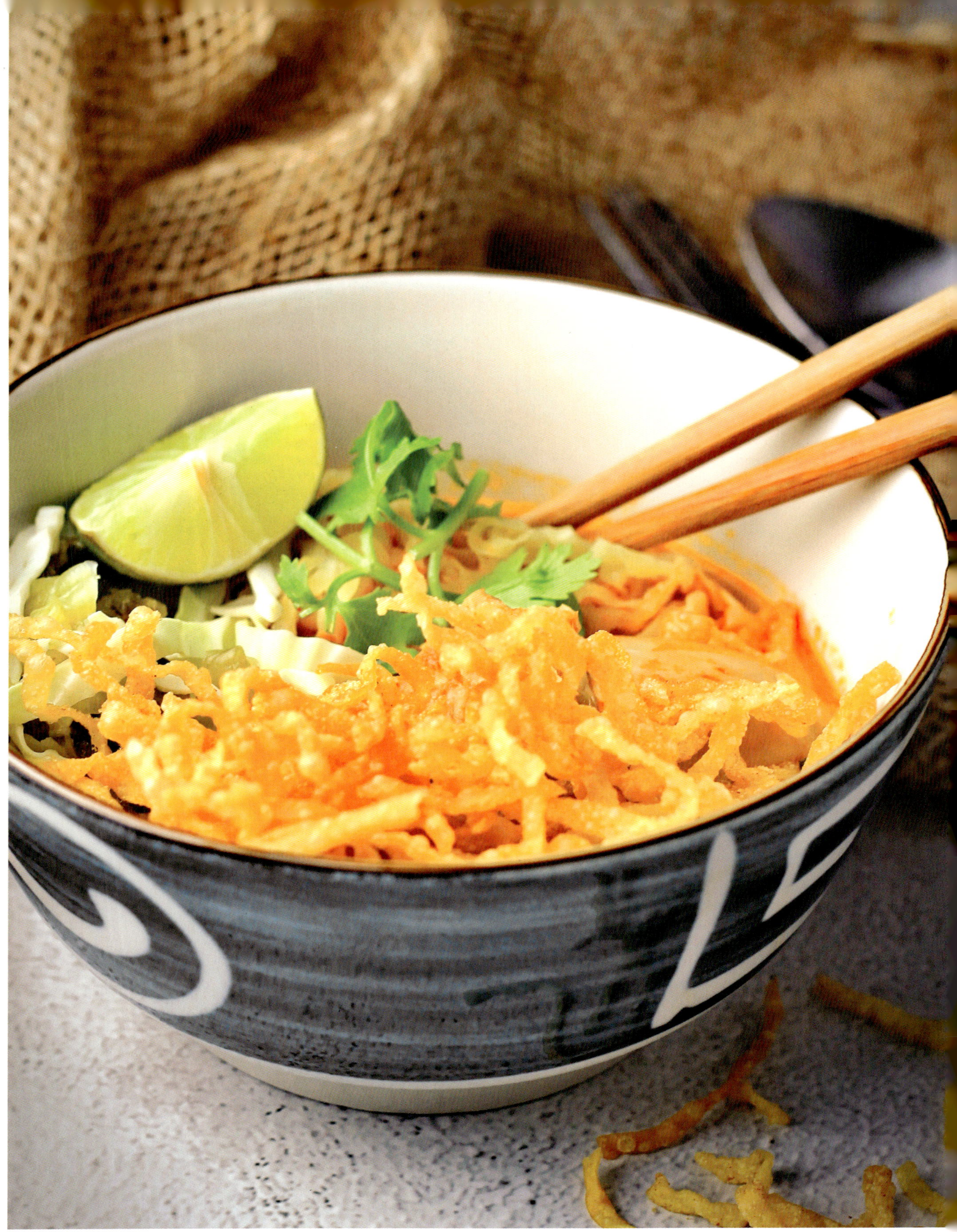

KHAO SOI GAI (COCONUT CURRY NOODLE SOUP)

1 tbsp + 1⅔ cups (400ml) vegetable oil

4 tbsps Thai red or yellow curry paste

2 tsps mild curry powder

1 tsp red chilli flakes

1 x 400ml can coconut milk

⅔ cup (150ml) coconut cream

¾ cup (200ml) vegetable or chicken stock

2 tbsps fish sauce

Juice of 2 limes

500g skinless, boneless chicken thighs, cut into bite-size pieces

300g Chinese dried egg noodles (medium or thin)

TO SERVE

1 cup (100g) shredded green cabbage

4 lime wedges

Handful of fresh coriander

STEPS

1. Heat 1 tablespoon oil in a large saucepan over medium heat. Add the curry paste and cook, stirring, for 5 minutes. Add the curry powder and chilli flakes and cook for 1 minute more, then add the coconut milk, coconut cream, stock, fish sauce and lime juice. Bring to a simmer.
2. Add chicken to the curry. Cook for 15 minutes or until tender.
3. Heat the vegetable oil in a wok or wide saucepan to 180°C (to test, dip in a wooden spoon and look for bubbles). Add 75g of the noodles to the wok in four batches until they bubble up and go crispy. Remove with a slotted spoon and drain on paper towels.
4. Cook the remaining noodles in a pan of boiling water according to the packet directions, until al dente, then drain.
5. Divide the boiled noodles between four bowls. Pour the curry over each and top with green cabbage, lime wedges, coriander and crispy noodles.

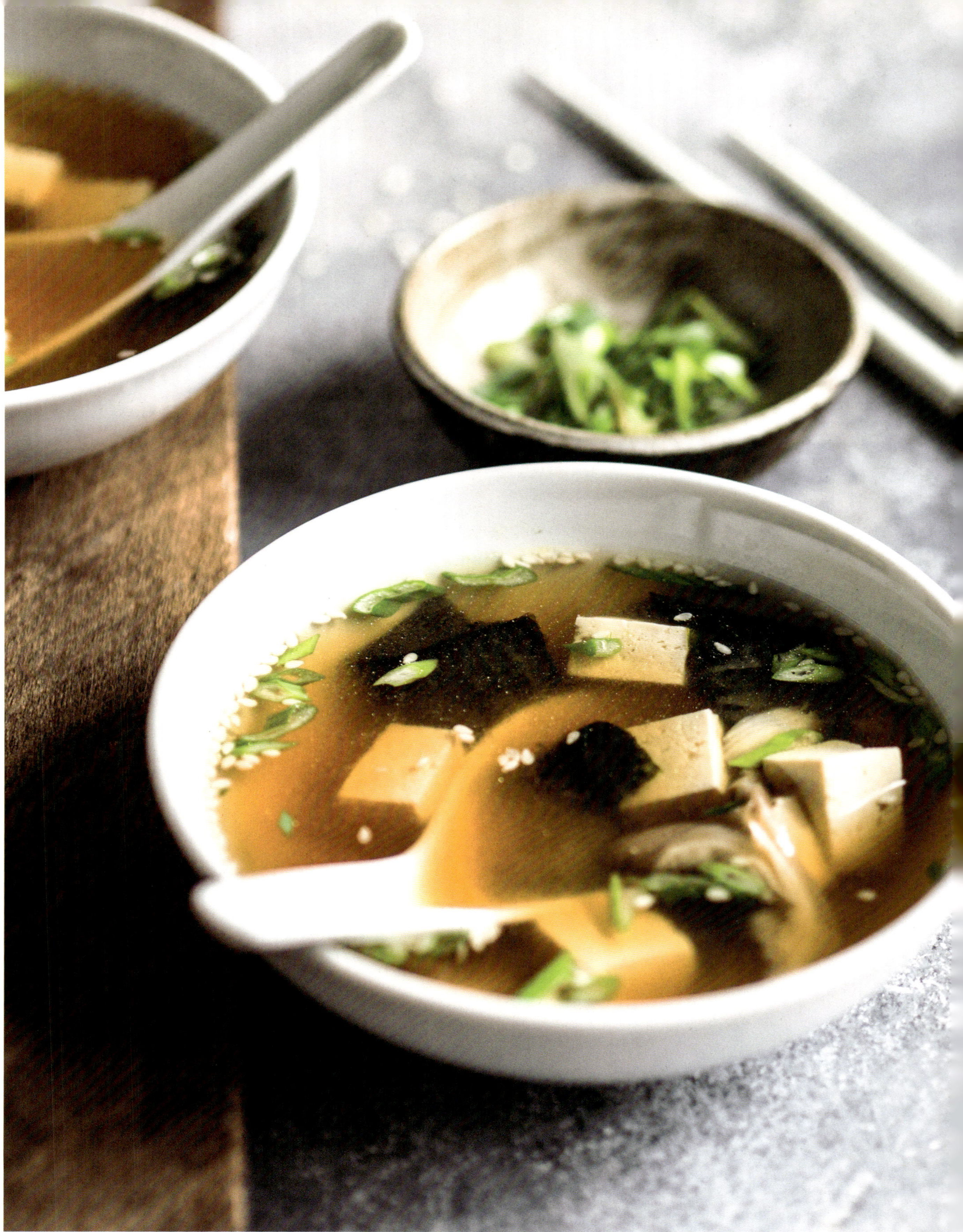

MUSHROOM MISO SOUP

SERVES 4 | PREP + COOK TIME: 30 MINS | DAIRY FREE |

DASHI

4 cups (1L) water

1 piece kombu (10 x 10cm)

1 cup (12g) dried bonito flakes (katsuobushi)

MISO SOUP

4-5 tbsps miso

½ cup (40g) oyster mushrooms, shredded

200g silken tofu, cut into 1½ cm cubes

1 tbsp dried wakame seaweed

1 spring onion, chopped

1 tsp sesame seeds

STEPS

1. Add the water and kombu to a medium saucepan over a medium-low heat. Slowly bring it to a boil and just before it reaches boiling point, remove the kombu and set it aside for another use. Add the katsuobushi to the kombu dashi and bring it back up to a boil. Reduce the heat, and simmer for 30 seconds, then turn off the heat and let the dashi sit for 10 minutes.
2. Strain the dashi through a fine mesh sieve into a saucepan.
3. Place the miso in a small bowl or cup. Add a ladleful of dashi and mix to dissolve the miso. Add the mixture to the saucepan of dashi.
4. Add mushrooms, tofu and wakame to the saucepan. Heat gently for a few minutes until the soup is just hot. Do not allow to boil.
5. Spoon into bowls and scatter with spring onions and sesame seeds to serve.

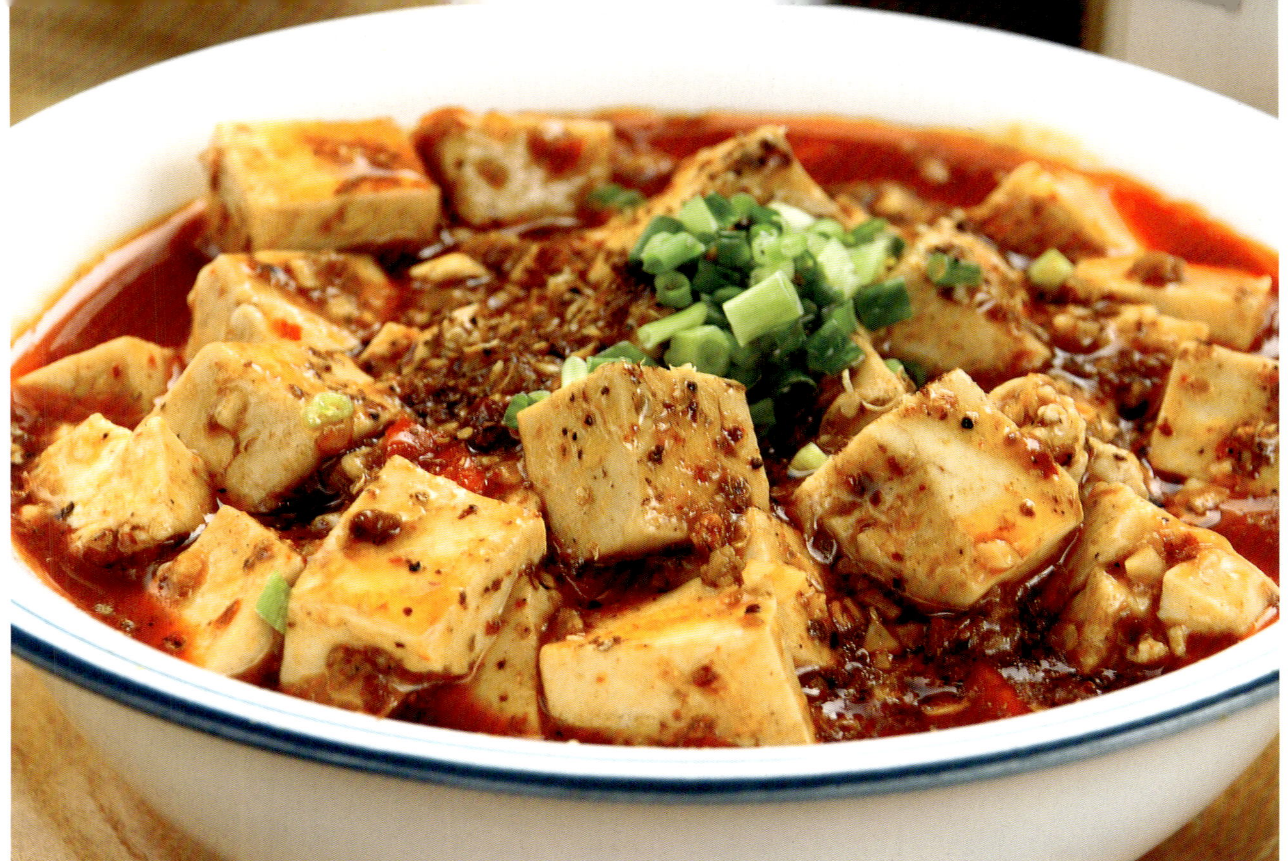

MAPO TOFU

1½ tbsps sesame oil

300g pork mince

800g firm tofu, patted dry with paper towels, cut into 1cm cubes

2 large cloves garlic, finely chopped

2 tbsps finely chopped fresh ginger

2 tbsps adzuki red bean paste

1 tbsp chilli bean paste (optional)

2 tbsps rice wine

1⅓ cups (350ml) chicken stock

2 tbsps soy sauce

¼ cup (10g) garlic chives, finely sliced

1 tbsp cornflour

¼ cup (60ml) water

Salt and pepper to taste

1 tsp Sichuan pepper, to garnish

STEPS

1. Heat the sesame oil in a large work over medium heat. Fry the pork and tofu for 4 minutes.

2. Add the garlic and ginger and stir for 1 minute. Next add the adzuki red bean paste and chilli bean paste, if using, and fry for 2 minutes, stirring constantly. Pour over the rice wine and mix until evaporated.

3. Add the stock and soy sauce and bring to a boil. Reduce heat to a simmer for 3 minutes. Stir through half the chives. Mix the cornflour and water and drizzle over the mapo, stirring continuously.

4. Gently stir until the sauce thickens. Bring to the boil again for 1 minute.

5. Season to taste and serve garnished with Sichuan pepper and the remaining chives.

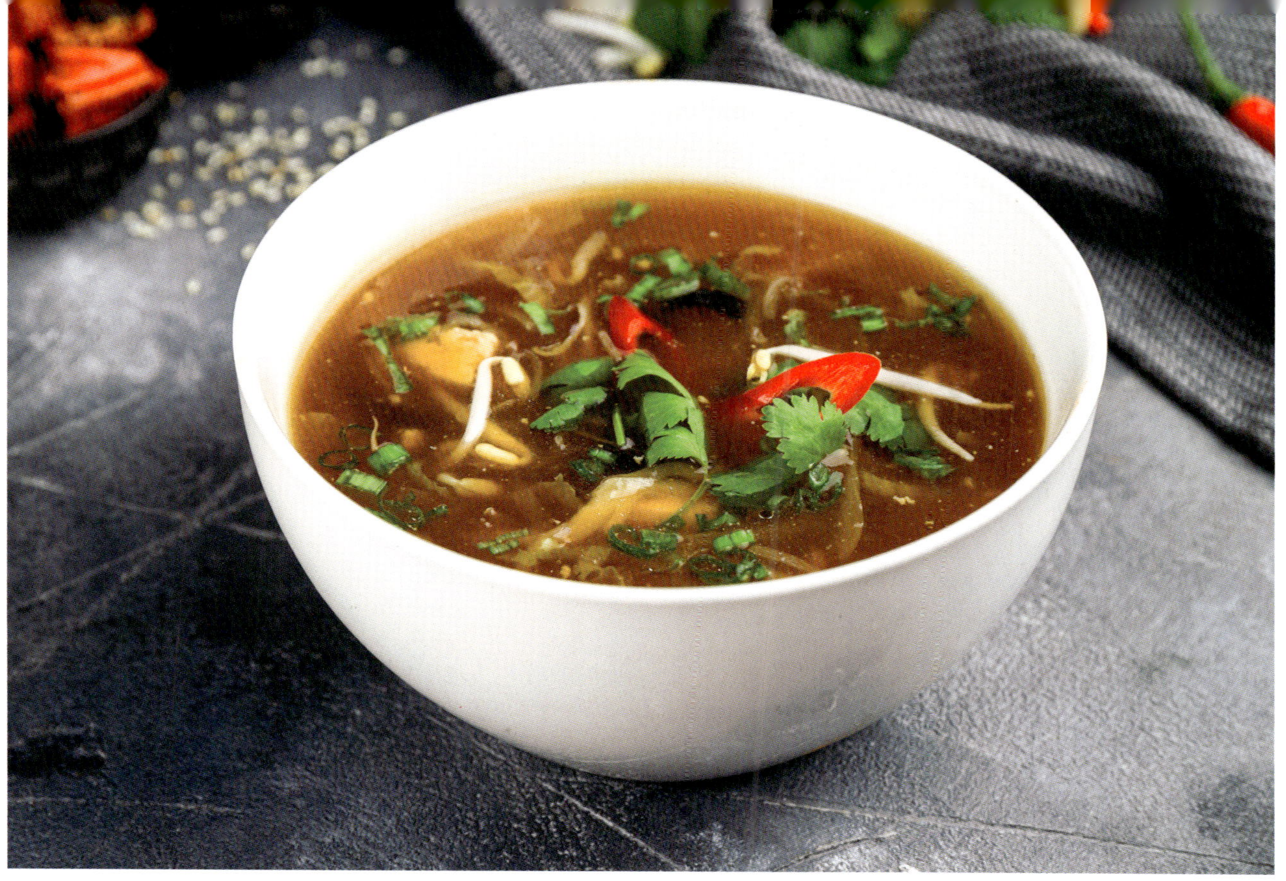

SERVES 4 | PREP + COOK TIME: 35 MINS | DAIRY FREE |

HOT & SOUR SOUP

6 cups (1.5L) chicken stock
Medium piece ginger, grated
1½ tbsps soy sauce
1 tsp dried chilli flakes
1 tsp pepper
1 tsp sugar
1 tsp sesame oil
220g chicken breasts
3 tbsps rice wine vinegar
250g shiitake mushrooms, sliced
1 x 225g can bamboo shoots, drained
150g firm tofu, diced
1 large egg, beaten
1 cup (110g) bean sprouts
2 spring onions, chopped
2 tbsps coriander leaves
1 red chilli, sliced

STEPS

1. Place chicken stock, ginger, soy sauce, chilli flakes, sugar, pepper and sesame oil in a large pot over medium-high heat.
2. Once simmering, add chicken, cover and simmer for 10 minutes. Remove chicken and shred.
3. Add vinegar, shiitake mushrooms, bamboo shoots, tofu and shredded chicken into the soup. Simmer for 10 minutes more.
4. Remove the soup from the heat. Using a chopstick, stir the soup in a one direction until you create a little whirlpool, then slowly add the beaten egg, stirring continuously to form thin ribbons.
5. Add the bean sprouts and spring onions. Serve into bowls and top with coriander leaves and sliced red chilli.

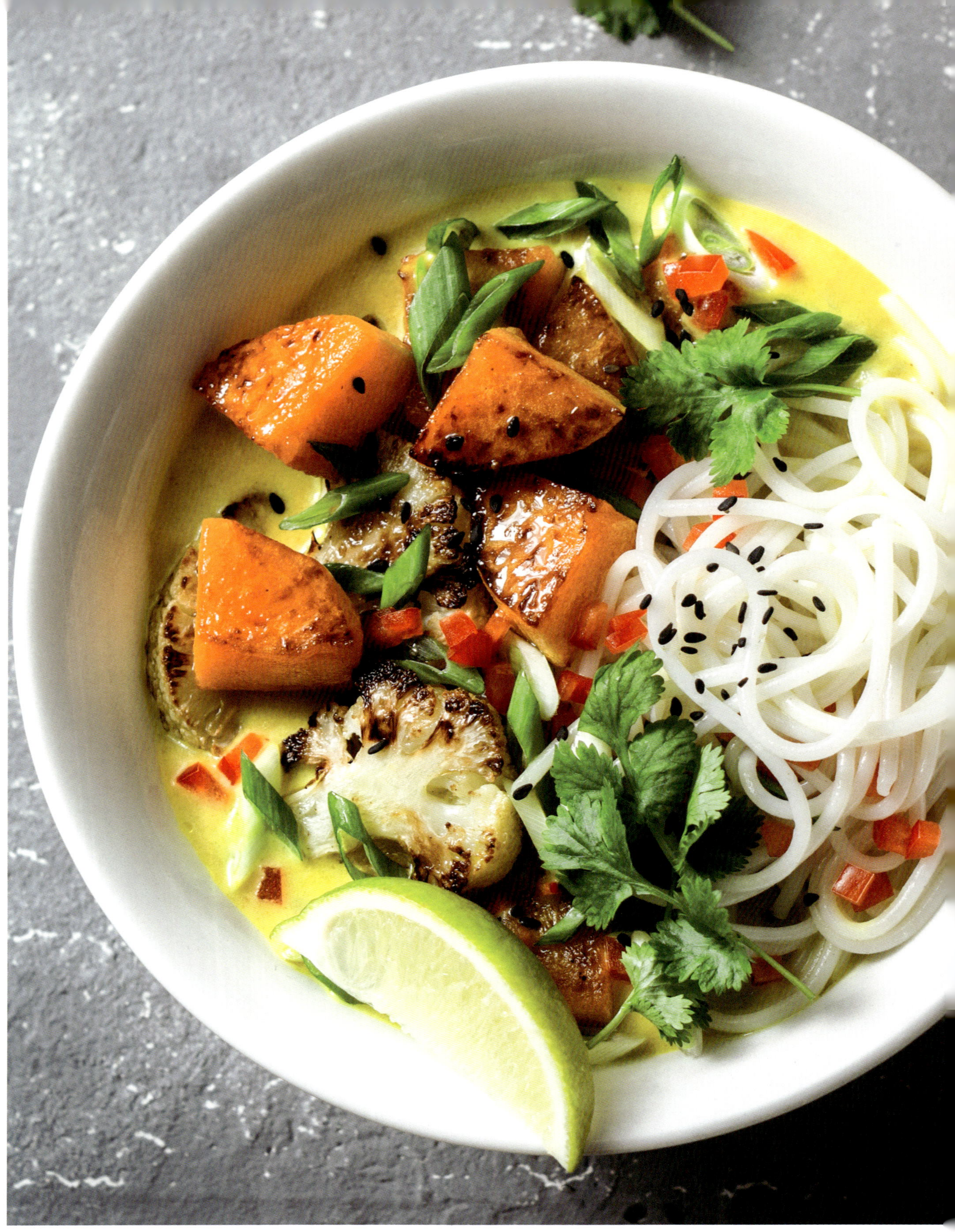

VEGAN KHAO SOI SOUP

PASTE

4 hot red chillies (fresh or dried)

6 cloves garlic

Medium piece ginger, roughly chopped

¼ cup (10g) chopped coriander stalks

2 stalks lemongrass, white inner part only, roughly chopped

2 Asian shallots, roughly chopped

½ tsp ground coriander

1½ tsps ground turmeric

1 tsp curry powder

4 tbsps water

SOUP

½ butternut pumpkin, peeled and cut into 3cm chunks

½ head cauliflower, cut into florets

3 tbsps peanut oil

2 tsps tamari

300g rice noodles

4 cups (1L) vegetable stock

1½ cups (375ml) coconut milk

3 tbsps vegan fish sauce

Juice of ½ lime

1-2 tbsps sugar

TO SERVE

Fresh coriander leaves

1 red chilli, finely chopped

2 spring onions, sliced

1 tsp black sesame seeds

Lime wedges

STEPS

Preheat oven to 225°C.

1. Place all the paste ingredients in a food processor, and process into a paste.
2. Toss butternut pumpkin and cauliflower with 2 tablespoons oil and tamari. Spread on a lined baking tray and bake for about 30 minutes, turning once or twice, until golden.
3. Meanwhile, cook noodles according to the packet instructions.
4. Heat 1 tablespoon of oil in a medium-size saucepan over medium heat. Add paste to the hot oil and stir-fry for about 4-6 minutes, until fragrant. Add vegetable stock and coconut milk and bring to a boil. Season with vegan fish sauce, fresh lime juice and sugar to taste.
5. Divided the soup between bowls and top with noodles, vegetables, coriander leaves, chopped chilli, spring onions and black sesame seeds. Serve with lime wedges.

SERVES 4 | PREP + COOK TIME: 40 MINS | VEG | GLUTEN FREE | DAIRY FREE |

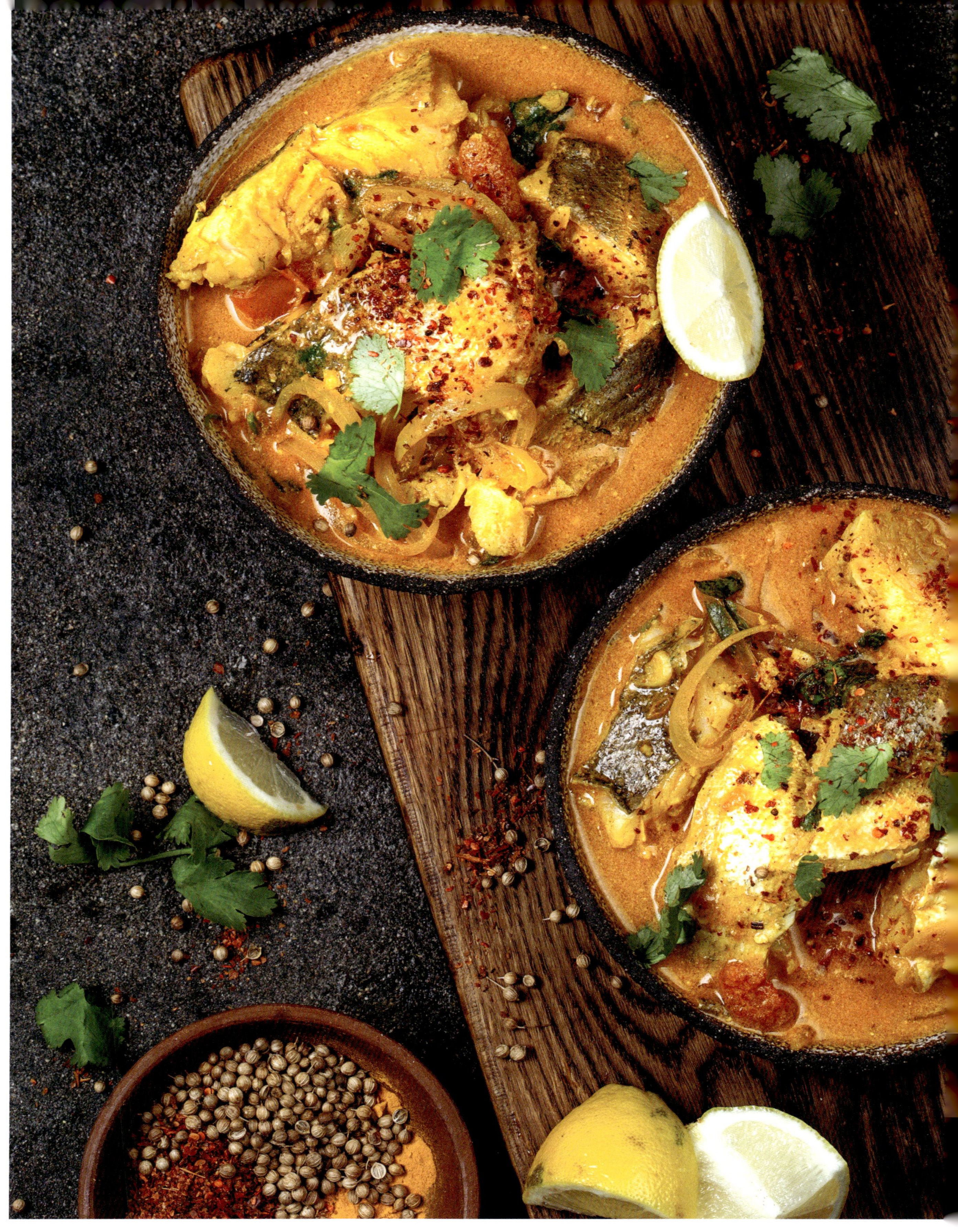

CLASSIC FISH CURRY

6 fish fillets (any firm white fish), skin on
2 tbsps lemon juice
1 tsp salt
5 cloves garlic
5 dried red chillies
3 ripe tomatoes
1 tsp cumin seeds
1 tbsp vinegar
1 tsp sugar
2-3 tbsps olive or sunflower oil
1 onion, sliced
1 cup (225g) tomato paste
Dried chilli flakes and coriander leaves, to garnish

STEPS

1. Marinate the fish fillets for 10-15 minutes in the lemon juice and ½ teaspoon of the salt.
2. Using a food processor or a pestle and mortar, grind together the garlic, red chillies, tomatoes, cumin seeds, remaining salt, vinegar and sugar to make a smooth paste.
3. Heat the oil in a deep frying pan. Fry the onion till light brown, approximately 5 minutes. Add the curry paste and fry for 2 minutes until aromatic. Add the tomato paste and cook for a further 2-3 minutes.
4. Add the fish fillets and enough water to almost cover the fish. Cover the pan and reduce the heat. Allow to simmer for 5-7 minutes or till the fish is tender. If the curry gets too dry, add a little more water. Cook uncovered another 2 minutes.
5. Scatter with chilli flakes and fresh coriander leaves to serve.

SERVES 6 | PREP + COOK TIME: 35 MINS + MARINATING | GLUTEN FREE | DAIRY FREE |

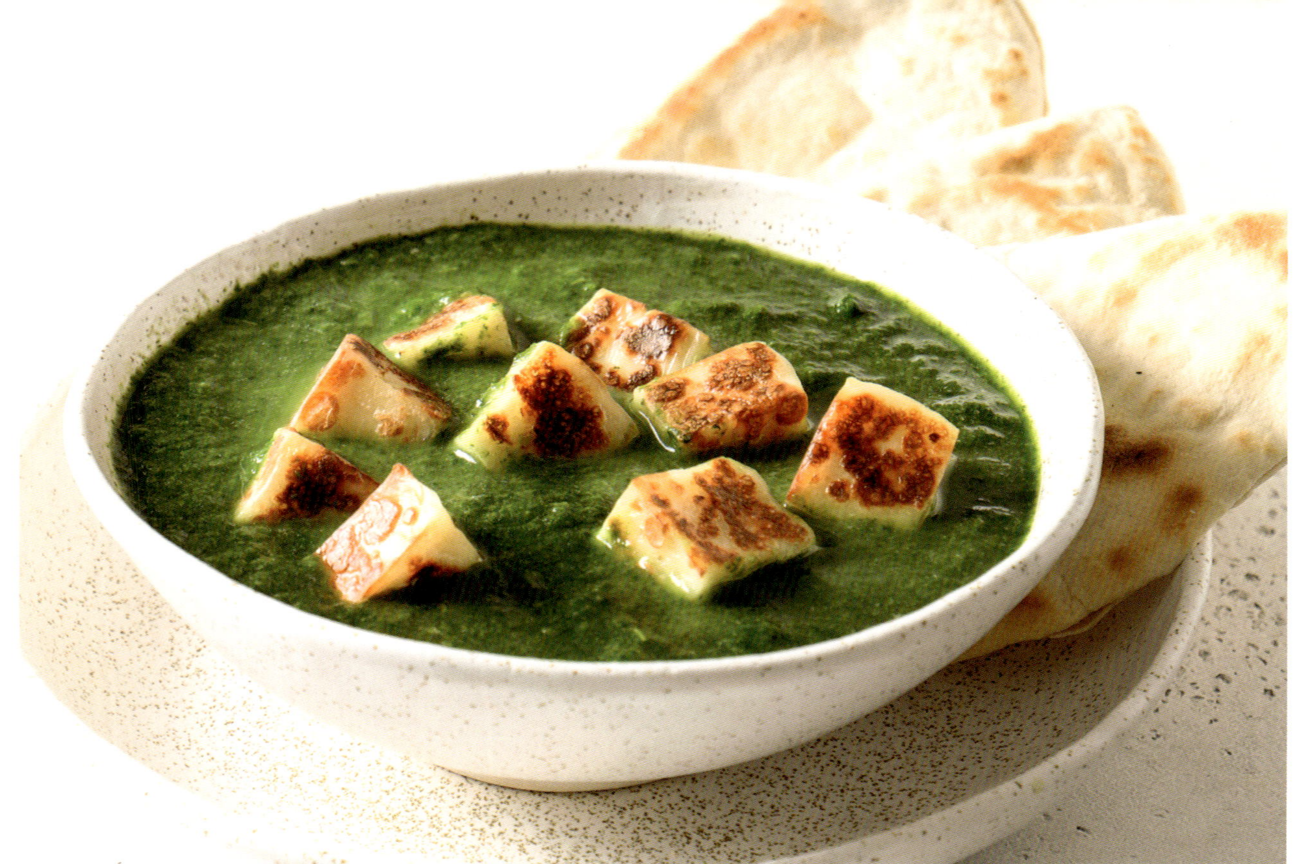

PALAK PANEER

PANEER

3 tbsps ghee

400g paneer, cut into 2cm cubes

Pinch of salt

SAUCE

500g baby spinach

2 tbsps ghee

1 onion, finely diced

Medium piece ginger, minced

4 cloves garlic, minced

1 long red chilli, deseeded and finely diced

1 tsp cumin seeds

2 tsps garam masala

¼ tsp ground turmeric

¼ tsp cayenne pepper

½ cup (125ml) thickened cream

1 tsp salt

STEPS

1. Heat half of the ghee for paneer in a large frying pan over medium heat. Add half of the paneer and sprinkle with salt. Fry for 2-3 minutes on each side until golden brown. Remove from the pan and set aside. Repeat with the remaining ghee and paneer.
2. Bring a large pan of water to a boil. Add spinach and cook for about a minute, until it wilts. Drain.
3. Blend spinach in a food processor until smooth.
4. Heat 2 tablespoons of ghee in a large frying pan over medium-high heat. Add onion and cook for 3-5 minutes until soft. Add ginger, garlic, chilli and cumin seeds and cook for 30 seconds. Then add garam masala, turmeric and cayenne pepper. Stir to coat the onions with the dried spices.
5. Add spinach to the pan along with the cream and salt. Cover with a lid, reduce heat to medium and simmer for 5 minutes. Add fried paneer and serve.

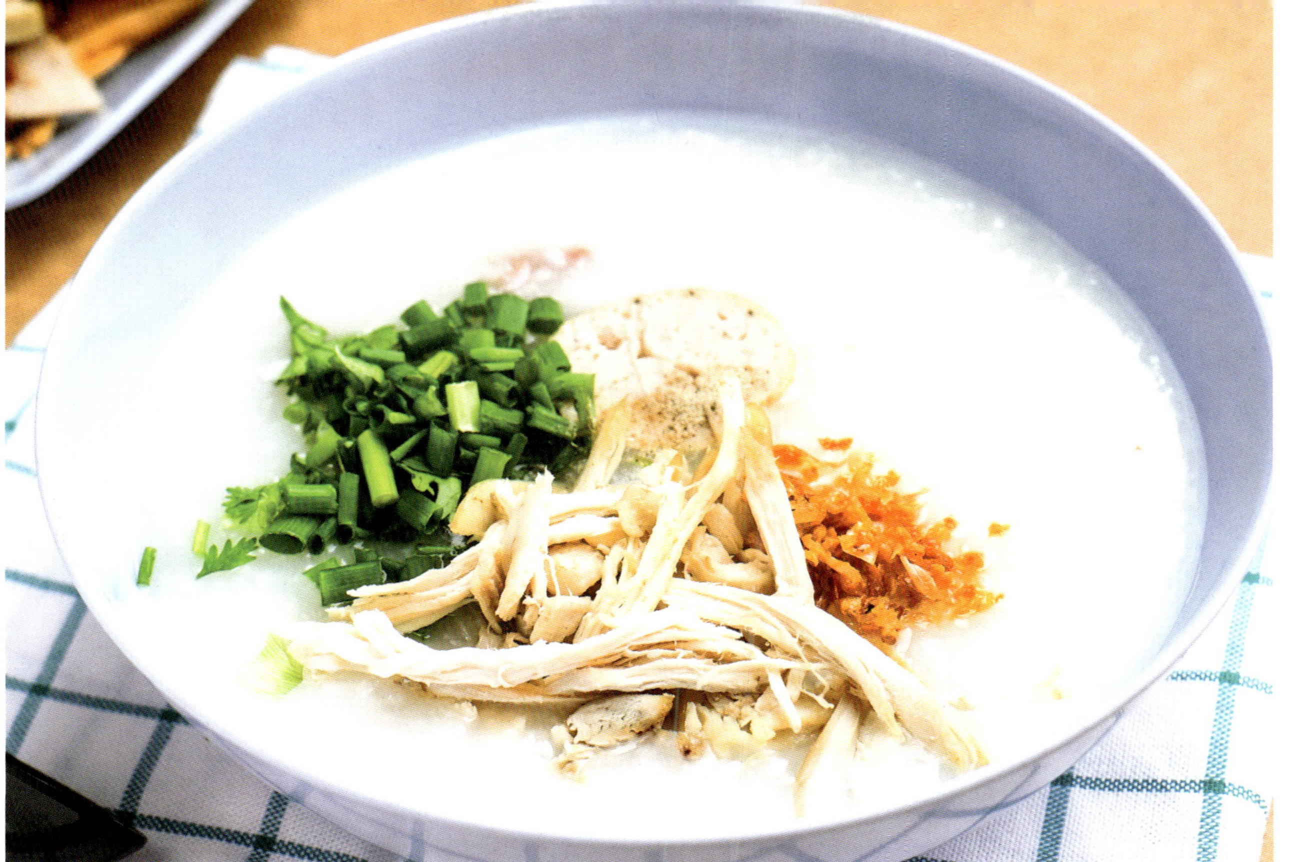

SERVES 4 | PREP + COOK TIME: 1 HOUR 15 MINS |

CHICKEN CONGEE

4 cups (1L) chicken stock
2 cups (500ml) water
4 slices fresh young ginger
1 tbsp butter
2 cloves garlic, minced
½ cup (80g) long-grain rice
1 tsp Shaoxing rice wine
Salt and ground white pepper
2 cups (250g) shredded barbecue chicken
2 tbsps finely sliced spring onion
2 tbsps crispy fried shallots
½ tsp sesame oil
Soy sauce to serve

STEPS

1. Bring the chicken stock, water and ginger to a boil over a high heat.
2. In a large, heavy-based saucepan melt butter over medium heat and saute garlic and rice for 2 minutes. Add hot stock, reduce heat and simmer steadily for 1 hour, covered, stirring occasionally, until thickened and most of the liquid has been absorbed.
3. Add the rice wine to the congee and season to taste with salt and pepper.
4. Serve the congee in bowls, top with chicken, spring onions and crispy fried shallots. Drizzle with sesame oil and serve with soy sauce on the side.

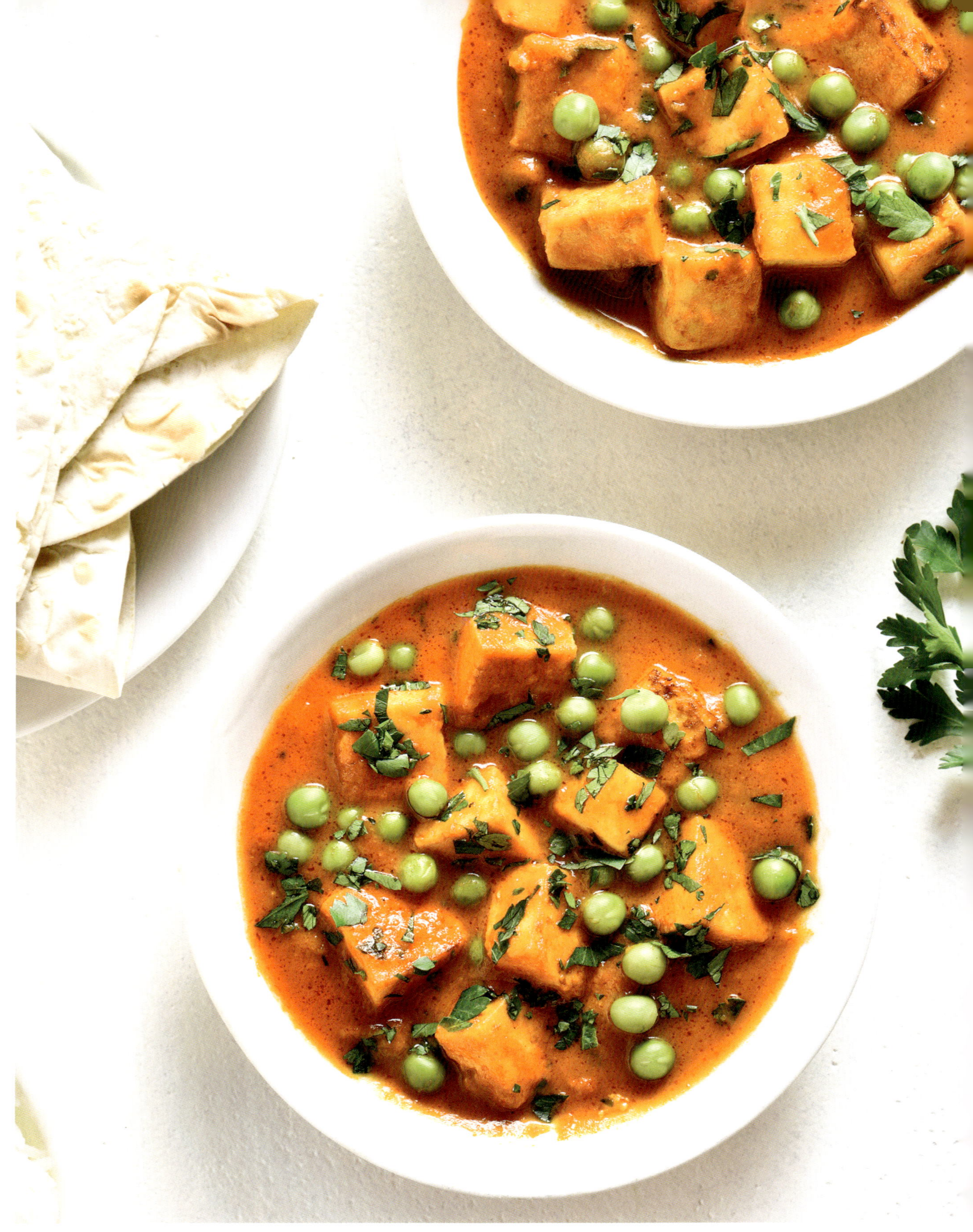

PANEER BUTTER MASALA

SERVES 4 | PREP + COOK TIME: 25 MINS | VEG | GLUTEN FREE |

- 2½ tbsps ghee
- ½ tsp cumin seeds
- 1 red onion, finely chopped
- Medium piece ginger, minced
- 4 cloves garlic, minced
- 1½ cups (375ml) tomato passata
- ¾ cup (185ml) water
- 1½ tsps garam masala
- ½ tsp Kashmiri red chilli powder
- 1½ tsps crushed kasuri methi (dried fenugreek leaves)
- Salt to taste
- 400g paneer, diced into 2cm cubes
- 1 cup (170g) peas
- 3 tbsps cream
- Chopped coriander to garnish

STEPS

1. Heat ghee in a large, deep frying pan over medium-high heat. Add cumin seeds and allow to crackle. Add onion and cook for 3-5 minutes until soft. Add ginger and garlic and cook for 1 minute until fragrant.
2. Add passata. Cover and simmer for 15 minutes until the sauce thickens.
3. Add water and return to a simmer. Add garam masala, red chilli powder and kasuri methi. Season with salt.
4. Add paneer and peas. Stir to coat in sauce. Cover and simmer for 5 minutes.
5. Add cream and stir through. Cook for 1 minute more. Garnish with coriander leaves to serve.

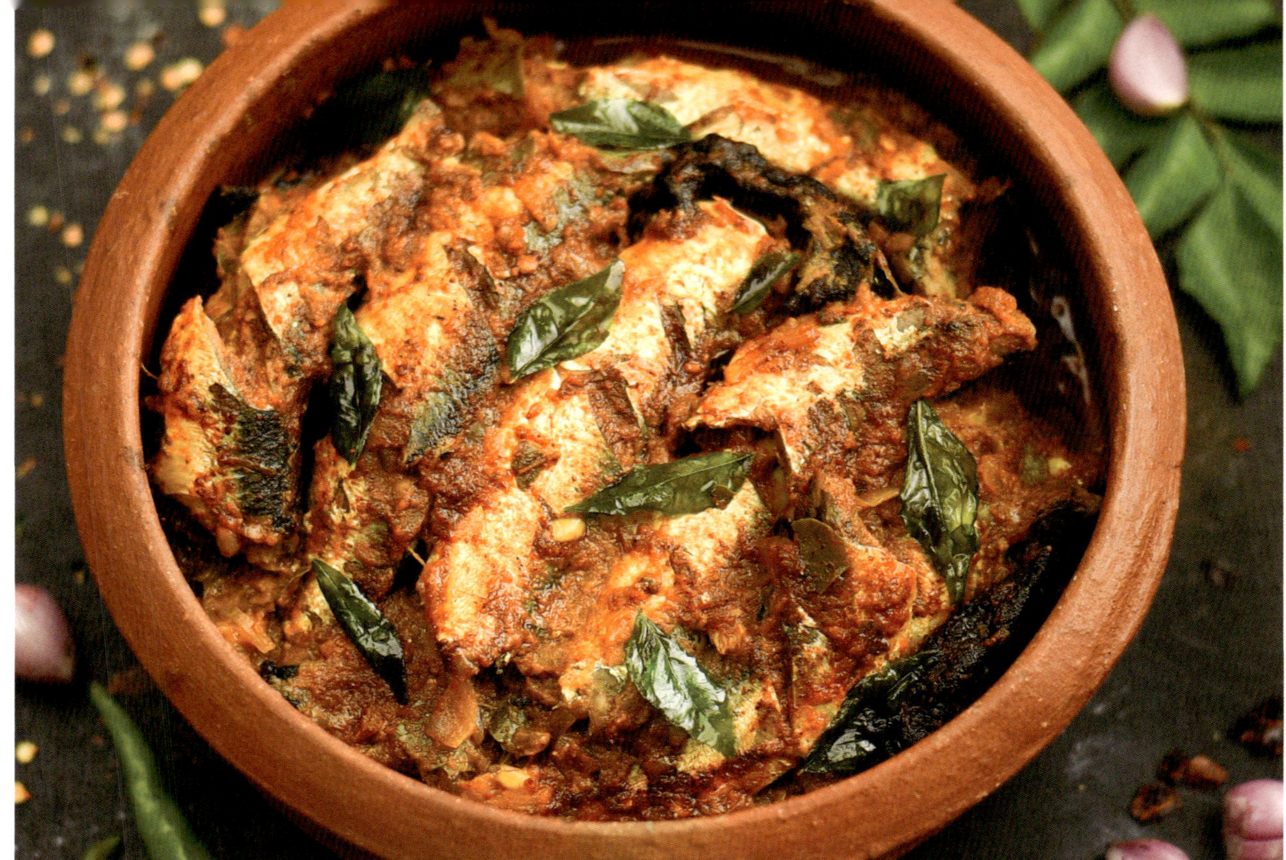

TOMATO & SARDINE CURRY

3 tbsps oil or use oil from canned sardines
½ tsp mustard seeds
1 onion, finely chopped
Small piece ginger, grated
2 cloves garlic, minced
1 cup (200g) chopped tomato
1 tsp red chilli powder
1 tsp ground coriander
½ tsp garam masala
¼ tsp ground turmeric
Salt to taste
1 cup (250ml) water or as needed
2 x 125g cans sardines in olive oil
1 sprig fresh curry leaves

STEPS

1. Heat oil in a saucepan over medium-high heat. Add the mustard seeds and heat for 1 minute until they begin to pop. Add onion and cook, stirring, for 3-5 minutes until soft and translucent. Add ginger and garlic and cook for 1 minute until fragrant.

2. Add chopped tomatoes and cook, stirring occasionally, for 5 minutes. Add red chilli powder, ground coriander, garam masala, ground turmeric powder and salt. Cook for a further 5 minutes.

3. Add water and bring to a boil. Reduce heat and simmer for 10 minutes.

4. Add the sardines and curry leaves and stir gently into the sauce. Cover and cook for 6-7 minutes or until the sardines are well cooked.

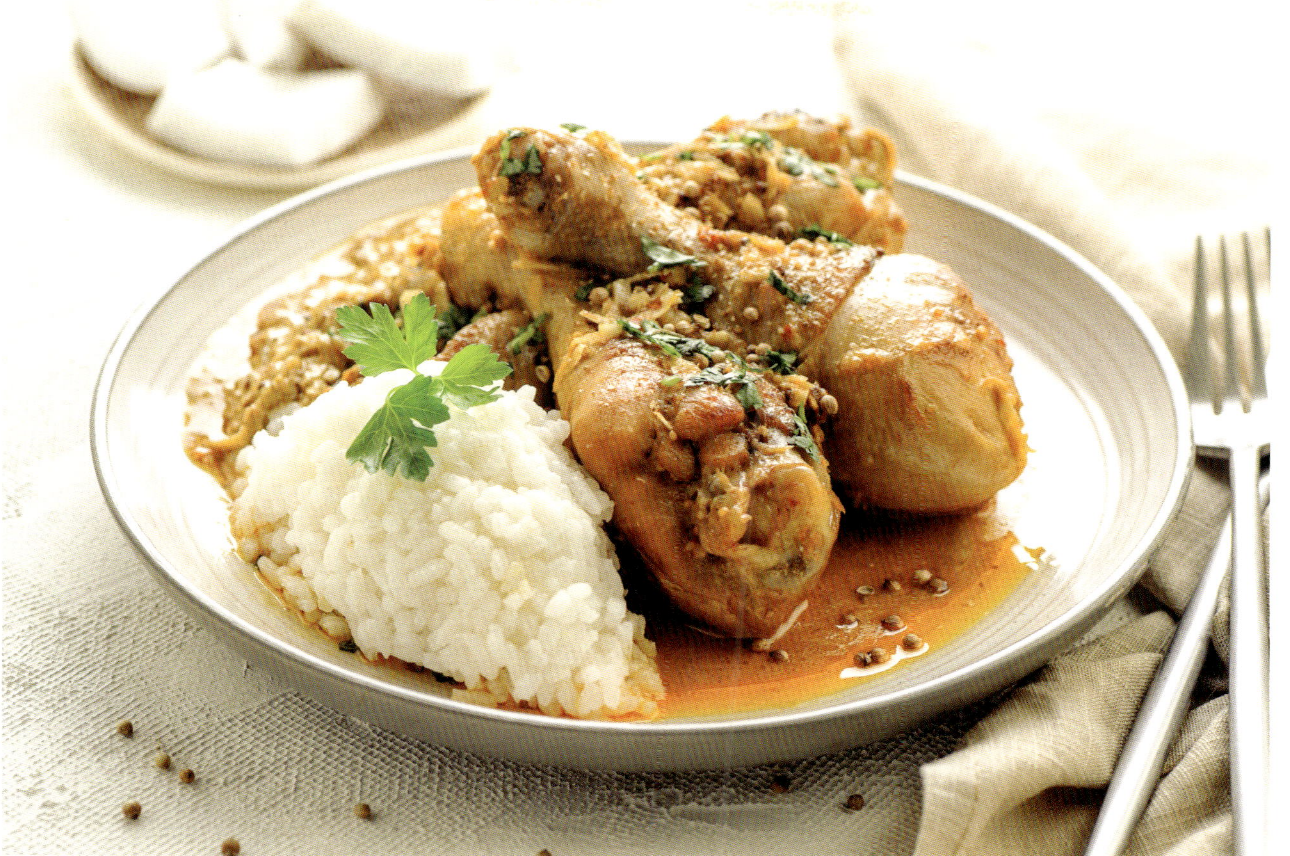

SERVES 4 | PREP + COOK TIME: 1 HOUR 15 MINS | GLUTEN FREE |

SPICED YOGHURT CHICKEN

- 8 chicken drumsticks
- Salt and pepper to taste
- 2 tbsps ghee
- 6 cloves garlic
- Medium piece ginger, thinly sliced
- 1 tbsp coriander seeds
- 1 tbsp cumin seeds
- ½ tsp dried chilli flakes
- 1 tsp ground turmeric
- 2 cups (500ml) plain yoghurt
- Chopped coriander leaves to serve
- Cooked rice to serve

STEPS

1. Season chicken all over with salt and pepper. Heat ghee in a large Dutch oven over medium heat. Arrange chicken drumsticks in pot skin-side down and cook for 10-15 minutes until skin is golden brown and crisp. Transfer to a plate and set aside.

2. Reduce heat to medium-low and add garlic and ginger to the pot. Cook, stirring occasionally, for 2 minutes. Add coriander, cumin and chilli flakes and cook, stirring often, for 1 minute until fragrant. Stir in turmeric followed by yoghurt and mix until smooth; season with salt.

3. Return chicken to pot, skin-side up, in a single layer and add water just until chicken is almost submerged. Bring to a very gentle simmer, and cook uncovered for 1 hour 15 minutes until very tender.

4. Scatter with chopped coriander leaves and serve with rice.

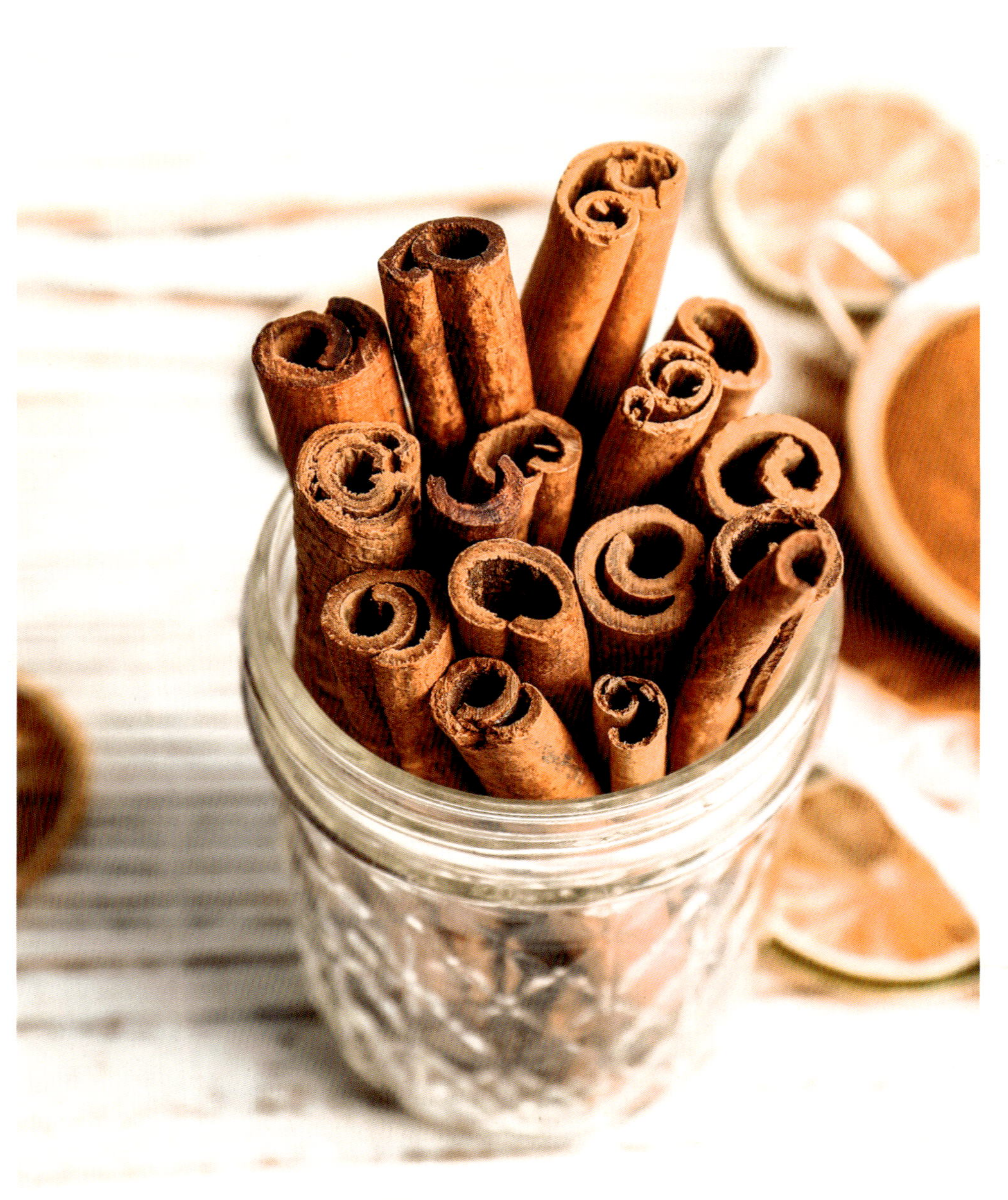

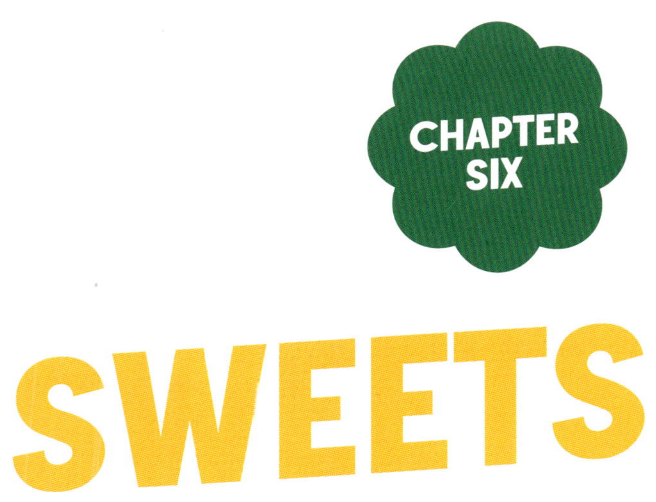

CHAPTER SIX

SWEETS

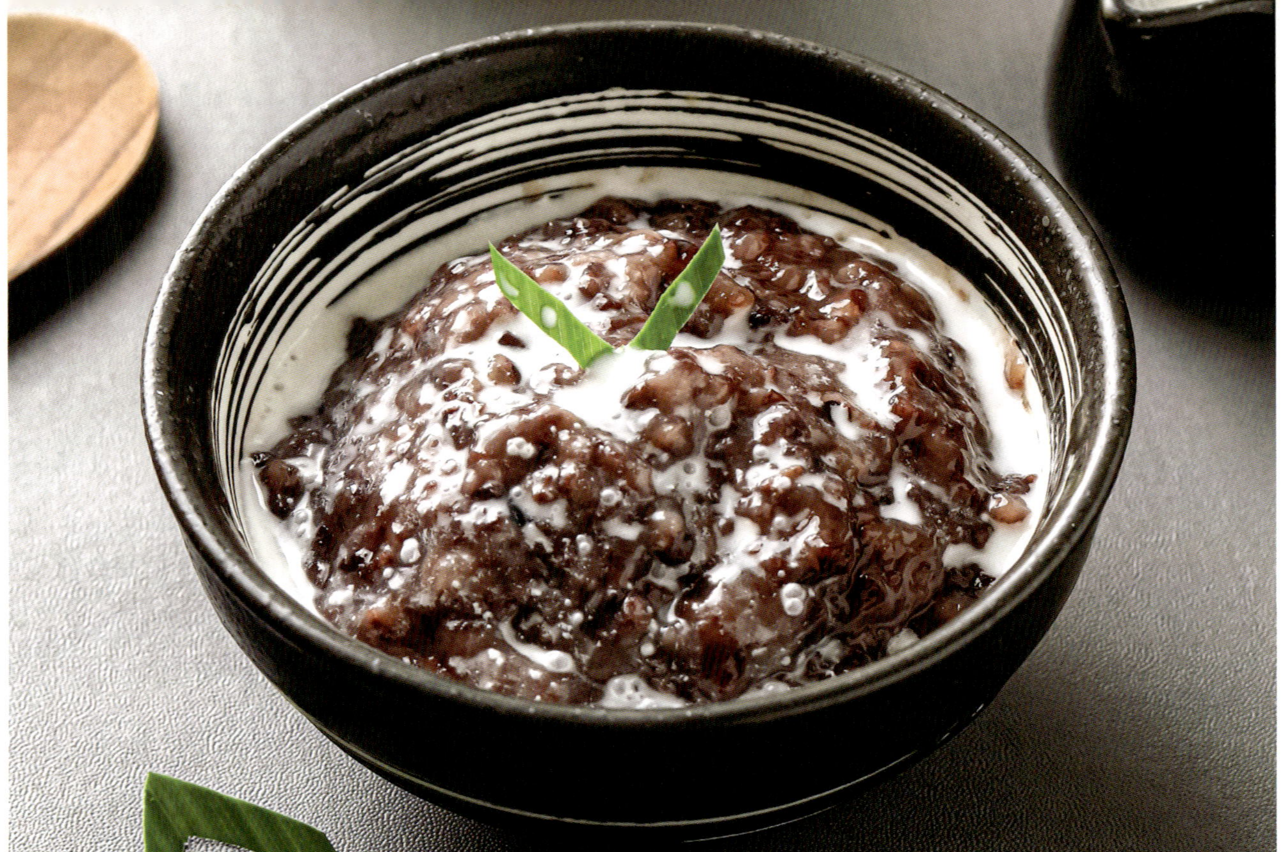

SERVES 4 | PREP + COOK TIME: 1 HOUR + SOAKING | VEG | GLUTEN FREE | DAIRY FREE |

BLACK STICKY RICE

1¼ cups (200g) black glutinous rice, soaked overnight

5 cups (1.25L) water

2 pandan leaves, tied in a knot

1 cup (150g) coconut sugar

Salt to taste

1 cup (250ml) coconut milk

STEPS

1. Drain soaked rice and place in a pan with water and pandan leaves. Place over medium-high heat.
2. Bring to the boil then reduce heat, cover and simmer for 30-45 minutes, stirring occasionally or until the rice is tender. Add the sugar and a pinch of salt. Stir thoroughly. Place the lid back on and simmer for another 5 minutes until all the water is absorbed or evaporated.
3. While the rice is cooking, heat the coconut milk over low heat. Add ½ teaspoon salt. Stir well and set aside.
4. Spoon rice into bowls and top with coconut milk.

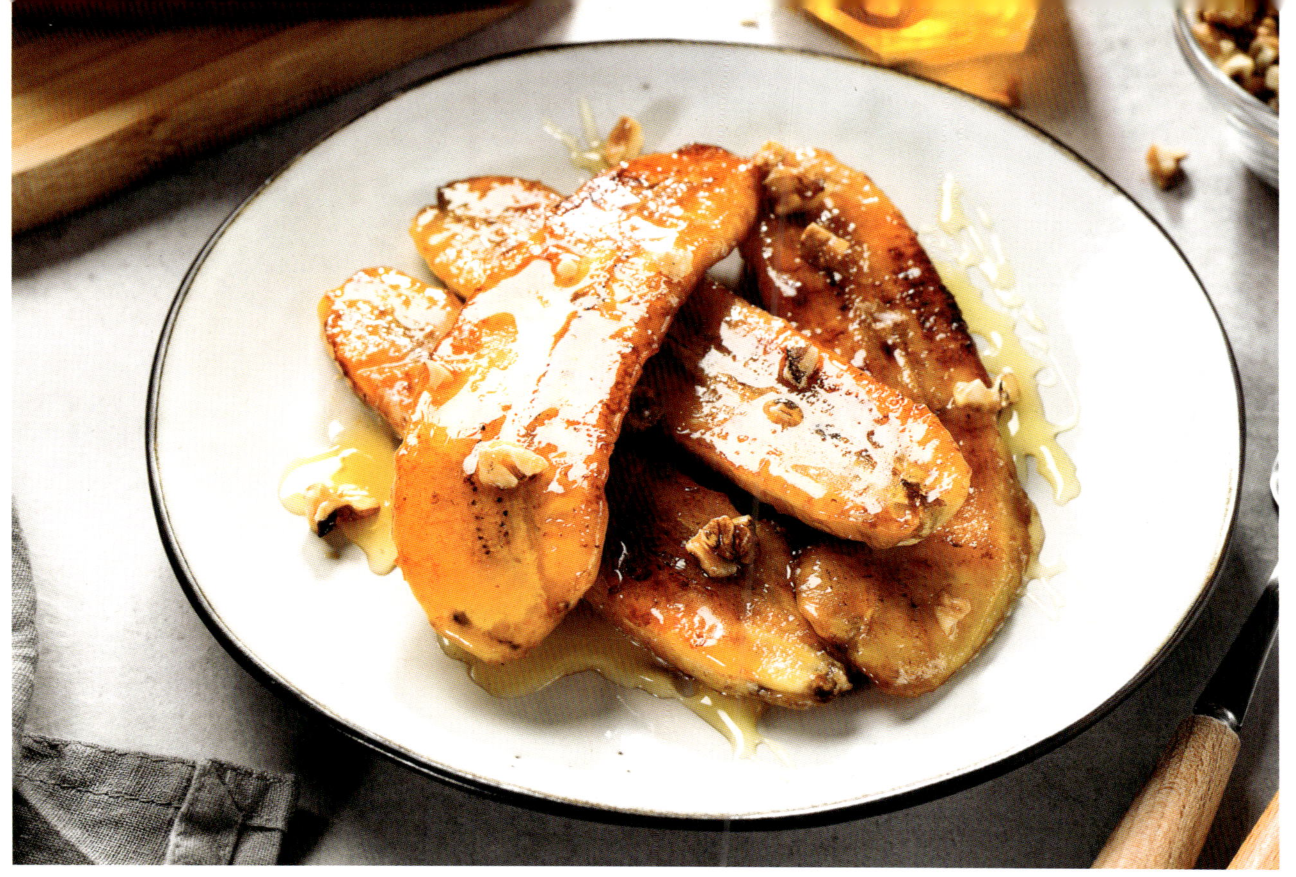

CARAMELISED BANANA

60g butter
3 tbsps maple syrup
3 tbsps brown sugar
½ tsp cinnamon
4 ripe, firm bananas, halved lengthways
¼ cup (30g) walnuts, roughly chopped

STEPS

1. Heat a large, heavy frying pan over medium-high heat.
2. Add the butter, maple syrup, sugar and cinnamon to the pan. When melted, tip to coat the pan evenly in the melted caramel.
3. Place the bananas cut-side down in the pan and reduce the heat to medium.
4. Let the bananas cook for at least 10 minutes until they have softened completely.
5. Serve bananas scattered with walnuts and with caramel sauce from the pan drizzled over the top.

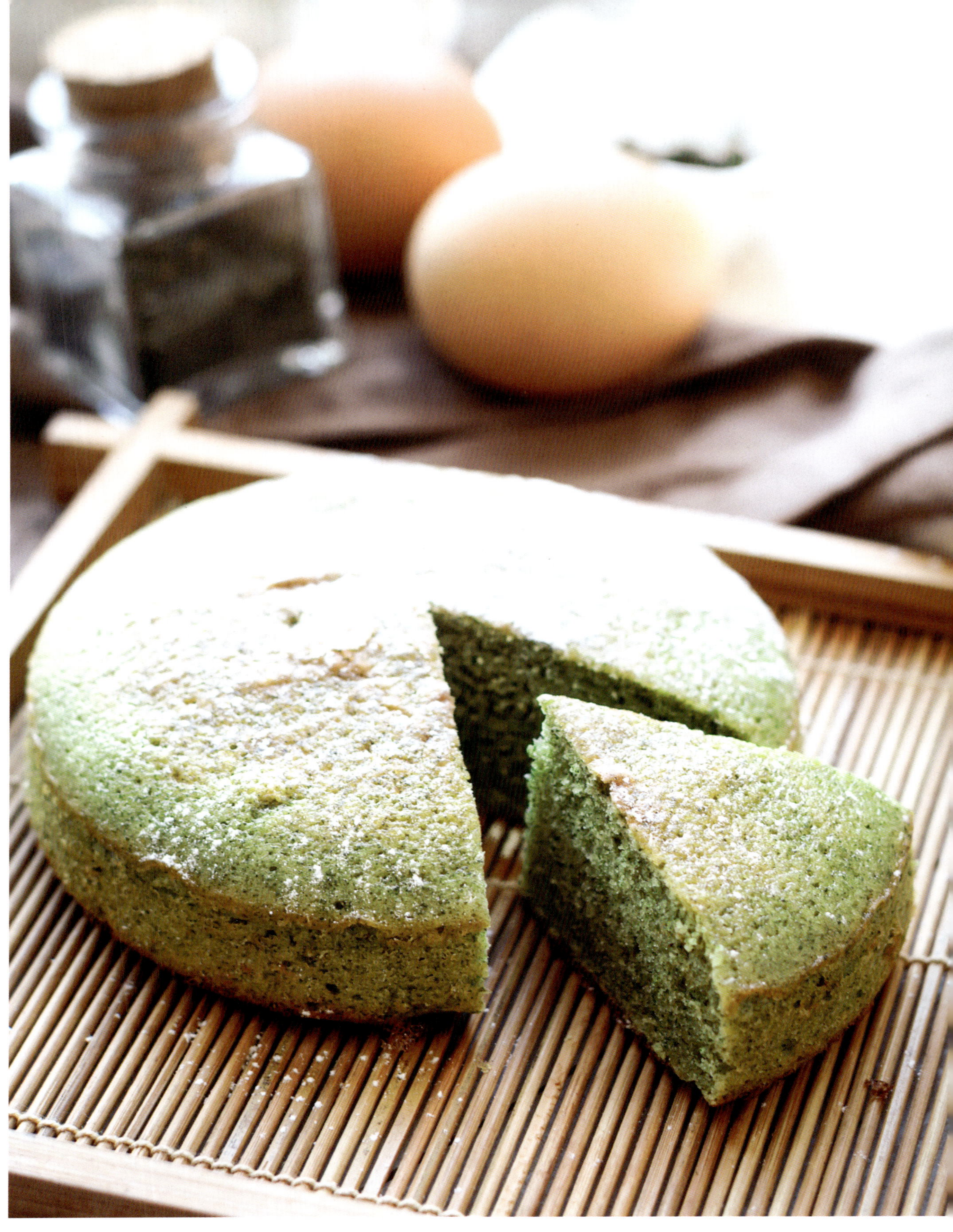

MATCHA GREEN TEA CAKE

1 cup (120g) plain flour
1 tsp baking powder
100g unsalted butter, softened
1 cup (220g) sugar
2 large eggs
1½ tbsps matcha powder
1 tsp vanilla extract
⅓ cup (80ml) buttermilk
Icing sugar for dusting

STEPS

Preheat oven to 160°C.

1. Grease and line a 22cm round cake tin.
2. In a medium bowl whisk together the flour and baking powder.
3. In another bowl, beat together the butter and sugar with an electric mixer until light and fluffy. Add the eggs, matcha powder and vanilla, and beat to combine. Add half of the flour mixture and stir to incorporate. Add all of the buttermilk, and stir again. Add the remaining flour mixture and stir until no streaks of flour remain.
4. Scrape the batter into the prepared tin, and bake for 30-35 minutes, until a skewer inserted in the centre comes out mostly clean with only a few moist crumbs attached.
5. Let the cake cool in the pan for about 15 minutes, before turning out onto a cooling rack to cool completely. Dust with icing sugar to serve.

SERVES 6 | PREP + COOK TIME: 1 HOUR | VEG |

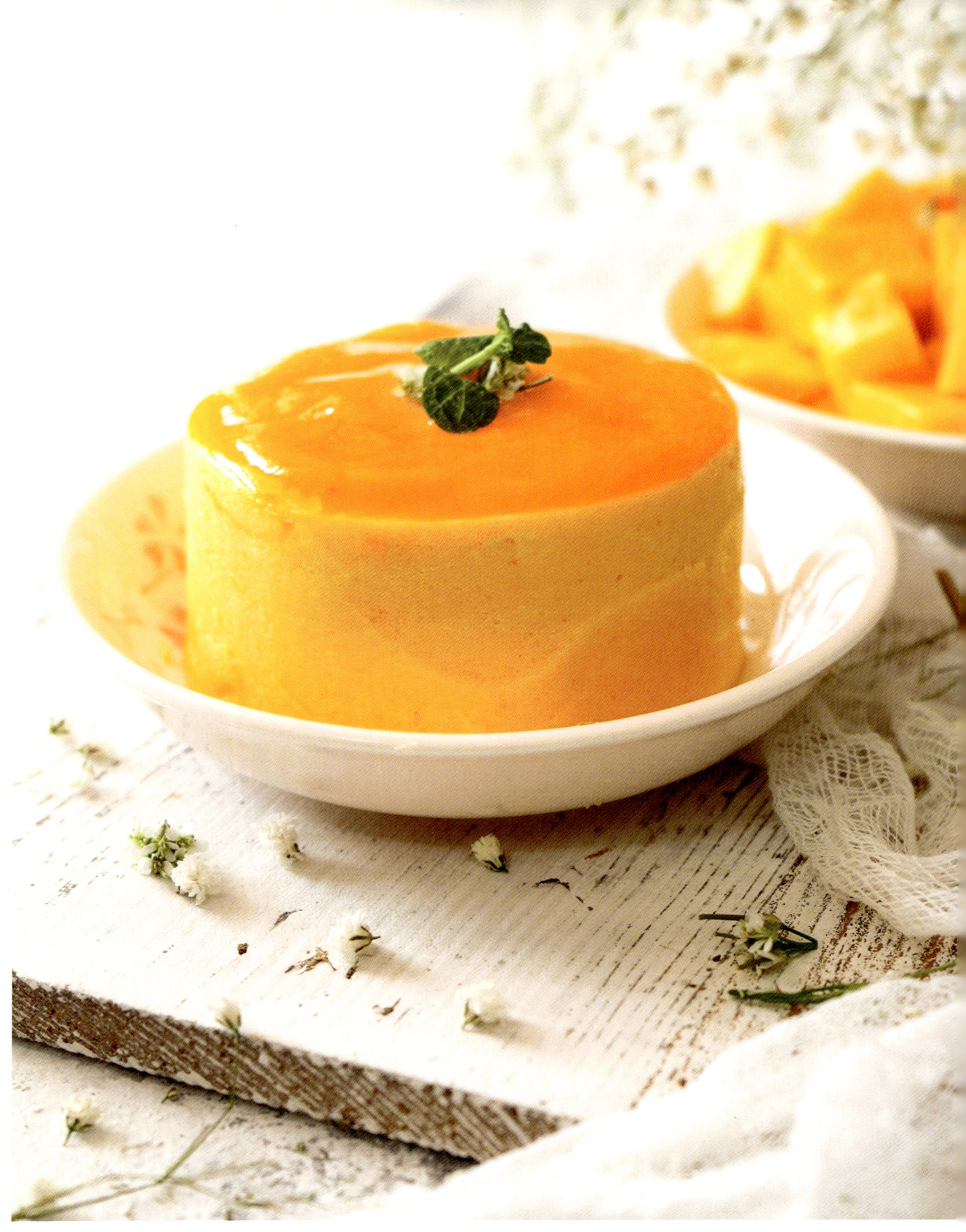

MANGO ORANGE PUDDING

1 tbsp + ½ tsp unflavoured gelatin

⅓ cup (70g) sugar

½ cup (125ml) water

½ cup (125ml) fresh strained orange juice

½ cup (125ml) coconut cream (use the thick cream from the top of an unshaken can)

1¾ cups (290g) pureed fresh mango

Mint leaves to serve

STEPS

1. Place the gelatin, sugar and water in a small saucepan and bring to the boil.
2. Reduce the heat to low, stir in orange juice, coconut cream and 1½ cups of the mango puree then remove from heat.
3. Lightly oil six small moulds with canola or vegetable oil.
4. Pour the mango mixture into the moulds. Chill for at least 3 hours until set.
5. Carefully turn out the puddings from the moulds onto small serving plates. Top with the remaining mango puree and mint leaves.

SERVES 6 | PREP + COOK TIME: 20 MINS + CHILLING | GLUTEN FREE | DAIRY FREE |

SERVES 4 | PREP + COOK TIME: 10 MINS + FREEZING | VEG | GLUTEN FREE |

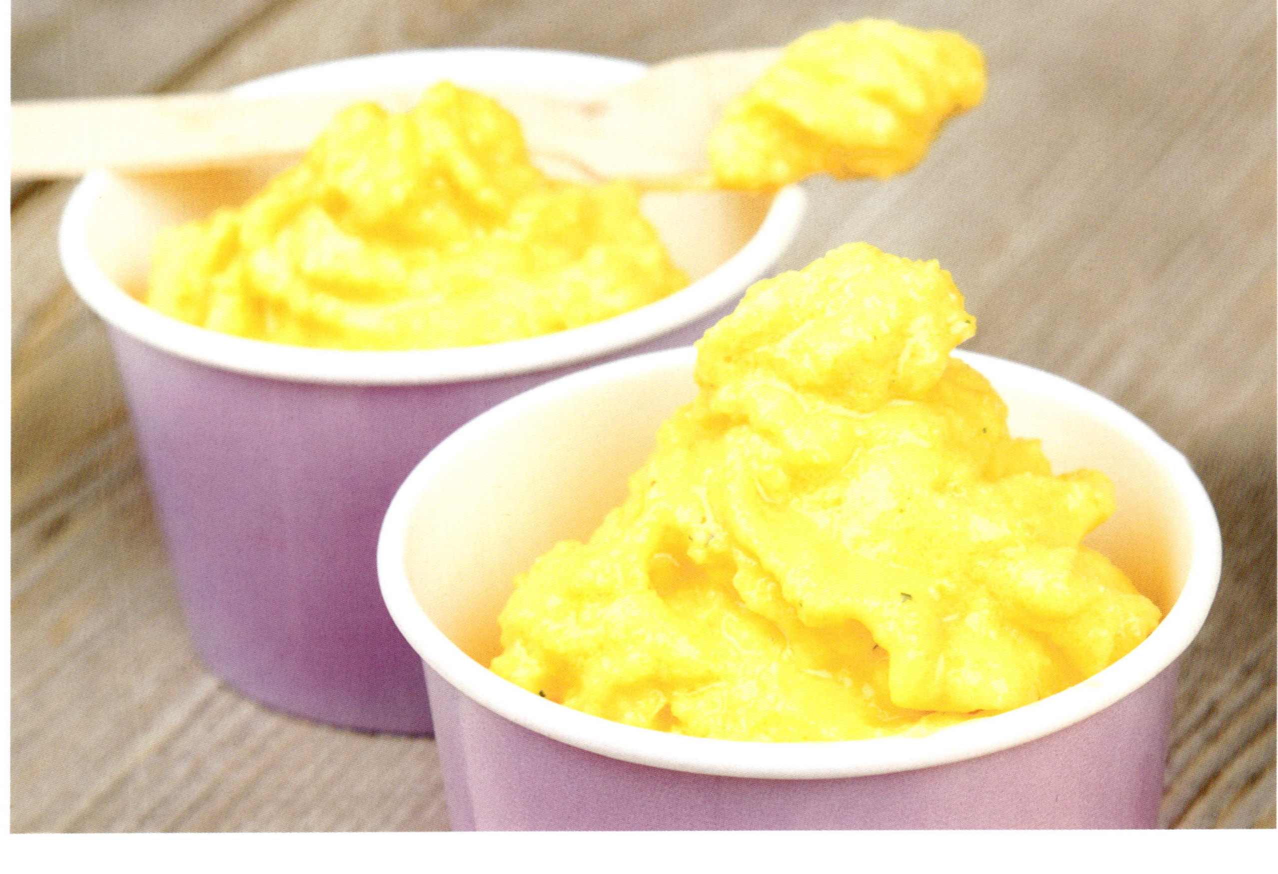

TROPICAL FROZEN YOGHURT

- 2 cups (500ml) Greek yoghurt
- 2 tbsps honey
- 2 tsps vanilla essence
- ¼ cup (5g) mint leaves (optional)
- 1 banana
- 1 fresh (or canned) mango
- 1 x 225g can pineapple in juice
- 1 tbsp brown sugar

STEPS

1. Place the yoghurt, honey, vanilla essence and mint, if using, in a food processor and blend until combined. Add the banana, mango and pineapple and process for 2-3 minutes or until smooth.
2. Transfer to a glass dish and place in the freezer for 4 hours.
3. Remove 10 minutes before serving to allow the dessert to soften slightly.

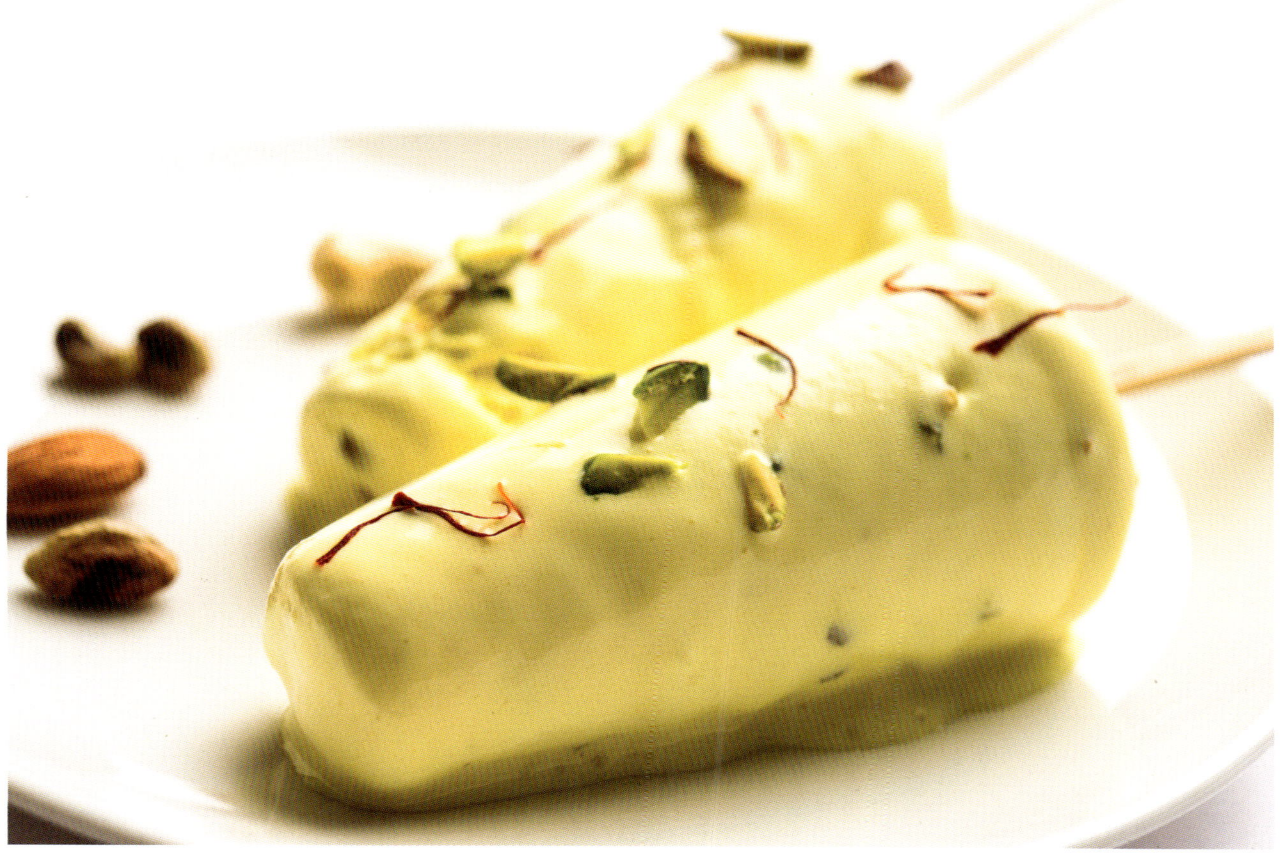

SERVES 4 | PREP + COOK TIME: 15 MINS + FREEZING | VEG | GLUTEN FREE |

QUICK KULFI

¼ cup (30g) mixed pistachios, almonds and cashews

3 cardamon pods

Pinch of saffron

1 cup (250ml) thickened cream

½ x 400g can condensed milk

TO SERVE (OPTIONAL)

1 tbsp roughly chopped pistachios

Small pinch of saffron threads

STEPS

1. Grind the pistachios, almonds and cashews in a food processor or spice grinder along with the cardamon pods and saffron until finely ground.
2. Whisk together the thickened cream, condensed milk and ground nut mixture until well combined.
3. Pour the mixture into popsicle moulds and add a popsicle stick. Transfer to the freezer and freeze for 6 hours or overnight, until set.
4. Run moulds under hot water to demould the kulfi. Scatter with chopped pistachios and saffron, if desired, to serve.

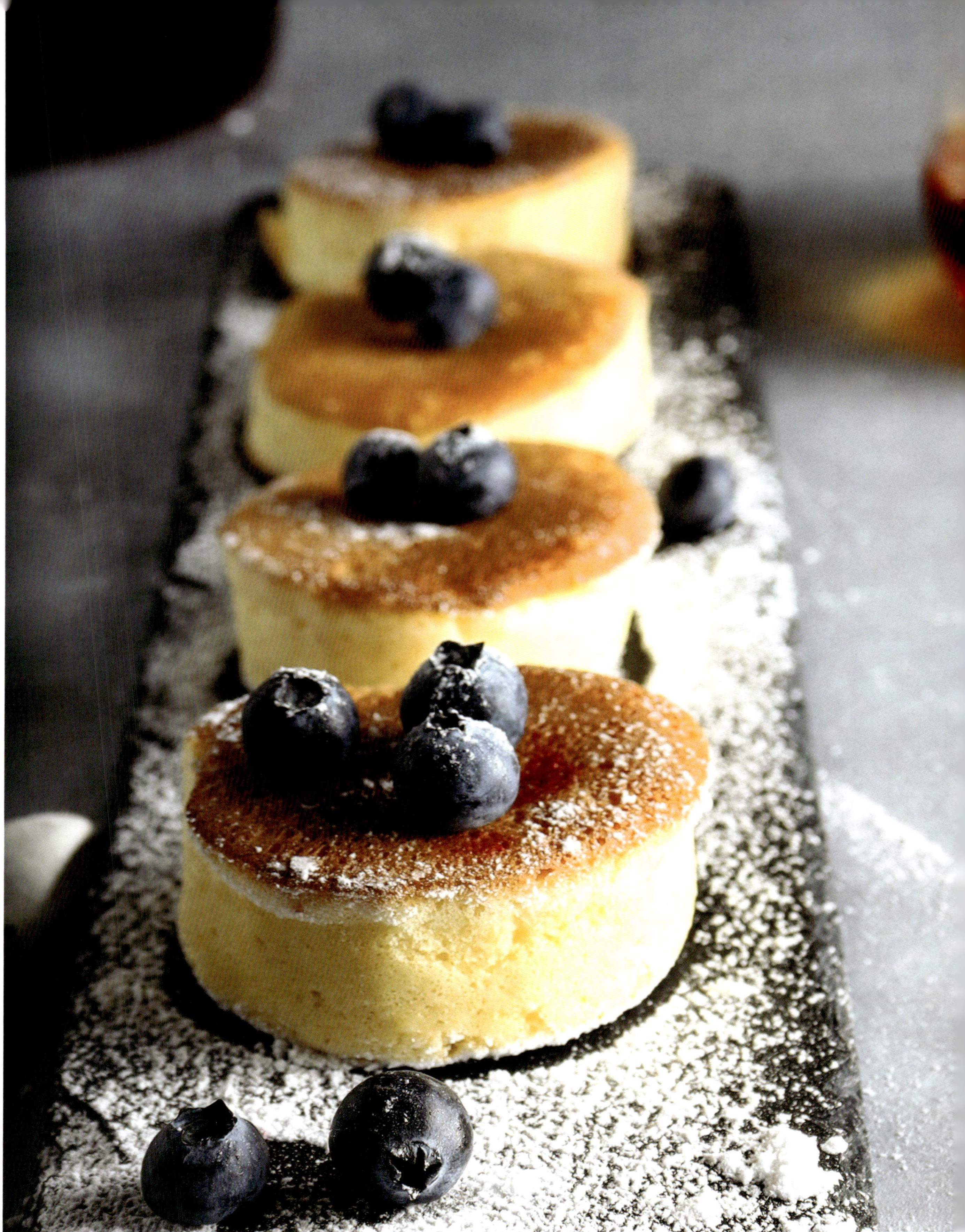

JAPANESE SOUFFLE PANCAKES

SERVES 4 | PREP + COOK TIME: 40 MINS | VEG |

2½ tbsps milk

1 tsp baking powder

¼ tsp vanilla extract

½ tbsp Kewpie mayonnaise

2 large eggs, separated

6 tbsps plain flour

3 tbsps sugar

1 tbsp water

Icing sugar and blueberries to serve

STEPS

1. Add milk, baking powder, vanilla, mayonnaise and egg yolks to a large bowl. Sift in flour. Whisk until smooth and pale yellow.

2. Using a clean whisk and bowl, whisk together egg whites and sugar until stiff peaks form.

3. Fold one-third of the egg white mixture into the batter until incorporated. Add remaining egg white and gently fold until no white streaks remain.

4. Grease a large lidded frying pan and the insides of two ring moulds. Place moulds in pan over low heat. Once pan is hot, half fill each mould with batter. Add ½ tablespoon of water to each side of the pan. Cover and cook for 3-4 minutes until the tops are almost cooked. Use a spatula to flip the pancakes, while still in their moulds. Cover and cook for 2-3 minutes until golden brown. Gently push out of the moulds and keep warm. Repeat with remaining batter.

5. Dust with icing sugar and top with blueberries. Serve warm.

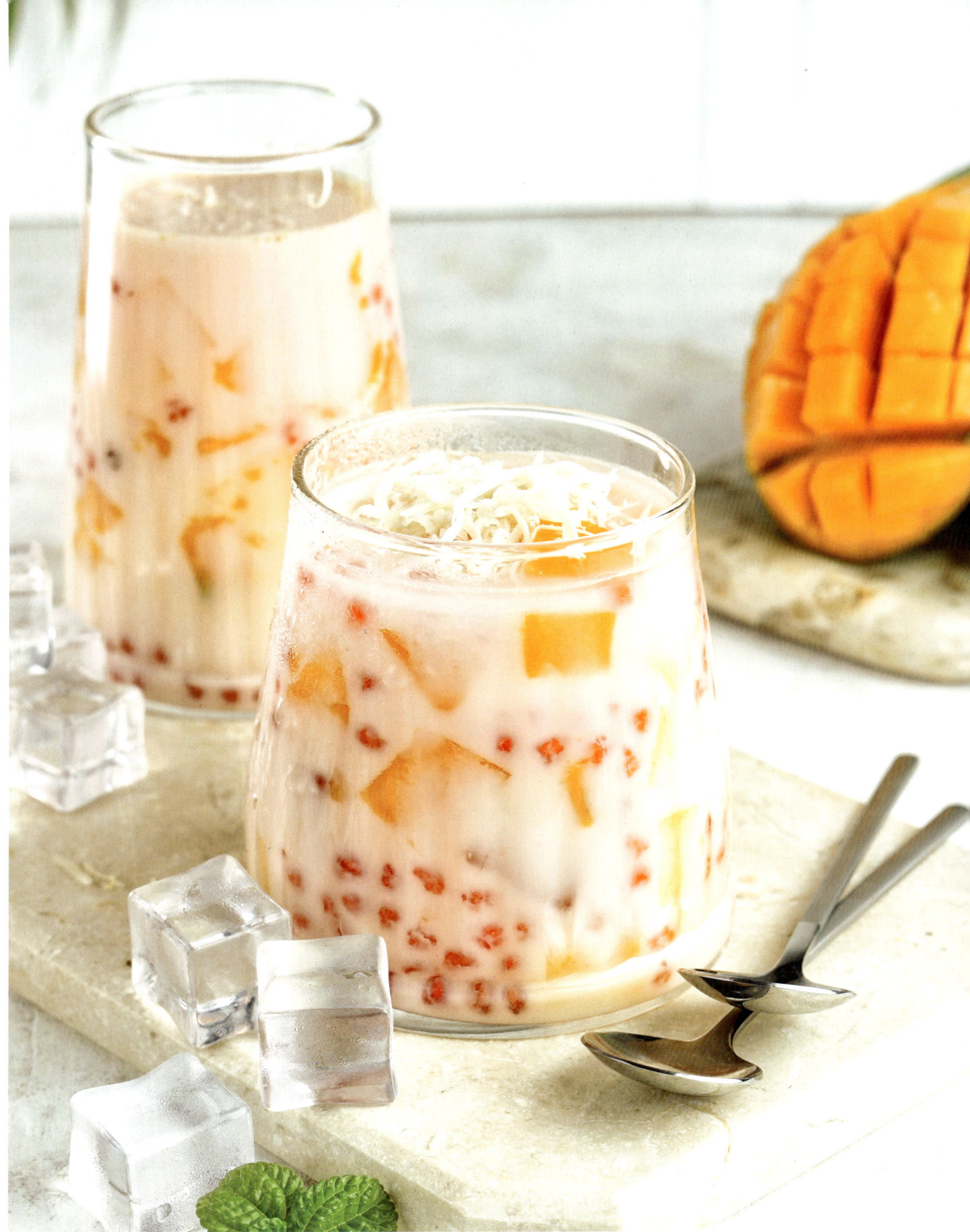

COCONUT MANGO TAPIOCA PUDDING

6 cups (1.5L) water

⅓ cup (50g) small pink tapioca pearls (or use regular tapioca pearls)

1 x 400g can coconut milk

2 tbsps honey

½ tsp vanilla extract

⅛ tsp salt

1 ripe mango, peeled and diced

¼ cup (20g) shredded coconut

Ice cubes

STEPS

1. Add the water to a large saucepan and bring to a rolling boil over high heat. Add the tapioca pearls, lower the heat and simmer for 15-20 minutes or until the tapioca is translucent, stirring frequently to avoid sticking.

2. Drain the tapioca into a sieve and run under cold water.

3. Pour the coconut milk into a saucepan and add the honey, vanilla and salt. Bring to a boil over high heat, stirring occasionally to dissolve the honey and salt. Turn off the heat and stir in the cooked tapioca.

4. Transfer to an airtight container and refrigerate for at least 2 hours.

5. When you're ready to serve, stir the pudding and spoon into 4 glasses. Add diced mango and a few ice cubes and stir to combine. Top with shredded coconut.

SERVES 4 | PREP + COOK TIME: 30 MINS + CHILLING | VEG | GLUTEN FREE | DAIRY FREE |

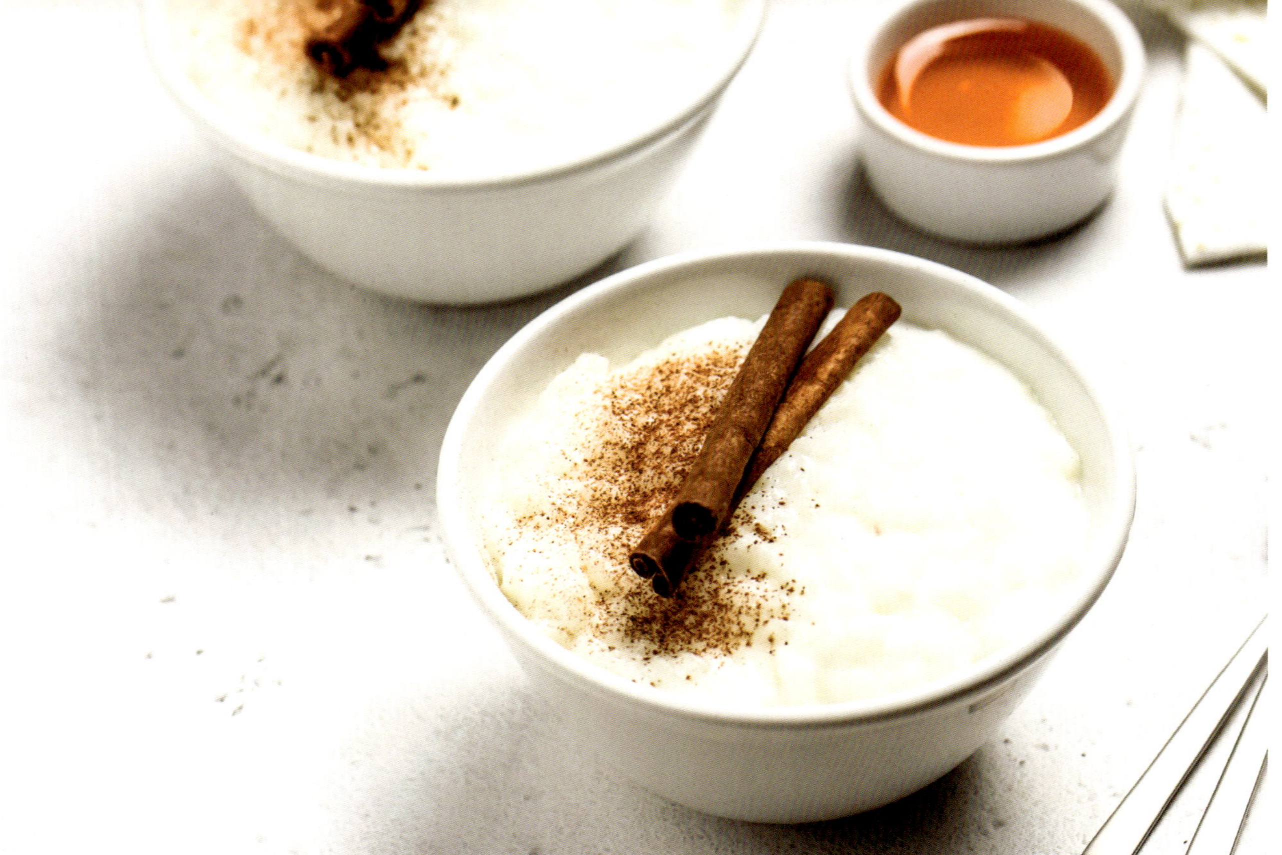

COCONUT RICE PORRIDGE

1½ cups (375ml) water
1 cardamon pod
Pinch of salt
¾ cup (120g) long-grain rice
1½ cups (375ml) coconut milk
2 tbsps agave syrup or maple syrup
¼ tsp vanilla extract
Cinnamon to serve

STEPS

1. Bring the water, cardamon pod and salt to a boil in a saucepan, add rice and return to a boil then cover and cook over low heat for about 20 minutes until water is absorbed.
2. Remove lid and fluff rice with a fork. Add coconut milk, syrup and vanilla extract and bring to a simmer over medium heat. Simmer for about 5 minutes until mixture thickens.
3. Dust with cinnamon to serve.

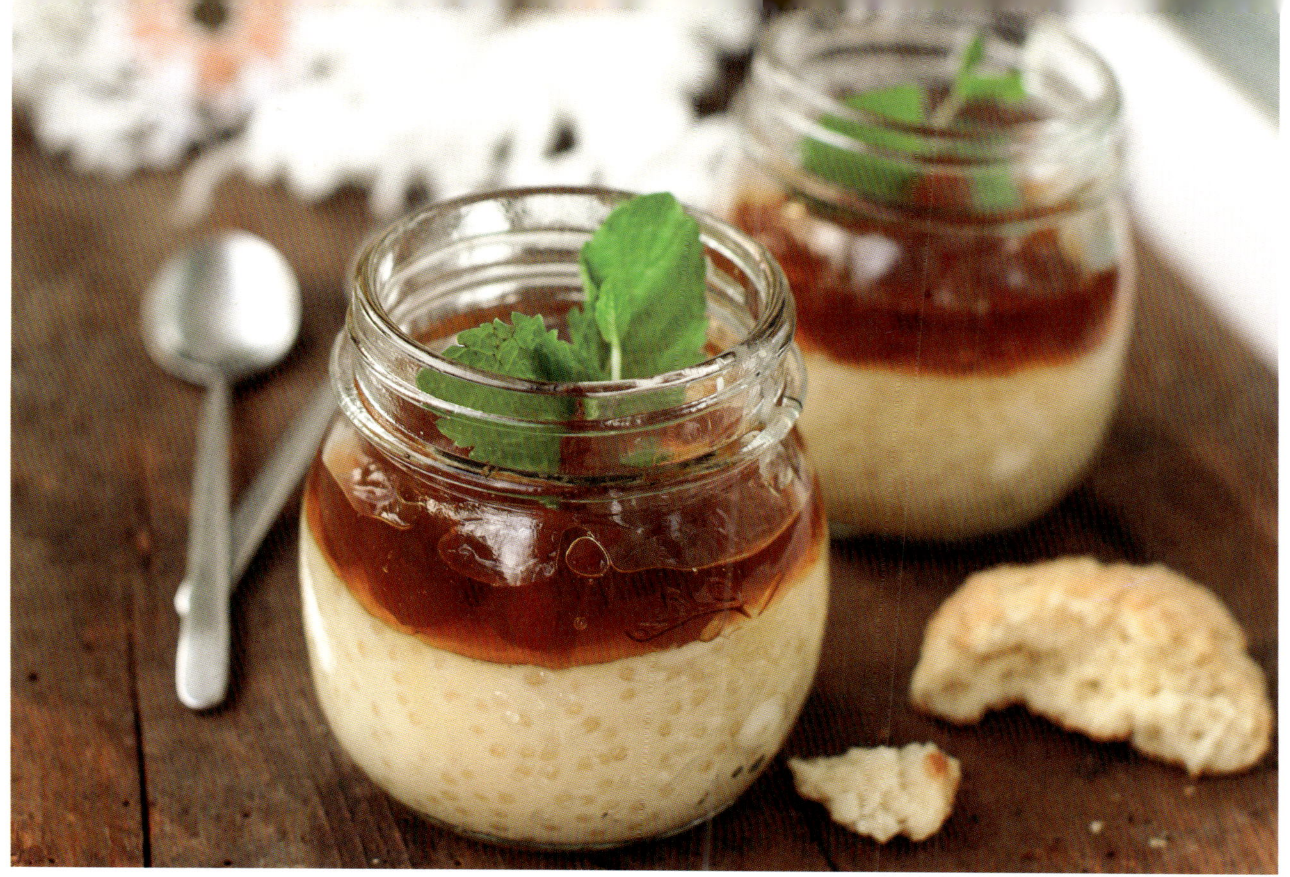

SERVES 4 | PREP + COOK TIME: 30 MINS | VEG | GLUTEN FREE |

TAPIOCA PUDDING

½ cup (75g) small pearl tapioca

3 cups (750ml) whole milk

¼ tsp salt

½ cup (110g) sugar

2 large eggs

1 tsp vanilla extract

½ cup (160g) jam of choice

STEPS

1. Place tapioca pearls in a pan with milk and salt. Cook over medium heat until simmering. Then reduce heat to low and start adding sugar a little at a time until the tapioca pearls increase in size.
2. Break the eggs into a heatproof bowl. Temper the eggs by adding a little of the hot tapioca mixture while whisking constantly.
3. Drizzle the tempered eggs mixture into the pan of tapioca mixture. Allow to simmer gently until thickened.
4. Cool for 15 minutes. Stir in vanilla.
5. Spoon into glasses and top with jam. Can be served warm or chilled.

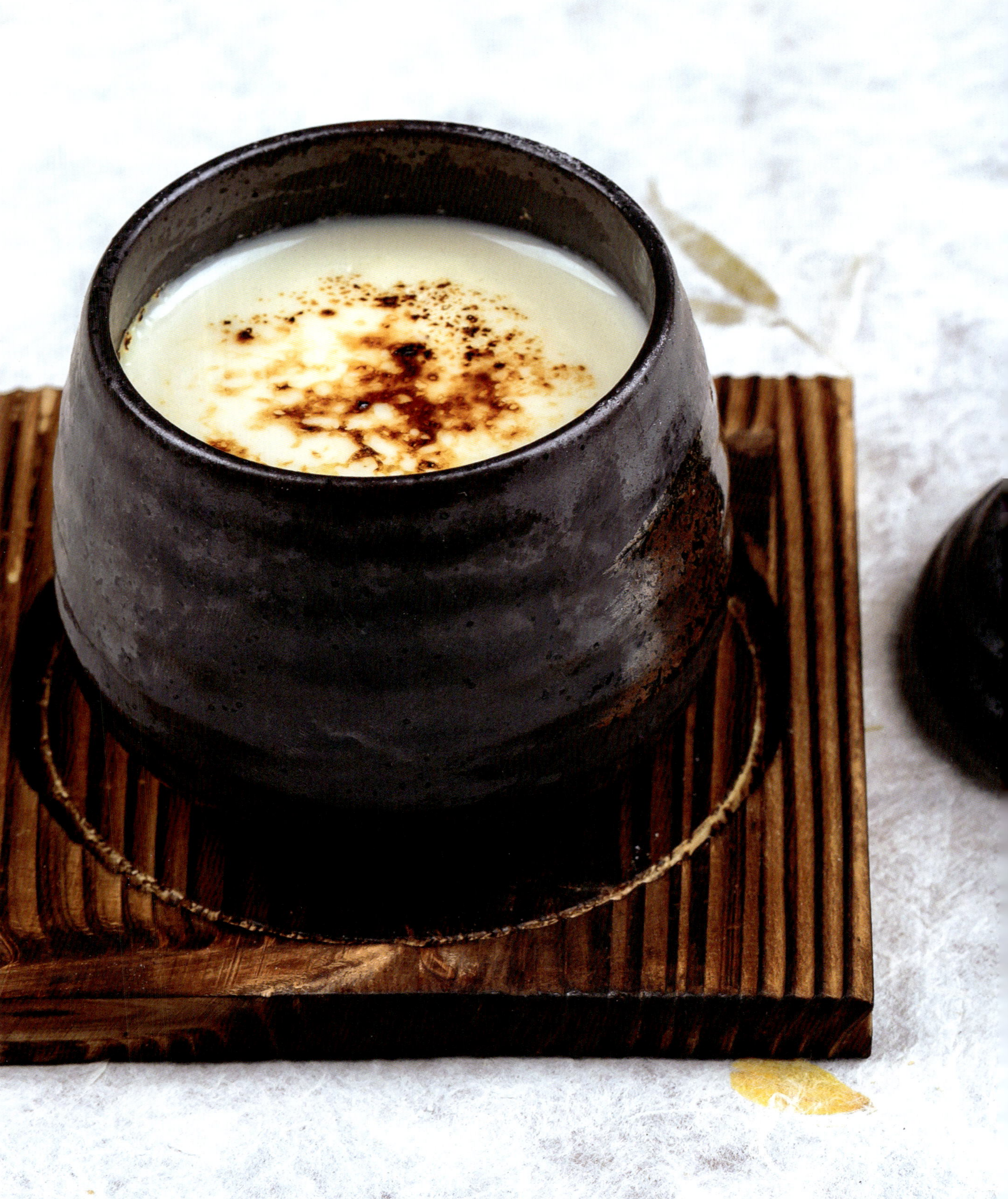

JAPANESE BAKED CUSTARD PUDDING

CARAMEL

½ cup (110g) sugar

1½ tbsps cold water

2 tbsps hot water

CUSTARD

1 cup (250ml) milk

1 cup (250ml) thickened cream

1 tbsp vanilla bean paste

4 egg yolks

⅓ cup (70g) sugar

STEPS

Preheat oven to 150°C.

1. In a small, deep saucepan, cook sugar and cold water over medium-low heat, stirring occasionally, until melted and a dark brown, caramel colour. Remove from the heat. Carefully, pour in the hot water, and stir to combine. Pour the caramel into four ramekins or heatproof containers and swirl to coat.
2. Pour milk and cream and vanilla bean paste into a medium saucepan. Heat mixture until warm, but before any bubbles appear.
3. In a bowl, whisk together the egg yolks and sugar. Gradually pour the warm milk into the egg mixture, whisking as you do so.
4. Pour custard into the ramekins. Place ramekins in a deep roasting tin and fill the tray about 4cm deep with boiling water. Cover tin with foil and bake for 20-25 minutes until custard is set.
5. Place ramekins on a wire rack to cool for 30 minutes, then transfer to the fridge. Chill for a minimum of 2 hours or overnight.

SERVES 4 | PREP + COOK TIME: 50 MINS + CHILLING | VEG | GLUTEN FREE |

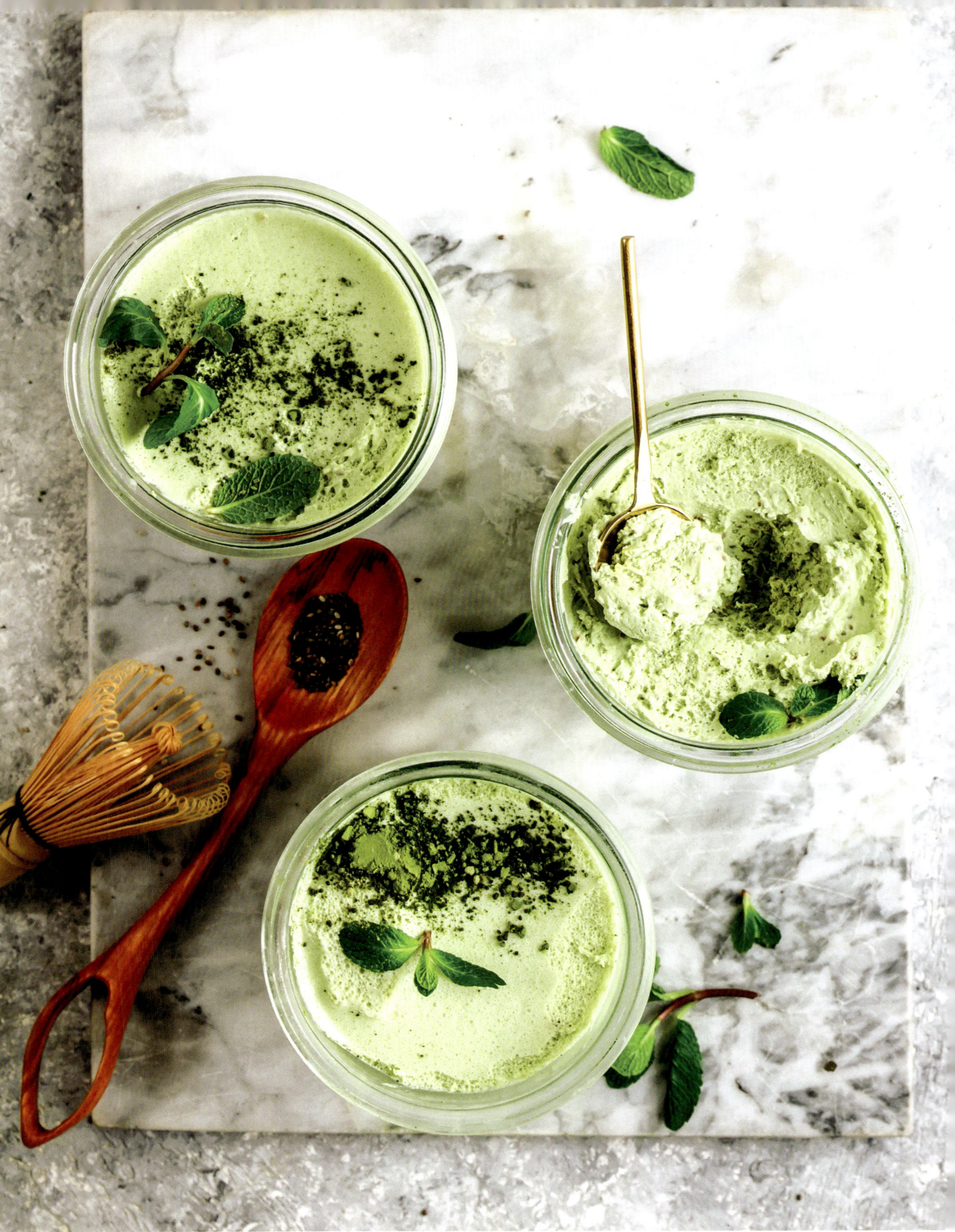

MATCHA & WHITE CHOCOLATE MOUSSE

1 tsp matcha powder

1 cup (250ml) thickened cream

125g white chocolate, coarsely chopped

1 tsp vanilla extract

1 tbsp chia seeds

TO SERVE

Matcha powder and mint sprigs (optional)

STEPS

1. In a heatproof bowl whisk the matcha powder with 4 tablespoons cream, until no lumps remain. Add the white chocolate and place over a pan of water over medium-low heat, stirring, until the chocolate is melted. Remove from the heat and let cool for 15 minutes, stirring occasionally, until cool to the touch.
2. In a large bowl, whisk the remaining cream and vanilla extract and beat until stiff peaks form. Combine half of the whipped cream with the melted white chocolate, and then fold in the remaining whipped cream and chia seeds. Spoon into four individual small bowls or glasses, cover, and chill in the fridge for 2 hours.
3. Dust with matcha powder and top with mint sprigs to serve.

SERVES 4 | PREP + COOK TIME: 15 MINS + COOLING AND CHILLING | VEG | GLUTEN FREE |

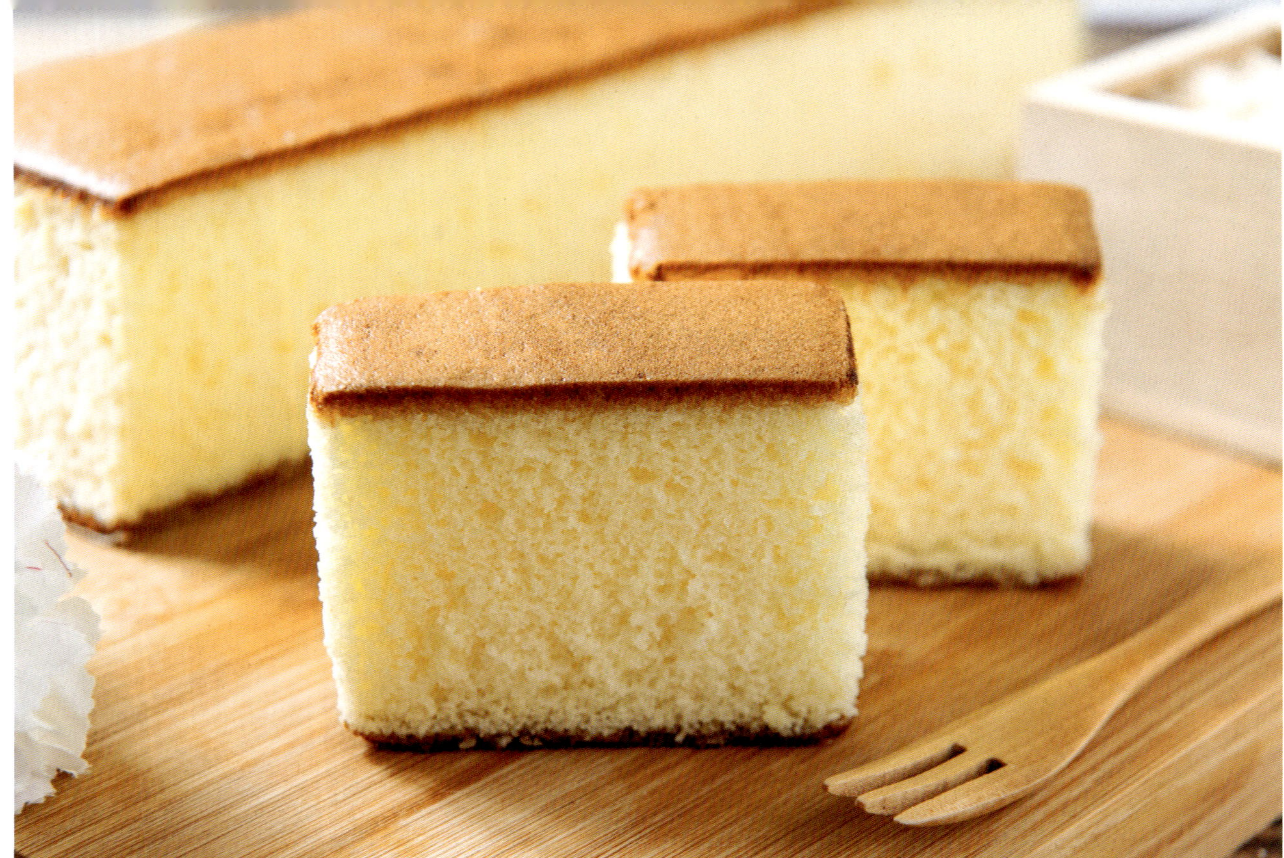

JAPANESE SPONGE CAKE

8 egg yolks, room temperature
6 egg whites, room temperature
1 cup (220g) caster sugar
¼ cup (50ml) milk
¼ cup (90g) honey
1 tbsp vegetable oil
1½ cups (185g) bread flour, sifted

STEPS

Preheat oven to 170°C.

1. Lightly grease and line a loaf tin with baking paper.
2. Beat the egg yolks and whites together on high for 4 minutes. Add the sugar and beat for a further 3 minutes.
3. Warm the milk and mix in the honey. Add to the batter with the oil and beat for 1 minute. Add the flour in thirds on low speed until completely mixed through.
4. Pour into the loaf tin. Bake for 60 minutes until golden brown on top or until a skewer inserted in the middle comes out clean.
5. Immediately wrap firmly in plastic wrap. Put in the refrigerator to rest for at least 12 hours to enhance the honey flavour. To serve, slice off the crust from the sides, then cut into slices.

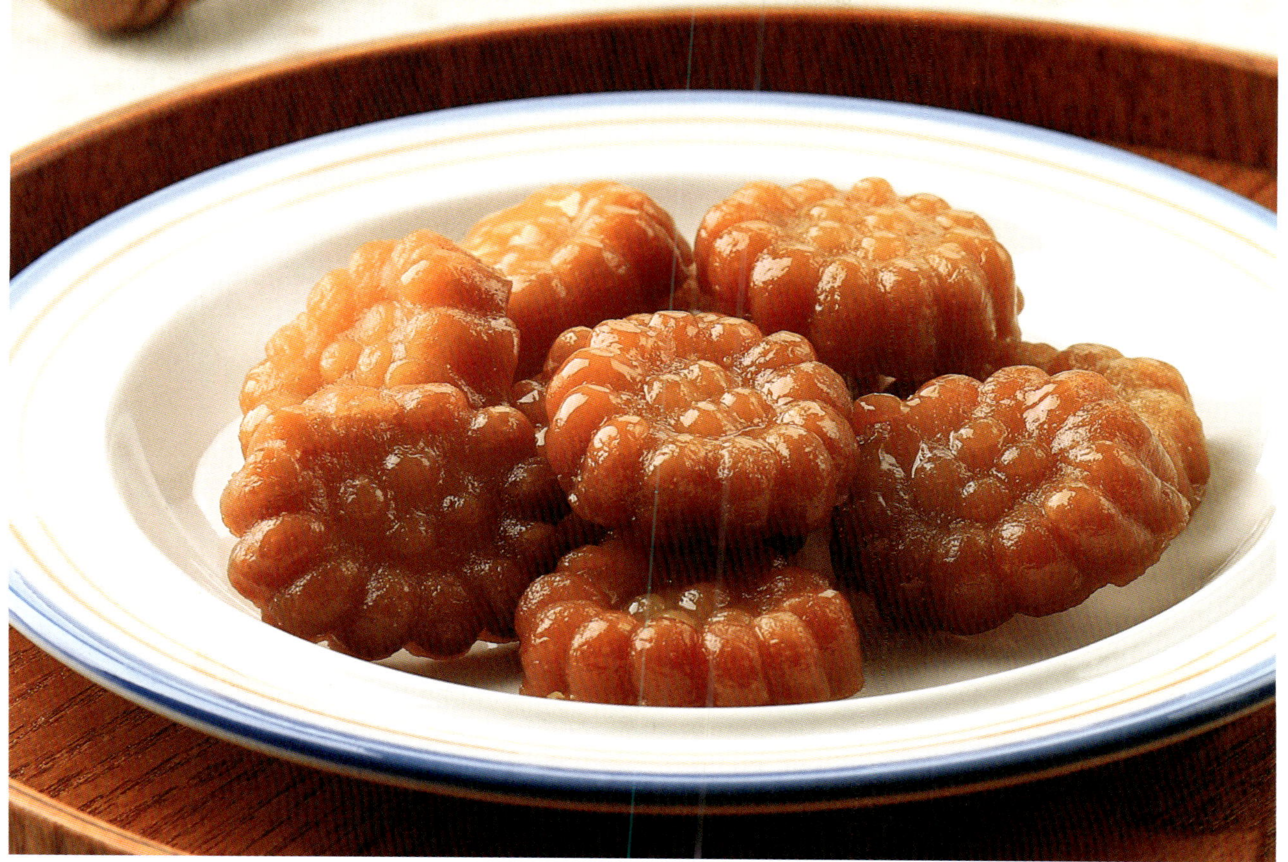

YAKGWA (HONEY COOKIES)

1 tsp baking powder

1⅔ cups (205g) plain flour

1 tbsp sesame oil

Pinch of salt

1 tbsp sugar syrup

1 tsp ground ginger

1¼ cups (440g) + 2 tbsps honey

4 tbsps rice wine

1 cup (250ml) + 2 tbsps water

½ tsp ground cinnamon

Small piece ginger, cut into matchsticks

2 tsps lemon zest

Vegetable oil for frying

STEPS

1. Mix baking powder, flour, sesame oil and salt in a large bowl. Add sugar syrup, ground ginger, 2 tablespoons honey, rice wine and 2 tablespoons water. Mix thoroughly then cover with plastic wrap and let sit for 1 hour.
2. Heat remaining honey with 1 cup water, cinnamon and fresh ginger in a small saucepan over medium heat for 5 minutes until simmering. Remove from heat, stir in lemon zest, strain out ginger. Let cool.
3. Roll dough out to 3cm thick, then fold in half. Repeat three times. Roll to 1cm thick. Cut into 4cm rounds (or use a yakgwa mould).
4. Heat 4cm of oil in a deep-sided pan over high heat. Add the biscuits in small batches and fry for 12 minutes until dark golden brown. Remove with a slotted metal spoon and drain on paper towels.
5. Soak in the syrup for 2 hours before serving.

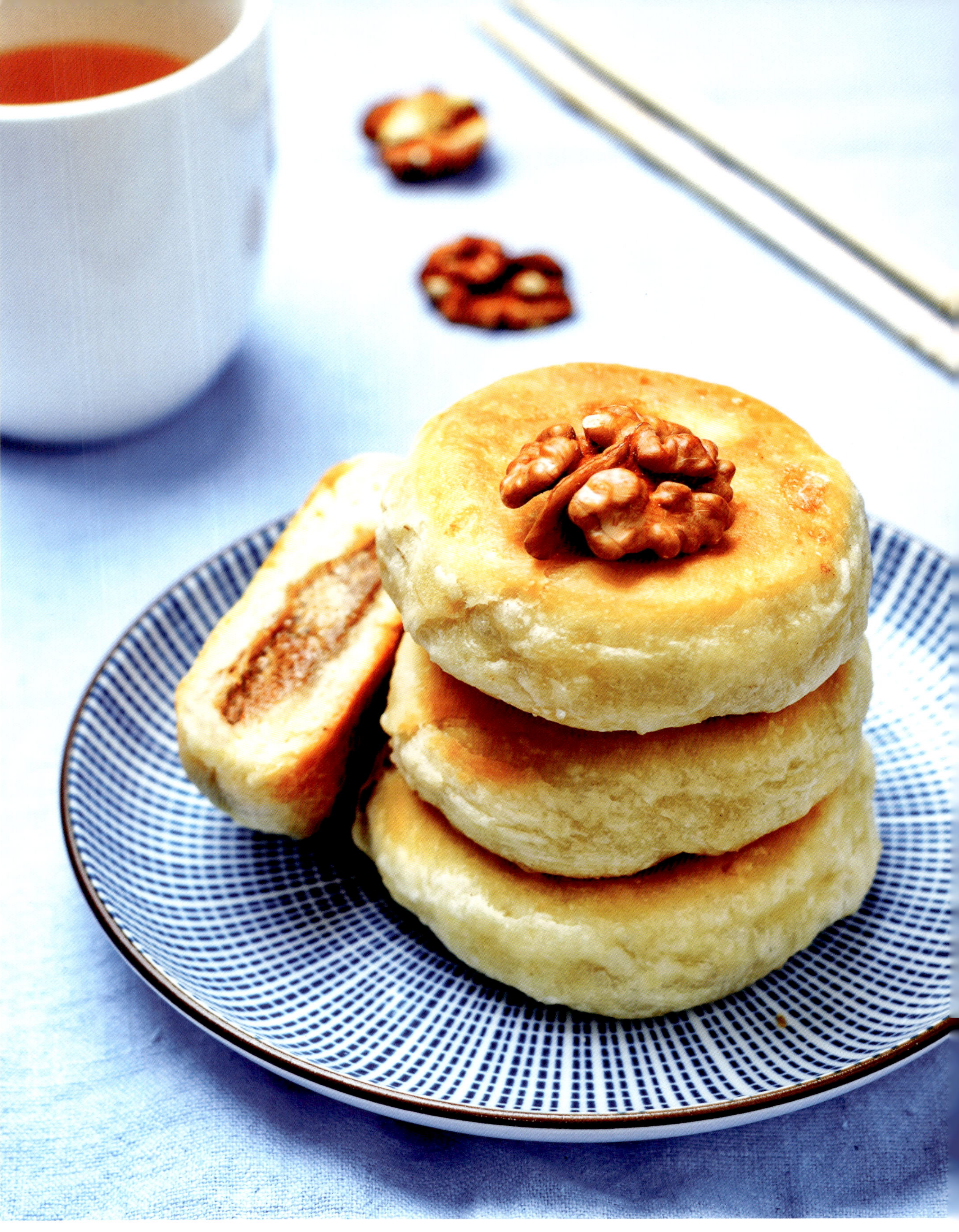

HOTTEOK (SWEET PANCAKES)

1½ tsps instant yeast
1½ tsps caster sugar
1 cup (240ml) warm water
1½ cups (240g) sweet rice flour
1½ cups (185g) plain flour
1 tsp salt
¾ tsp ground cinnamon
⅔ cup (80g) walnuts, roughly chopped
¾ cup (120g) brown sugar
Vegetable oil for frying

STEPS

1. Place the yeast, caster sugar and warm water in a small bowl and stir gently. Let sit for 10 minutes until it is bubbling.

2. Mix together the rice flour, plain flour and salt in a large mixing bowl and make a well in the middle. Pour in the yeast mix and incorporate into the flour. Cover with plastic wrap and let it sit at room temperature for 3 hours.

3. Place the cinnamon, walnuts and brown sugar in a food processor and blend into a smooth mixture.

4. Divide the dough into thirds and cut each third into five sections. Lightly oil your hands and shape the dough into flat rounds around 10cm in diameter. Place 2 teaspoons of the walnut mix in the centre and seal the dough around it into a little round cake.

5. Heat 4 tablespoons of oil in a large, deep-sided frying pan over medium heat. Add the hotteoks in batches and gently press down with an oiled spatula to flatten them. Fry for 3-4 minutes until edges start to brown.

MAKES 15 | PREP + COOK TIME: 50 MINS + PROVING | VEG | DAIRY FREE |

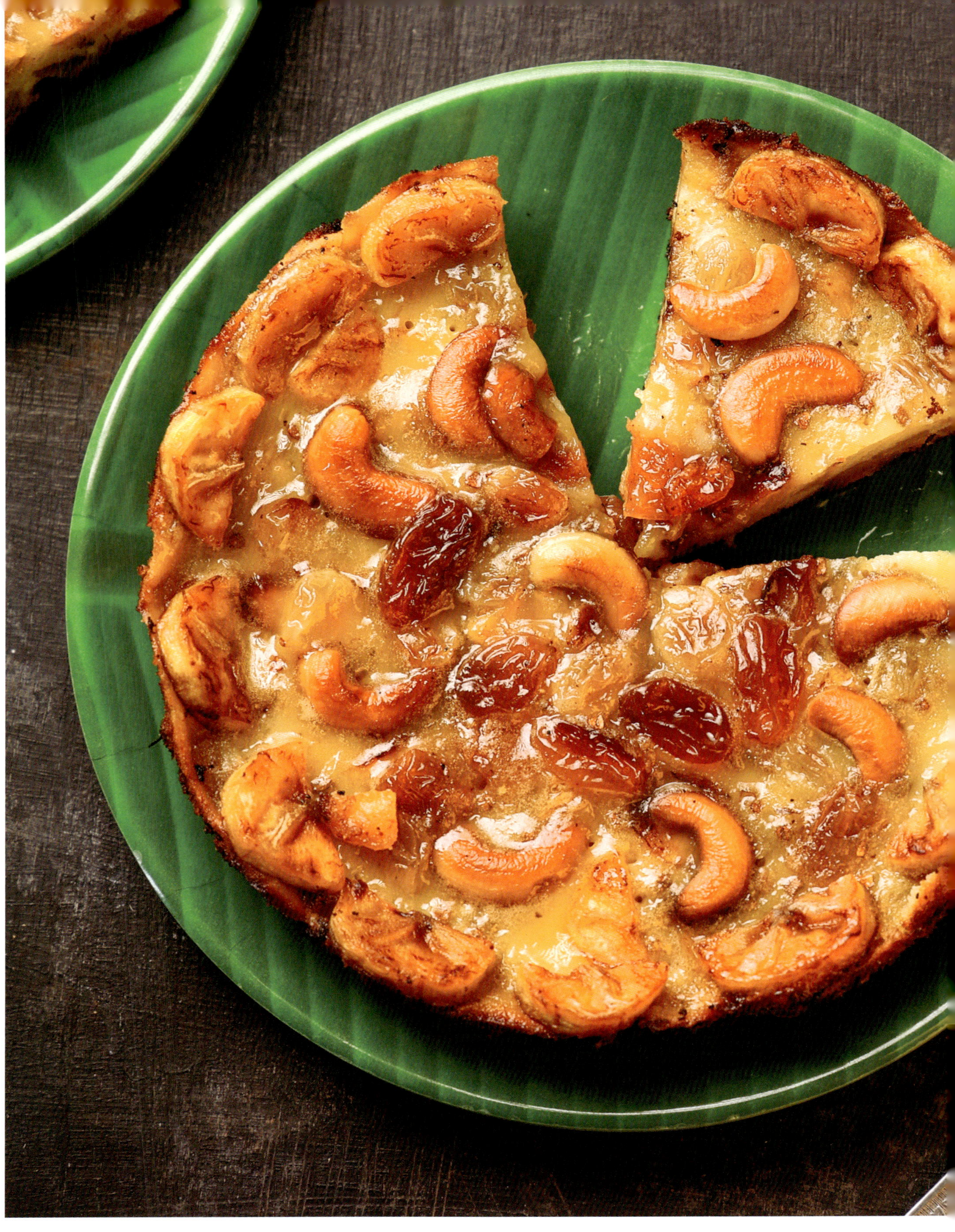

BANANA & CASHEW CAKE

3 tbsps ghee + more for greasing
3 ripe bananas; 2 finely chopped, 1 sliced
2 eggs
½ cup (125ml) milk
3 tbsps sugar
2 tbsps raw cashews
2 tbsps golden raisins

STEPS

1. Heat 2 tablespoons ghee in a nonstick saucepan over medium heat. Add chopped banana and saute for 4-5 minutes until golden brown.
2. Beat the eggs, milk and sugar with an electric mixer until light and fluffy. Add the fried chopped banana chunks, 1 tablespoon raw cashews and 1 tablespoon raisins and stir well.
3. Grease a medium nonstick frying pan with ghee and place over low heat. Pour in the banana mixture and cover with a lid. Cook, covered, for 10 minutes. Remove the lid and cook for a further 10 minutes, until cooked through. Remove from the heat.
4. Heat 1 tablespoon ghee in a saucepan over medium heat. Add sliced banana and remaining cashews and raisins and saute for 4-5 minutes until golden brown.
5. Transfer cake to a serving plate and top with fried banana slices, cashews and raisins.

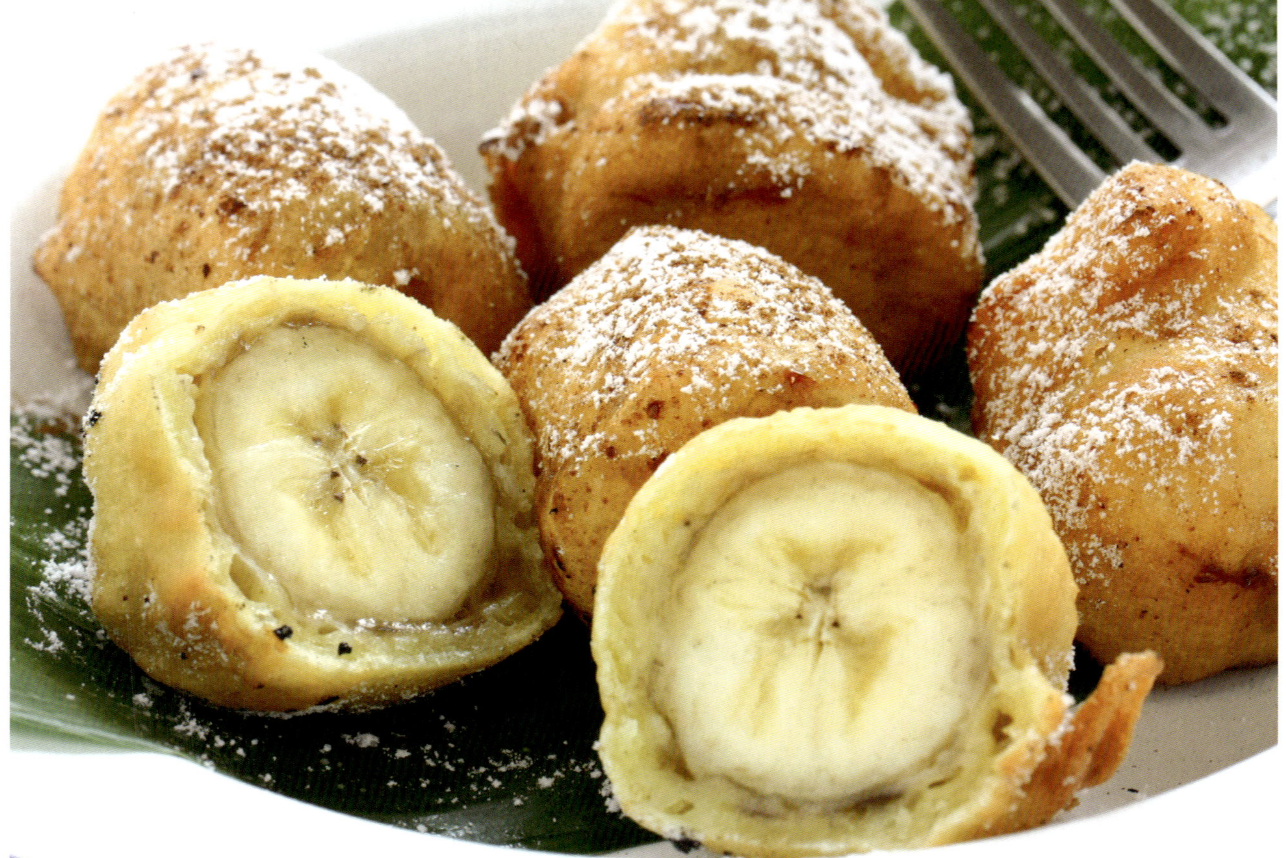

GORENG PISANG (BANANA FRITTERS)

2 tbsps rice flour

¾ cup (90g) plain flour

2 tsps brown sugar

1 tsp baking powder

1 tsp salt

½ cup (125ml) water or as needed

1 tsp vanilla extract

6 ripe bananas, cut into 3cm sections

Vegetable oil for frying

Icing sugar for dusting

STEPS

1. Whisk together the rice flour, flour, sugar, baking powder and salt in a large bowl. Add enough water to make a batter that thinly coats the back of a spoon. Stir in the vanilla extract, then cover and place in the refrigerator for 1 hour to chill.

2. Heat at least 5cm of oil in a deep-sided saucepan over high heat.

3. Dip the banana in the batter and carefully drop into the oil in small batches. Fry for 4 minutes or until golden brown all over. Drain on a wire grill over paper towels and serve warm dusted with icing sugar.

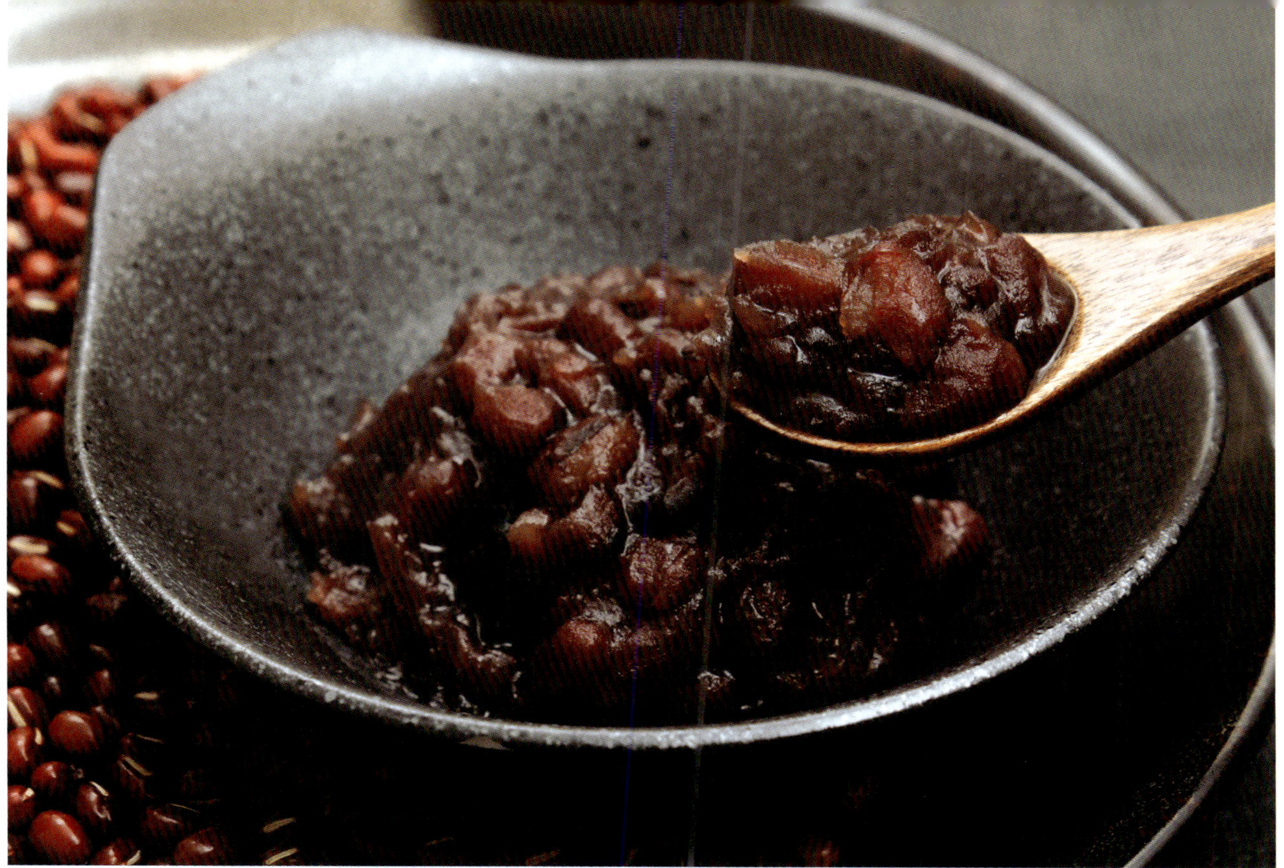

ADZUKI RED BEAN PASTE

200g dried adzuki beans

9 cups (2.25L) water + more as needed

½ cup (100g) caster sugar

⅔ cup (100g) brown sugar

STEPS

1. Soak the beans overnight in plenty of water.
2. Drain and place the beans in a large pot with 4½ cups of water. Boil for 5 minutes, then drain and rinse.
3. Return the beans to the pot with another 4½ cups of water and again bring to a boil. Reduce heat to low and simmer, covered, for at least 2 hours. Add more water as needed to ensure the beans are completely covered.
4. Drain, then return the softened beans to the pot. Add the sugars and stir over medium heat for 12 minutes until the sugar is incorporated and the mixture forms a paste that is slightly shiny.
5. Serve warm or cold over your favourite pudding.

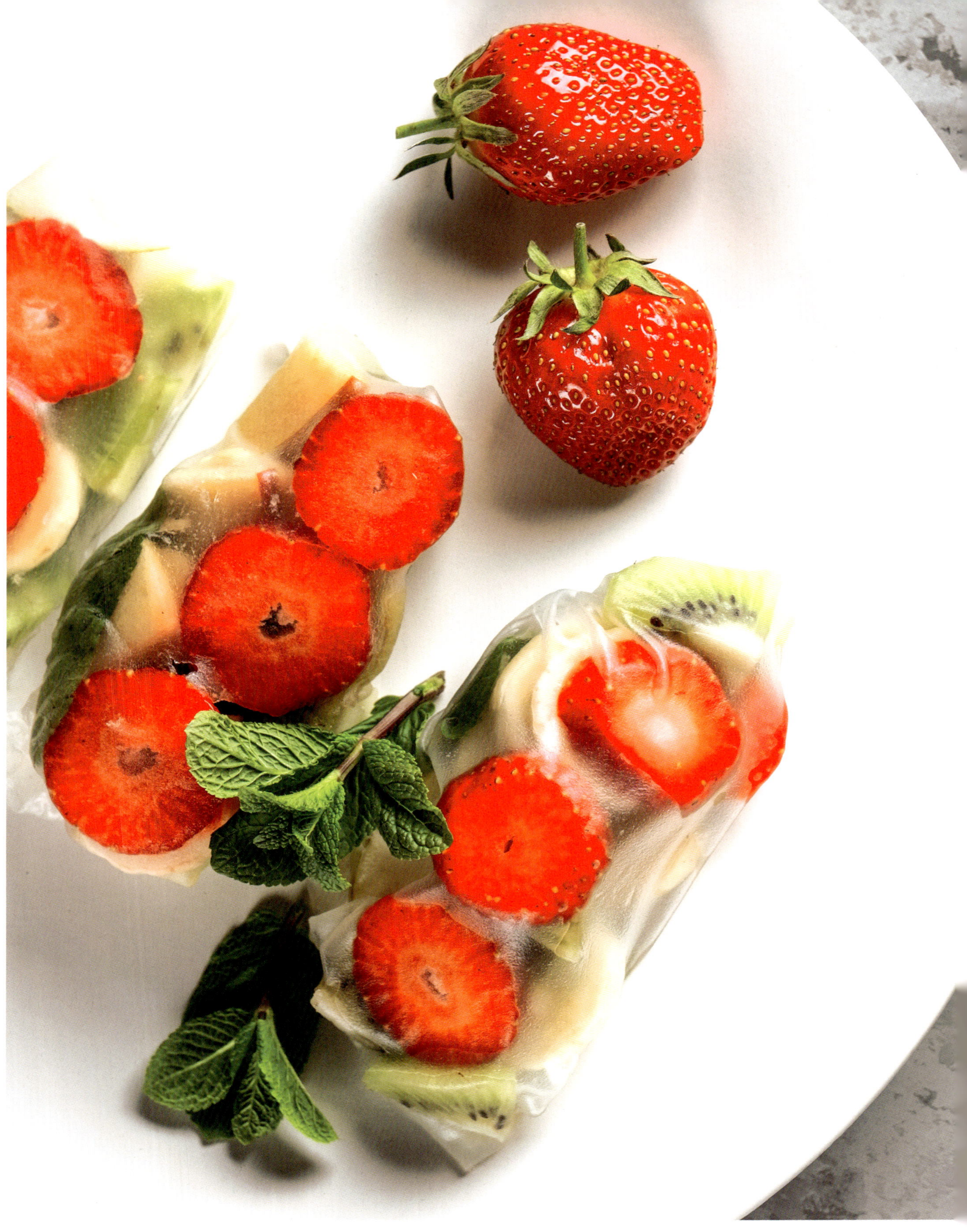

STRAWBERRY, KIWI & BANANA ROLLS

3 heaped cups (600g) sliced banana

3 heaped cups (540g) kiwi fruit, sliced into half moons

2 heaped cups (400g) sliced strawberries

½ cup (110g) white sugar

1 cup (15g) fresh mint leaves, roughly torn

18 rice paper wrappers

STEPS

1. Toss the fruit together with the sugar and mint leaves in a large bowl.
2. Dip a sheet of rice paper into a large bowl of hot water very quickly to soften it. Let it sit for about 30 seconds to dry. Place a heaped ⅓ cup of fruit mix in a strip along the side of the sheet, leaving 3cm free at both ends.
3. Fold up the free ends over the fruit, then roll up starting from the fruit side and sit the roll on the fold. Repeat with the rest of the sheets and the filling.
4. Serve immediately or chill until ready to serve.

MAKES 18 | PREP + COOK TIME: 30 MINS | VEG | GLUTEN FREE | DAIRY FREE |

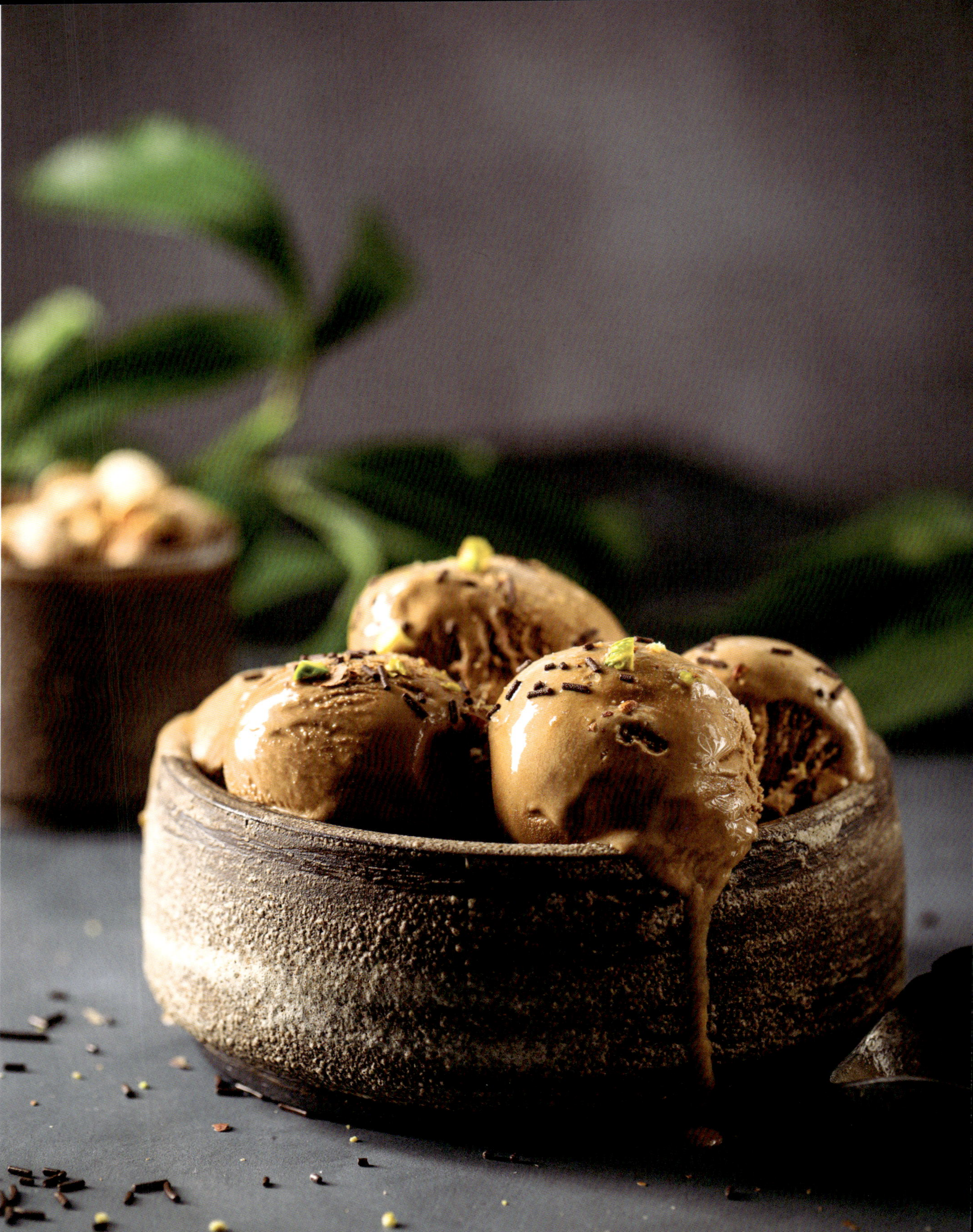

HOMEMADE COFFEE ICE CREAM

2½ cups (600ml) thickened cream

½ cup (125ml) coconut cream

1 cup (250ml) full cream milk

1 tbsp instant coffee powder

6 large egg yolks

1 tsp vanilla extract

¼ cup (50ml) maple syrup

⅓ cup (60g) brown sugar

STEPS

1. Bring the cream, coconut cream, milk and coffee to a simmer in a large saucepan. Remove from the heat.

2. Whisk together the yolks, vanilla, maple syrup and sugar in a large bowl until creamy.

3. Drizzle ¼ cup of the cream mixture into the yolks and whisk through. Pour this tempered mixture back into the remaining warm cream mixture and whisk until thick.

4. Heat over medium heat for 10 minutes until the mixture coats the back of a spoon. Remove from heat, cover and allow to cool in the refrigerator for 1 hour.

5. Pour into an ice-cream machine and churn according to instructions. Serve immediately or transfer to a container and chill in the freezer until ready to serve.

SERVES 4 | 1 HOUR + CHILLING AND FREEZING | VEG | GLUTEN FREE |

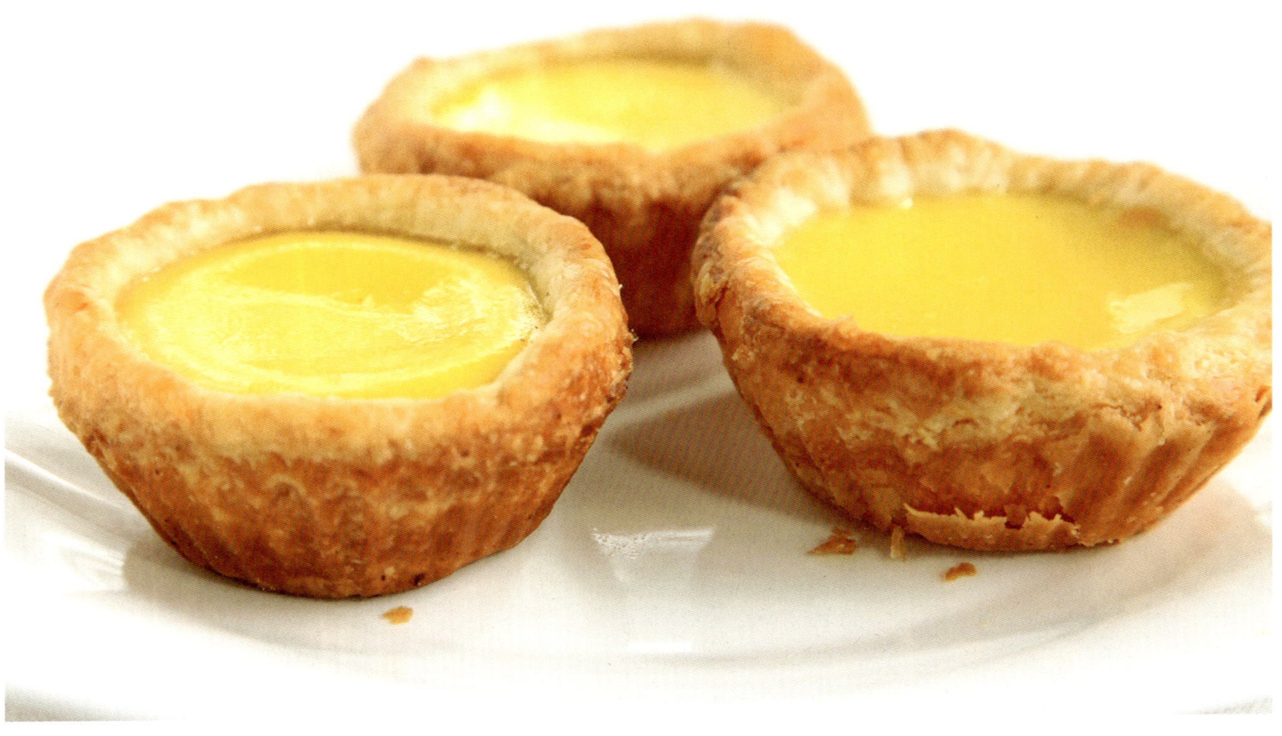

CHINESE CUSTARD TARTS

6 egg yolks
½ cup (100g) caster sugar
⅔ cup (150ml) cream
½ cup (125ml) milk
2 tsps vanilla extract
2 sheets frozen puff pastry, thawed

STEPS

Preheat the oven to 180°C.

1. Grease a 12-hole muffin tin.
2. In a large jug, whisk together the egg yolks, sugar, cream, milk and vanilla until smooth. Set aside.
3. Place the pastry on a lightly floured surface. Cut out 10cm circles using a round pastry cutter.
4. Press each pastry circle into a greased hole of the muffin tin, then pour in the egg mixture.
5. Bake for 18-20 minutes until puffed at the edges and pale golden on top. Remove from oven and allow to cool slightly before serving.

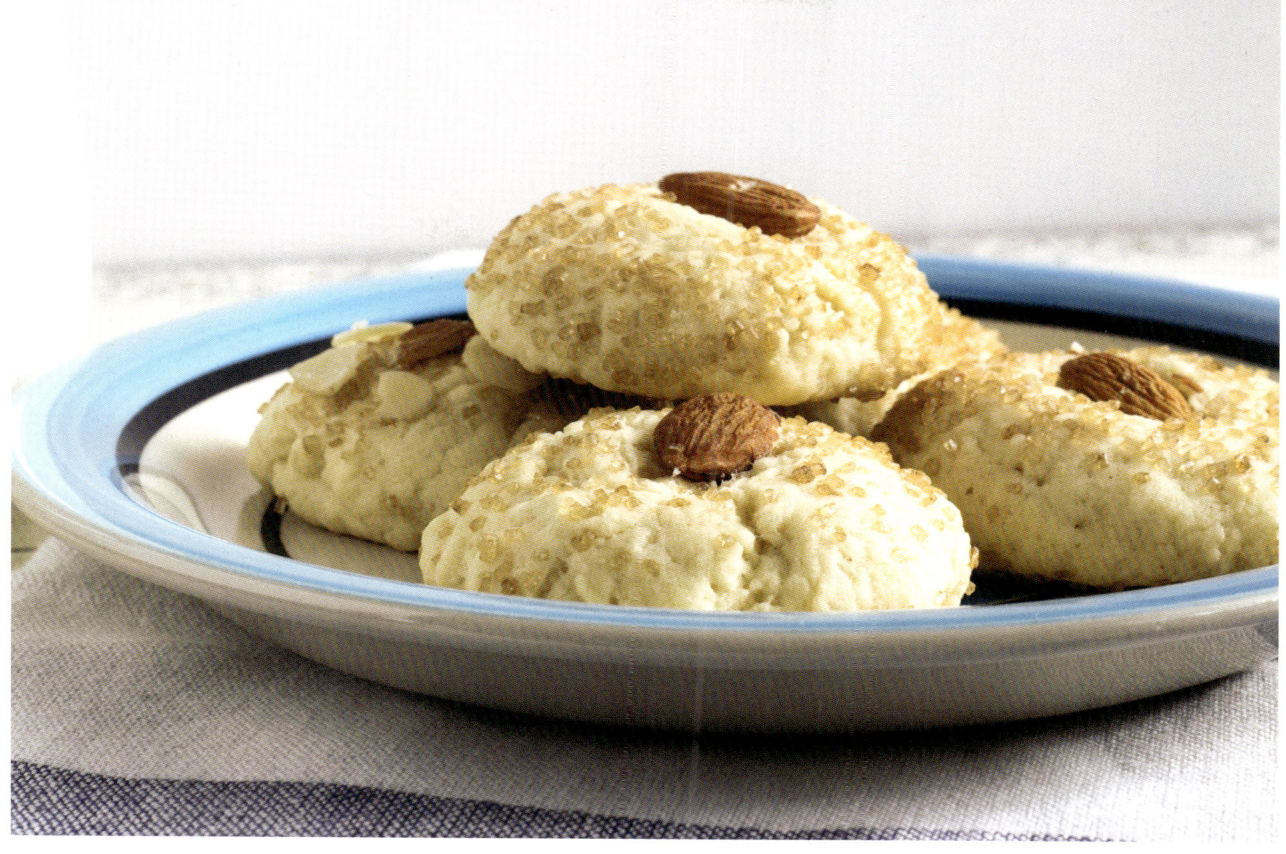

MAKES 44 | PREP + COOK TIME: 50 MINS | VEG |

CHINESE ALMOND COOKIES

250g unsalted butter
1 cup (220g) caster sugar
¼ tsp vanilla extract
1 tbsp almond extract
¼ tsp salt
3 cups (375g) plain flour
2 tbsps water
1 egg yolk
¼ cup (55g) brown sugar
44 whole almonds

STEPS

Preheat the oven to 150°C.

1. Line two large baking trays with baking paper.
2. Cream the butter and caster sugar, then mix through the vanilla and almond extracts and salt. Add the flour in thirds, mixing until combined each time.
3. Shape dessertspoons of mixture into round domes on the baking trays, leaving 3cm between each.
4. Whisk together the water and egg yolk and glaze each cookie with a small amount. Sprinkle cookies with brown sugar and press an almond into the centre of each one.
5. Bake for 30 minutes or until the cookies are just browned on the edges. Remove from the oven and transfer to a rack to cool.

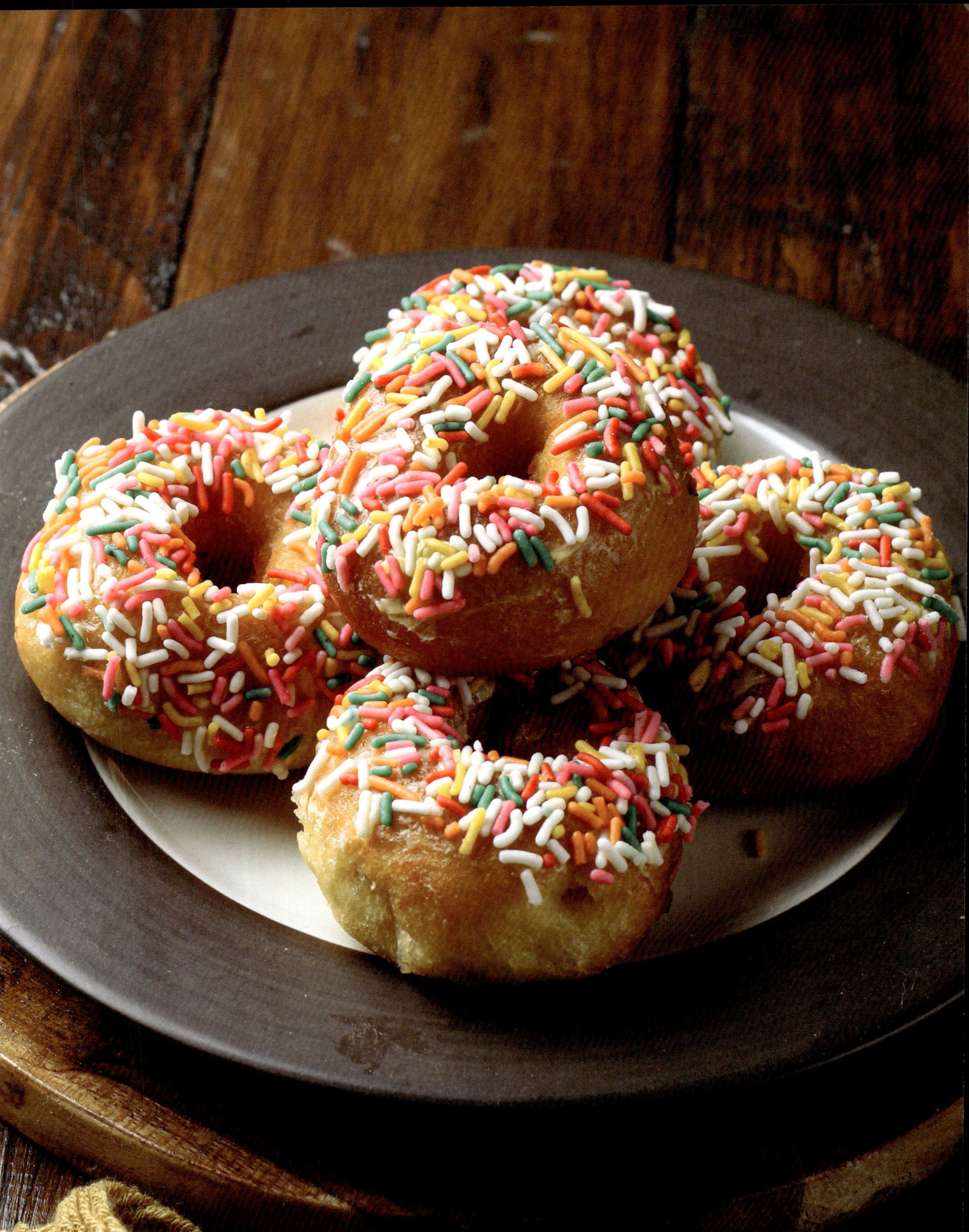

SWEET POTATO DOUGHNUTS

600g cooked and mashed sweet potato

¼ cup (40g) rice flour

1 cup (120g) plain flour + extra for dusting

¾ tsp salt

1 tbsp butter, melted

⅔ cup (150g) raw sugar

¼ cup (50ml) water

Vegetable oil for frying

2 tbsps sugar sprinkles (optional)

STEPS

1. Mix together the sweet potato, flours, salt and butter in a large bowl until thoroughly combined and smooth. Lightly dust your hands with flour and shape the mixture into doughnut rings and dust them with flour.

2. Heat the sugar and water in a small saucepan over medium heat. Bring to a boil, then simmer until it has thickened slightly. Remove from the heat.

3. Heat at least 10cm of oil a deep saucepan over high heat. Deep-fry the doughnuts, two or three at a time, for 3 minutes until golden brown. Drain on a wire rack over paper towels.

4. Drizzle the glaze over the doughnuts and scatter with sprinkles if desired.

SERVES 4 | PREP + COOK TIME: 50 MINS | VEG |

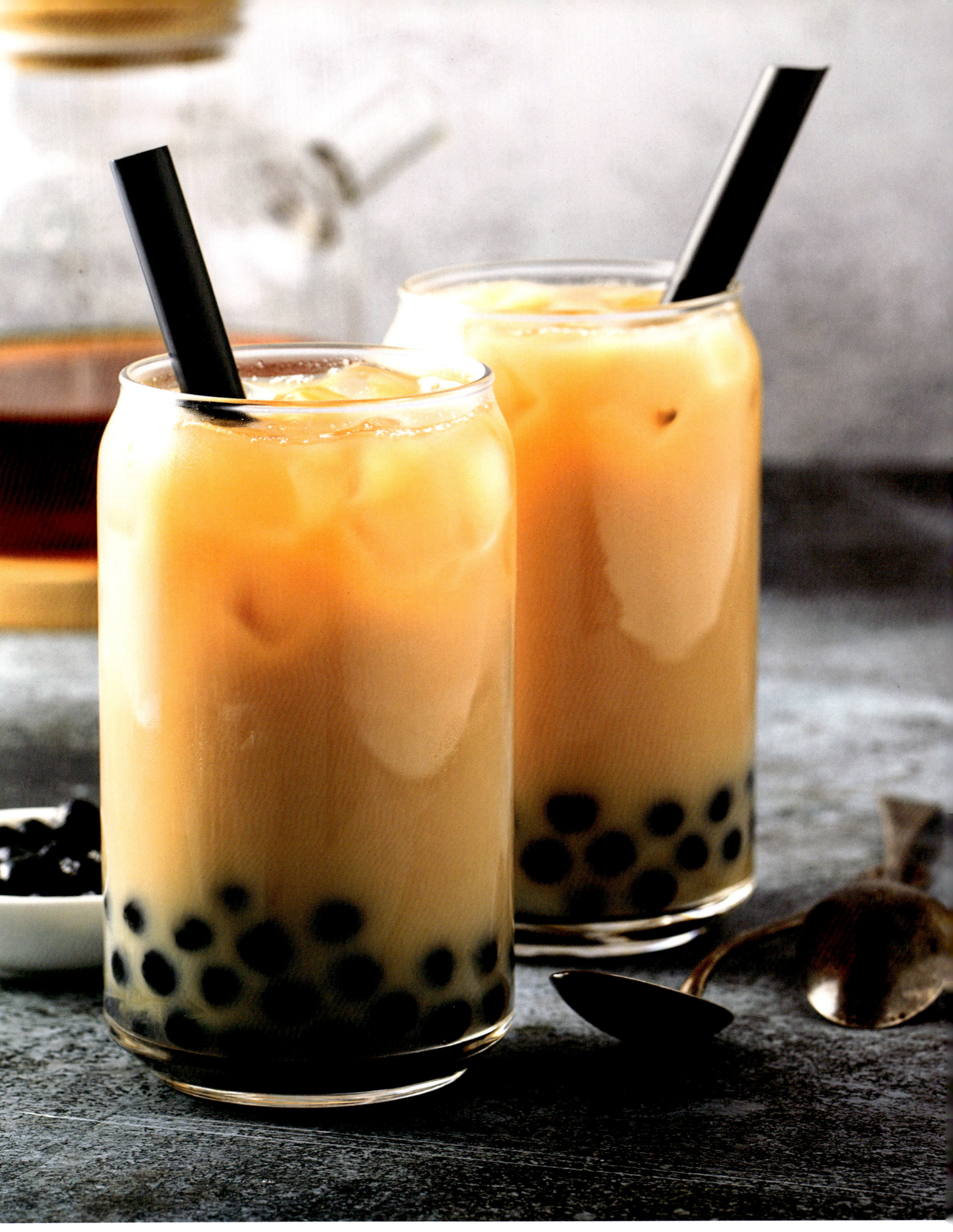

MILK BUBBLE TEA

4 cups (1L) boiling water

8 bags of black tea

4 cups (1L) cold water

¾ cup (110g) quick-cooking black tapioca pearls

Ice cubes to serve

6 tbsps milk or more to taste

SIMPLE SYRUP

½ cup (125ml) water

½ cup (110g) sugar

STEPS

1. Pour the boiling water onto the teabags in a large jug. Leave the tea to steep until the water cools completely. Remove the tea bags from the cooled water.

2. To make the syrup, heat the water and sugar in a saucepan over medium-high heat. Heat, stirring once or twice, until the water boils and the sugar completely dissolves. Remove from heat and allow to cool.

3. Bring the 4 cups cold water to a boil and add the tapioca pearls. Stir in the pearls and wait for them to float to the top. Then, cook for another 5 minutes until the pearls are soft. Use a slotted spoon to remove the pearls from the hot water. Quickly rinse with cold water. Transfer the pearls into a bowl, and mix the pearls with a few tablespoons of simple syrup to taste.

4. Divide the cooked tapioca pearls into four large glasses. Add a few ice cubes to each glass. Pour 1 cup of the tea into each glass. Add 1½ tablespoons of milk and 1½ tablespoons of simple syrup into each glass. Add more milk or simple syrup to taste.

5. Serve immediately.

SERVES 4 | PREP + COOK TIME: 10 MINS + COOLING | VEG | GLUTEN FREE |

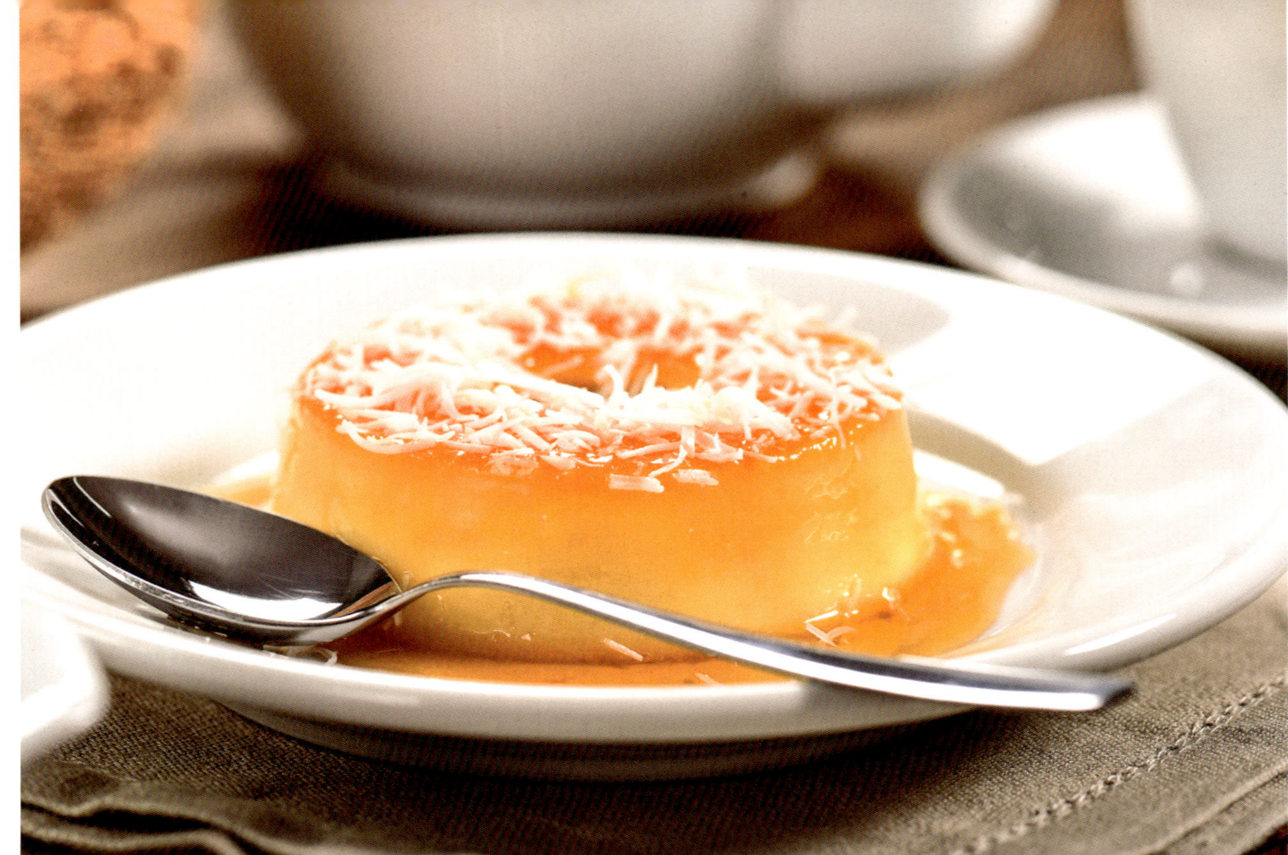

COCONUT CREME CARAMEL

1 cup (225g) white sugar
⅓ cup (80ml) water
1 x 400ml can coconut milk
1½ cups (375ml) milk
6 eggs, lightly whisked
½ cup (100g) brown sugar
1 tsp vanilla bean paste
Shredded coconut to serve

STEPS

Preheat oven to 160°C.

1. Heat white sugar and water in a saucepan over low heat, stirring, for 2 minutes until sugar dissolves. Increase heat to high. Boil, without stirring, for 3-4 minutes until golden. Pour into eight ramekins.
2. Whisk together coconut milk, milk, egg, brown sugar and vanilla bean paste. Pour into ramekins.
3. Place ramekins in a large roasting tin. Pour enough boiling water into the tin to reach halfway up the sides of the ramekins. Bake for 35-40 minutes until the custards are just set.
4. Cool ramekins on a wire rack for 30 minutes, then transfer to the fridge. Chill overnight.
5. Run a knife around the inside edge of the ramekins and carefully turn onto serving plates. Sprinkle with shredded coconut to serve.

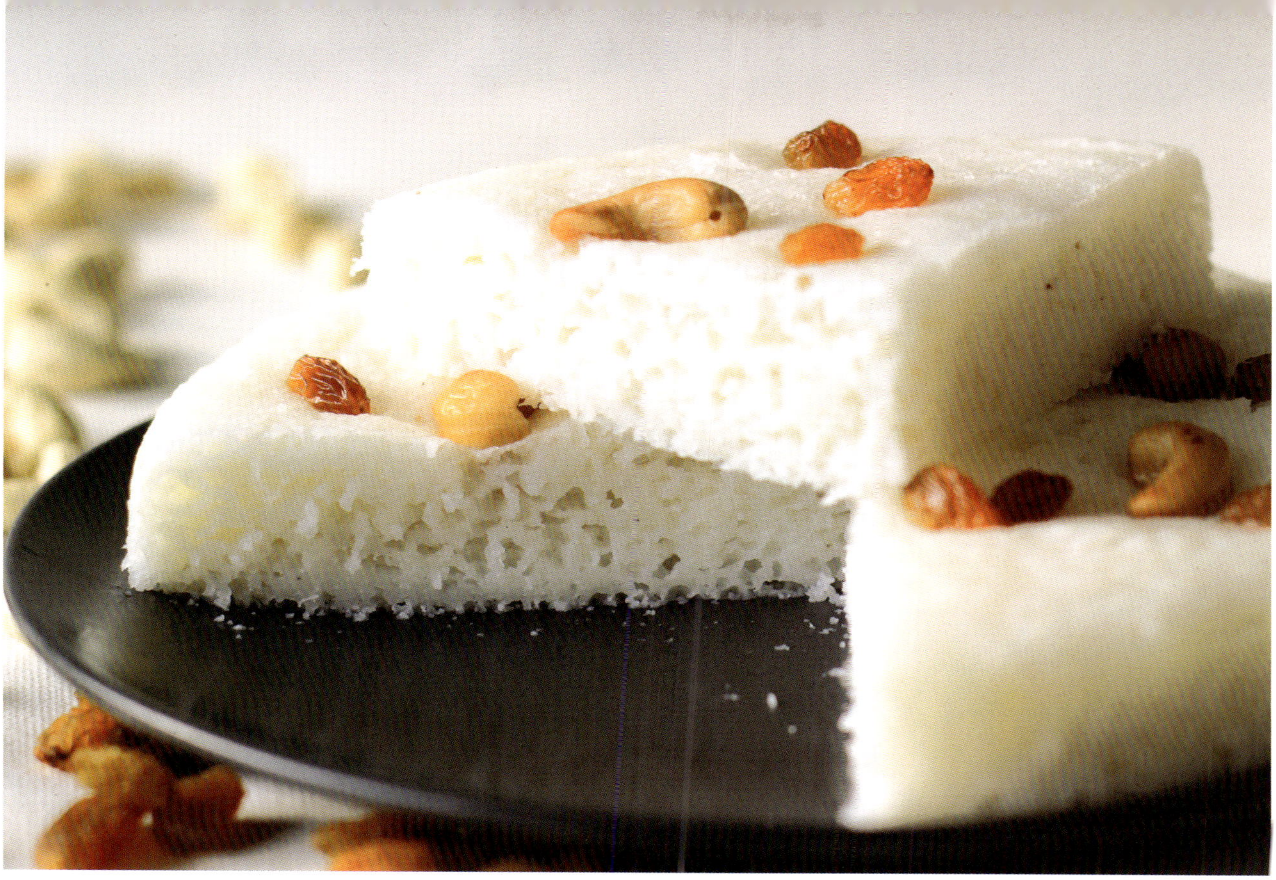

VATTAYAPPAM

SERVES 8 | PREP + COOK TIME: 40 MINS + SOAKING AND FERMENTING | VEG | GLUTEN FREE | DAIRY FREE |

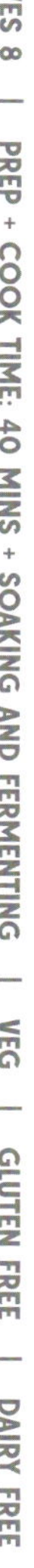

½ tsp yeast

½ cup (110g) + ¼ tsp sugar

2 cups (500ml) + 1 tbsp water

1 cup (155g) rice, soaked for 6-7 hours

¾ cup (65g) desiccated coconut

¼ cup (40g) cooked rice

¼ tsp ground cardamon

¼ tsp ground cumin

¼ cup (40g) raisins/sultanas and cashews, to decorate

STEPS

1. Combine yeast, ¼ teaspoon sugar and 1 tablespoon water in a bowl. Set aside for 10-15 minutes to ferment.
2. Meanwhile, blend soaked rice, coconut, cooked rice and 2 cups water together in a high-speed blender to make a smooth, thick batter. Add in yeast mixture, ½ cup sugar and ground cardamon and cumin. Mix well.
3. Leave the batter in a warm place to ferment for 7-8 hours.
4. Pour the batter into a greased, small round cake tin. Decorate with cashews and raisins. Place the cake in a steamer and steam for 15-20 minutes.
5. Allow to cool before slicing and serving.

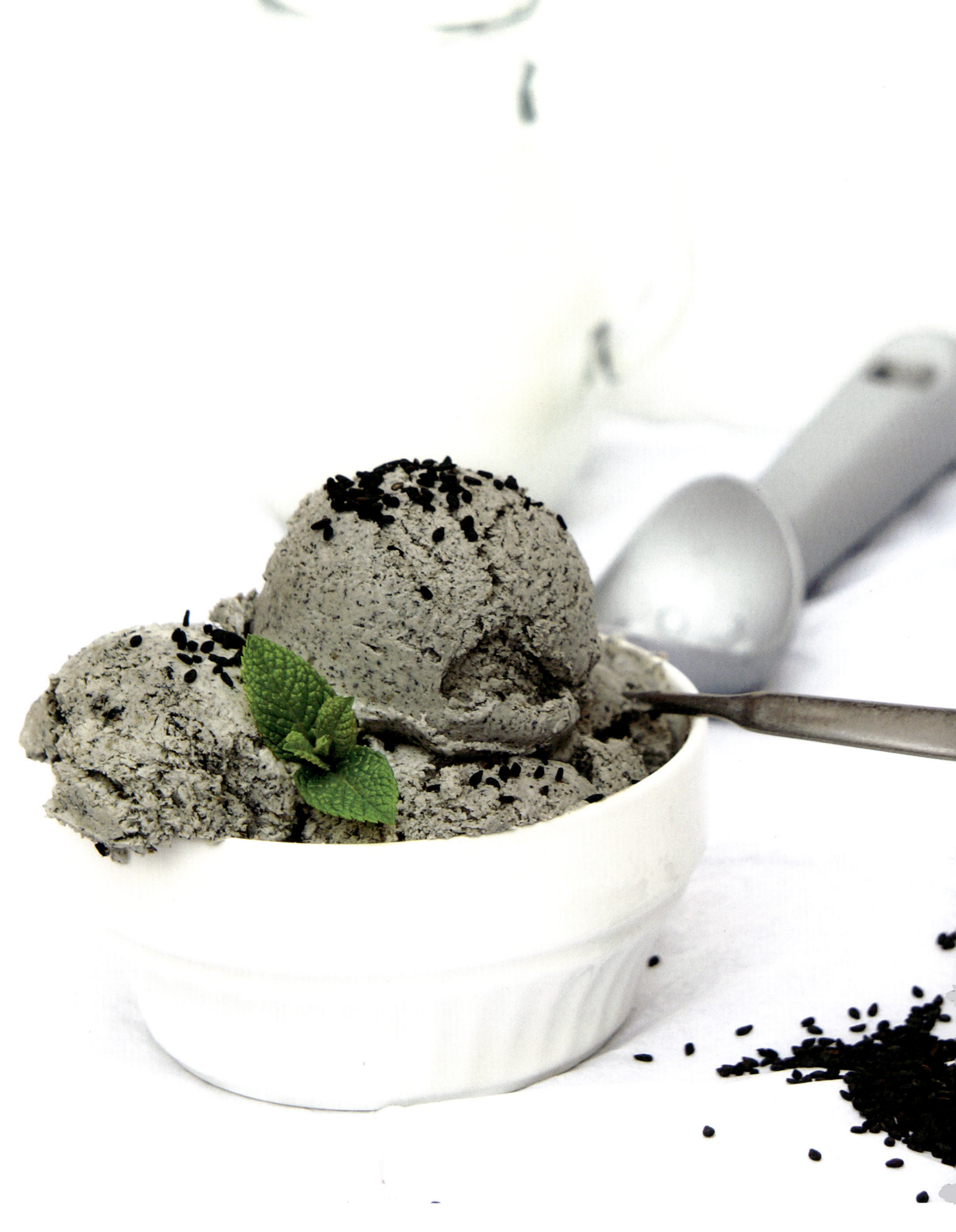

BLACK SESAME ICE CREAM

SERVES 4 | PREP + COOK TIME: 15 MINS + COOLING AND FREEZING | VEG | GLUTEN FREE |

½ cup (115g) black tahini

1 cup (240ml) thickened cream

½ cup (110g) sugar

1 tsp xanthan gum

2 cups (480ml) whole milk

STEPS

1. Place the black tahini and cream in a blender and blitz until smooth. Add the sugar, xanthan gum and milk to the blender and blend until the mixture is very smooth and slightly thickened.

2. Pour into a bowl, cover and refrigerate for 1-2 hours until completely chilled.

3. Pour into an ice-cream machine and churn according to instructions. Serve immediately or transfer to a container and chill in the freezer until ready to serve.

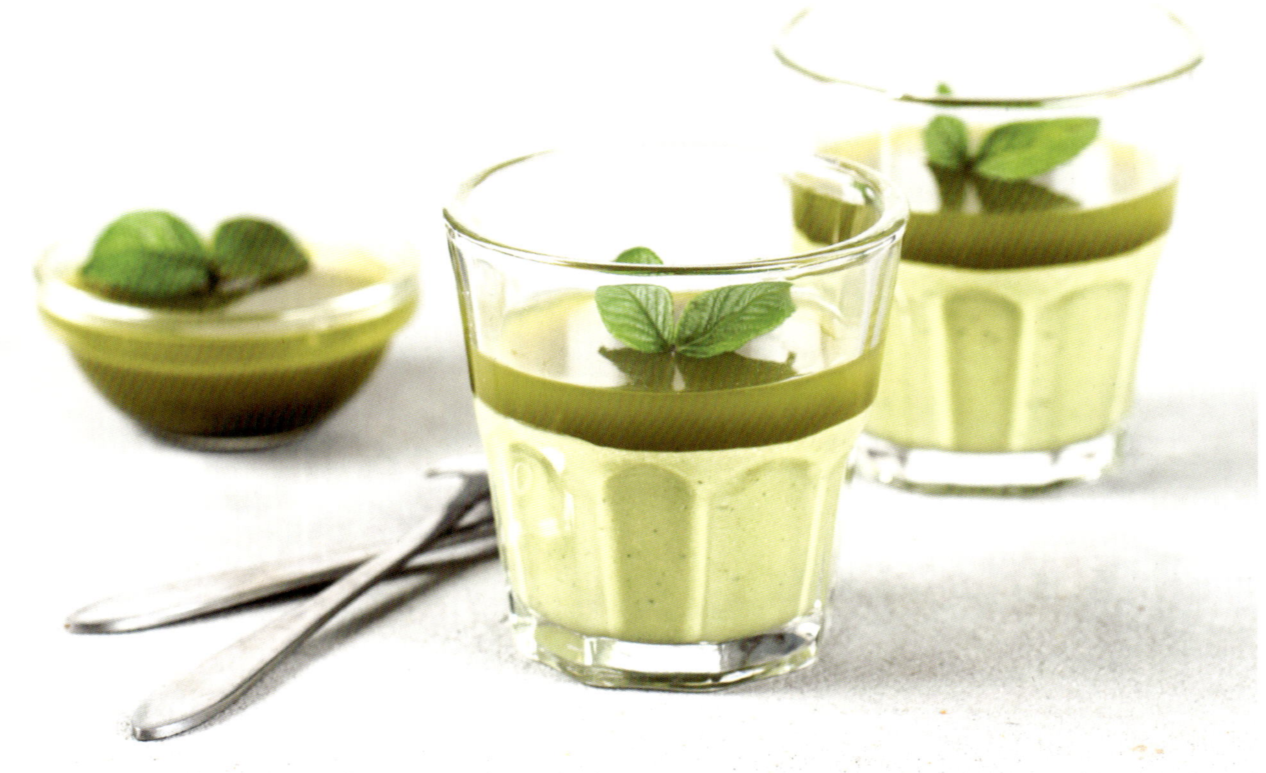

GREEN TEA PANNA COTTA

PANNA COTTA

4 tbsps water

15g gelatin powder

1½ cups (375ml) cream

1½ tbsps matcha powder

4 tbsps sugar

JELLY

½ tbsps matcha powder

½ cup (125ml) + 3 tbsps boiling water

4 tbsps sugar

7g gelatin

STEPS

1. To make the panna cotta whisk together water and gelatin in a small bowl. Let sit for 5 minutes.
2. In a saucepan, heat cream over medium-low heat. Add gelatin mixture and whisk for 2 minutes until smooth. Add matcha powder and whisk until dissolved. Remove from heat and stir in sugar.
3. Strain through a sieve and pour into six individual ramekins or glasses. Set aside for 30 minutes.
4. In a small saucepan dissolve matcha powder in 3 tablespoons of boiling water. Place over medium heat and add sugar, gelatin and remaining boiling water, whisking as you do so. Continue whisking until sugar and gelatin are dissolved. Allow to cool for 15 minutes.
5. Pour jelly on top of panna cottas. Let cool to room temperature then set in the fridge for at least 2 hours or until firm.

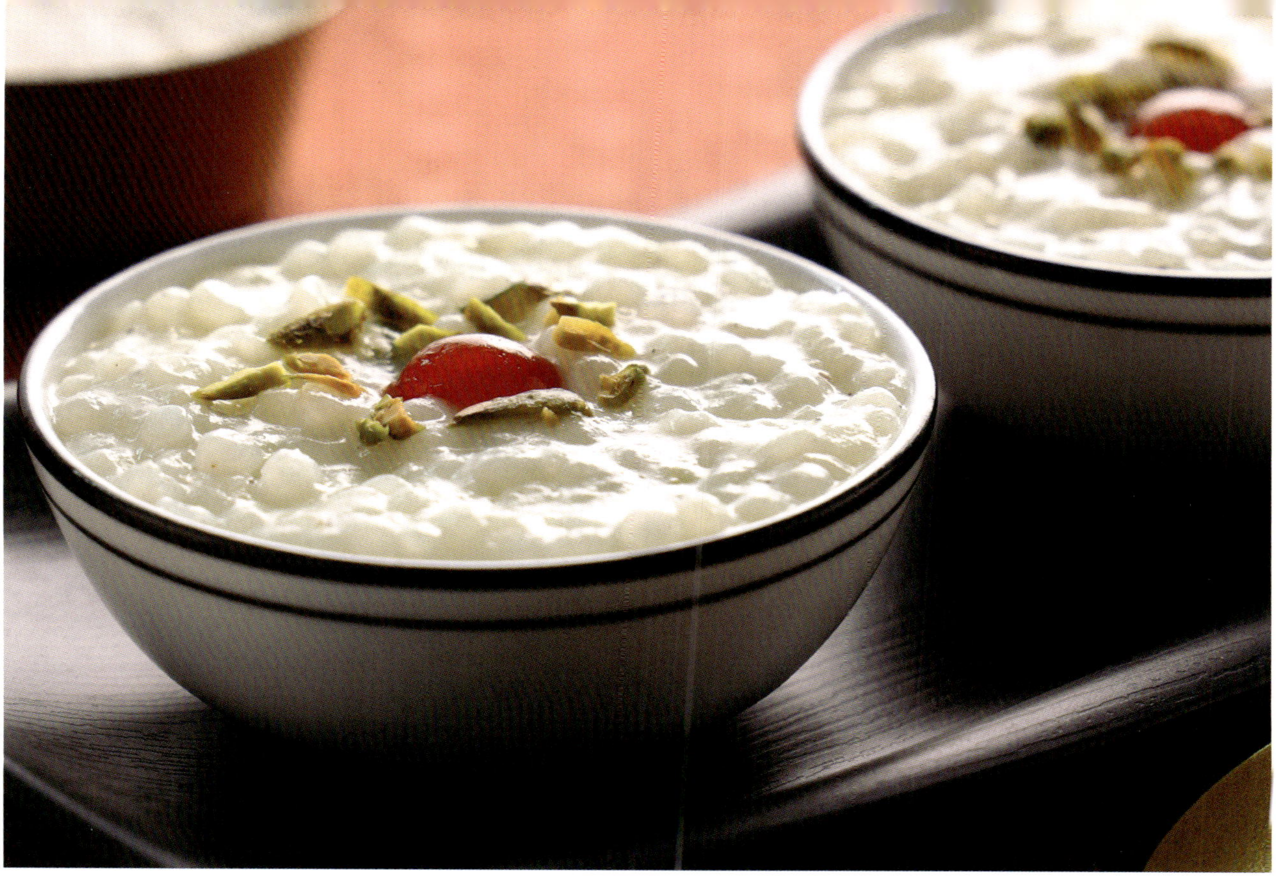

COCONUT SAGO PUDDING

SERVES 4 | PREP + COOK TIME: 20 MINS + SOAKING | VEG | GLUTEN FREE | DAIRY FREE |

1 x 400ml can coconut cream

1 x 400ml can coconut milk

¾ cup (110g) sago (or tapioca) pearls

1 cup (250ml) water

⅓ cup (70g) caster sugar

1 tsp vanilla bean paste

2 tbsps chopped pistachios to serve (optional)

4 glace cherry halves to serve (optional)

STEPS

1. Place coconut cream, coconut milk, sago and the water in a medium saucepan. Set aside to soak for 30 minutes.

2. Place saucepan over moderate heat. Cook and stir until the mixture comes to the boil. Reduce heat to very low; simmer, stirring occasionally, for 10 minutes or until sago is tender. Remove from heat. Stir in sugar and vanilla. Cool slightly.

3. Spoon into bowls. Top with chopped pistachios and glace cherry halves to serve. Serve warm or allow to cool to room temperature, refrigerate and serve chilled.

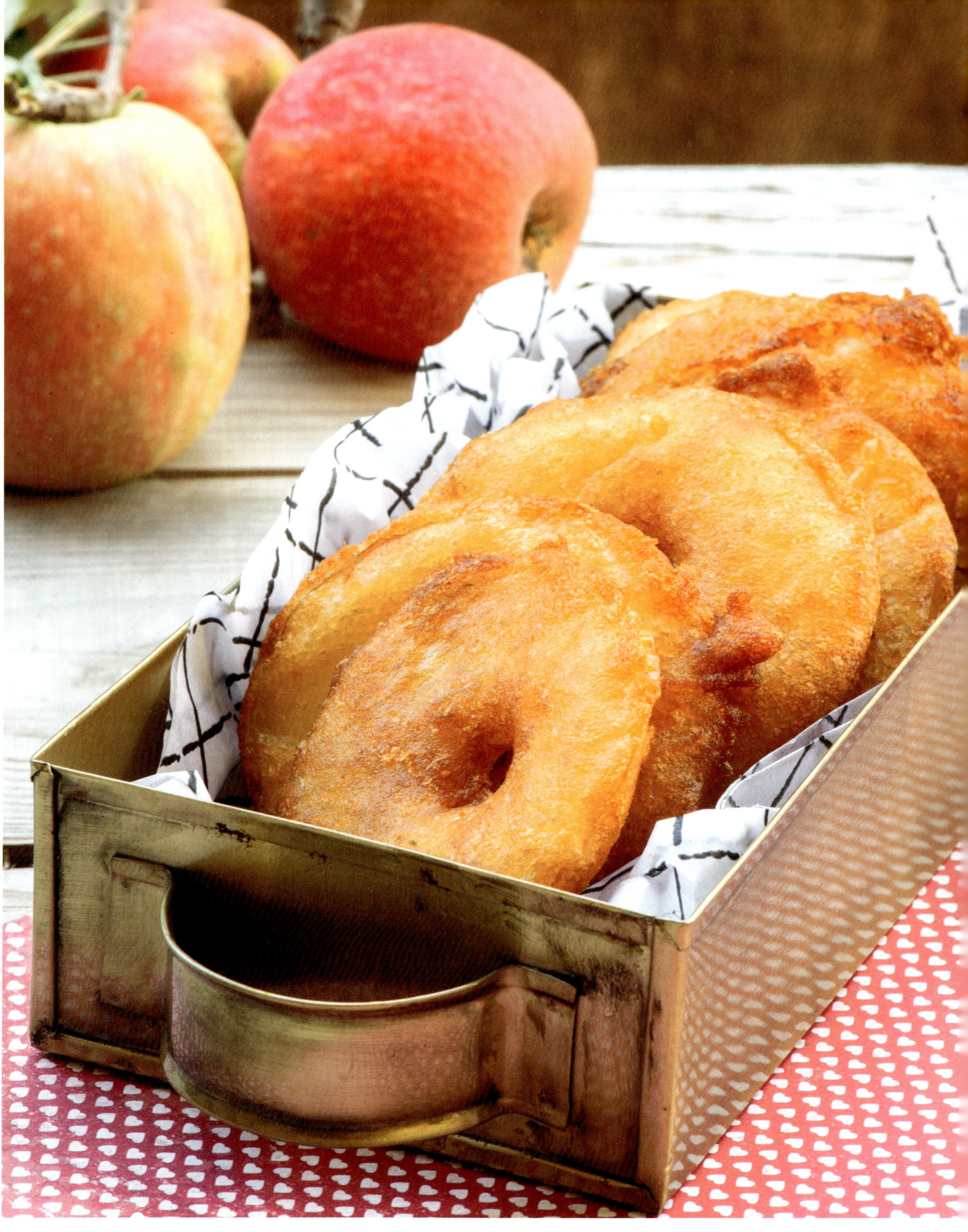

TEMPURA APPLE RINGS

1 cup (125g) flour

½ tsp salt

¼ tsp cayenne pepper

1 egg

½ cup (125ml) apple juice

½ cup (125ml) sparkling water

Canola oil for frying

2 apples, cored and thinly sliced into rings

1 tbsp cinnamon

1 cup (220g) sugar

STEPS

1. Whisk flour, salt and cayenne pepper in a large bowl.
2. In another bowl beat egg with apple juice and sparling water. Add to dry ingredients and mix until just until just combined. Refrigerate.
3. Pour about 10cm of canola oil into a heavy-bottomed saucepan and place over medium-high heat. Heat to 180°C.
4. Dip apple slices into batter and fry in the oil until golden.
5. Drain on a paper towels. Dust with cinnamon and sugar to serve.

SERVES 2–4 | PREP + COOK TIME: 15 MINS | VEG | DAIRY FREE |

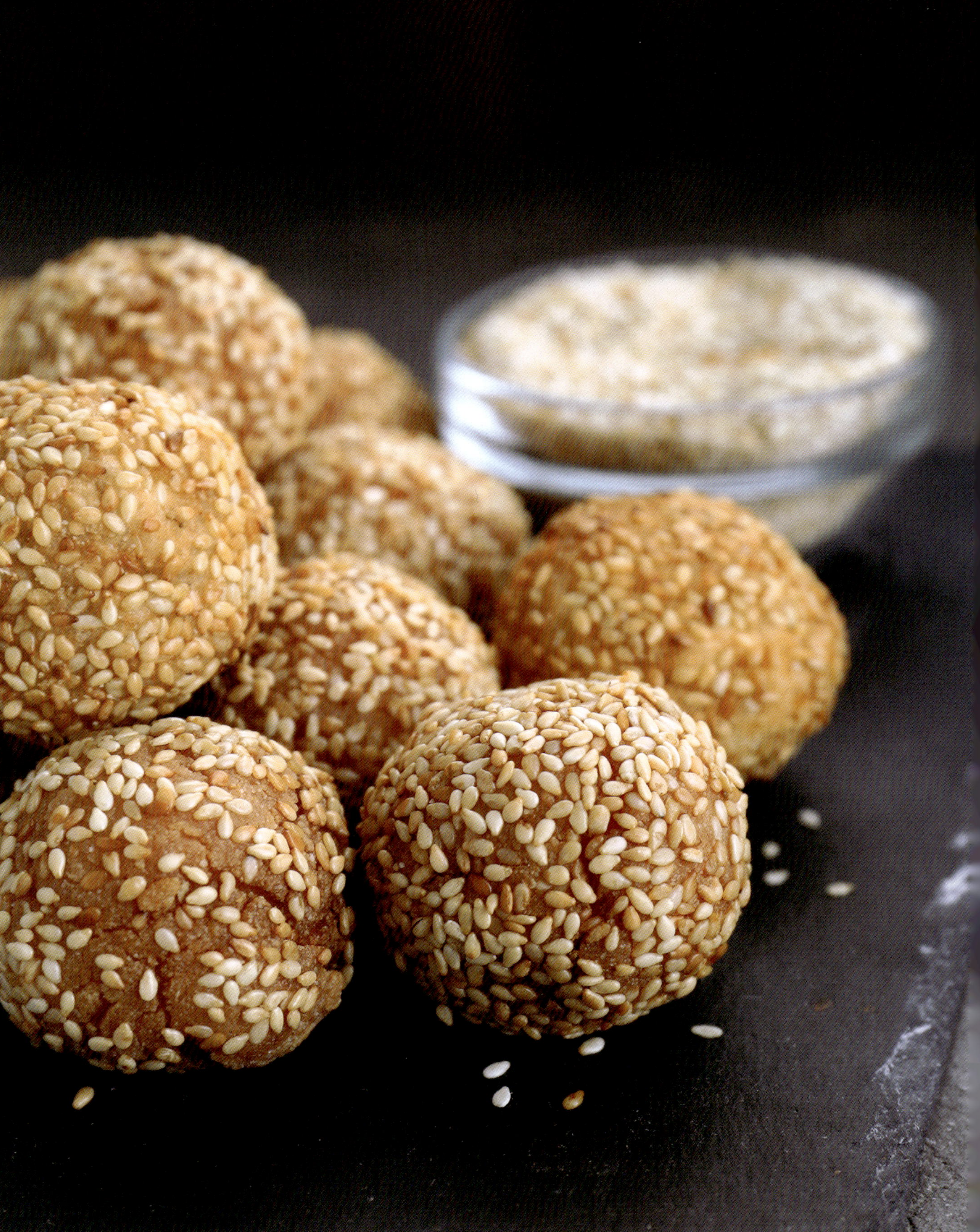

SESAME BALLS

MAKES 8 | PREP + COOK TIME: 30 MINS + COOLING | VEG | GLUTEN FREE | DAIRY FREE |

⅔ cup (160ml) hot water

½ cup (100g) light brown sugar

2 cups (320g) glutinous rice flour + more for dusting

8 tsps adzuki red bean paste (see recipe page 297)

½ cup (80g) sesame seeds

7 cups (1.75L) vegetable oil

STEPS

1. In a small bowl, whisk the hot water with the brown sugar until the sugar dissolves.
2. Add the glutinous rice flour to a medium bowl and create a small well in the centre. Pour the sugar syrup into the well and stir for 5 minutes, until the dough is well combined and no longer sticks to the bowl.
3. Dust a clean work surface with glutinous rice flour. Knead the dough for 5 minutes, until it forms a smooth, round ball. Divide dough into 8 pieces and roll each piece into a 1¼ cm-thick disc.
4. Place 1 teaspoon of red bean filling in the centre of each piece of dough. Fold in the edges to cover the filling, then roll into a ball. Roll the ball in the sesame seeds until the dough is covered. Repeat with the remaining ingredients.
5. Heat the vegetable oil in a large saucepan until it reaches 180°C. Fry the sesame balls for 15 minutes, stirring frequently, until golden brown. Transfer to a wire rack set over a baking tray to drain and let cool for 15 minutes before serving.

INDEX

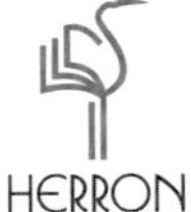

First Published in 2023 by Herron Book Distributors Pty Ltd
14 Manton St
Morningside
QLD 4170
www.herronbooks.com

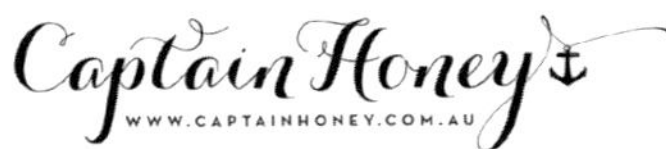

Custom book production by Captain Honey Pty Ltd
12 Station St
Bangalow
NSW 2479
www.captainhoney.com.au

Cataloguing-in-Publication. A catalogue record for this book is available from the National Library of Australia

ISBN 978-1-922944-31-3

Printed and bound in China.

5 4 3 2 1   23 24 25 26 27

NOTES FOR THE READER

All reasonable efforts have been made to ensure the accuracy of the content in this book. Information in this book is not intended as a substitute for medical advice. The author and publisher cannot and do not accept any legal duty of care or responsibility in relation to the content in this book, and disclaim any liabilities relating to its use.